Fast-Track in Cardiac Anesthesia

Giuseppe Sepolvere • Simona Silvetti
Editors

Fast-Track in Cardiac Anesthesia

Cardiac Surgery in the Era of ERAS

Springer

Editors
Giuseppe Sepolvere
Anesthesia and Cardiac Surgery ICU
San Michele Hospital
MADDALONI, Caserta, Italy

Simona Silvetti
Department of Cardiac Anesthesia and
Intensive Care, Cardiovascular Network
IRCCS Ospedale Policlinico San Martino
Genoa, Italy

ISBN 978-3-031-70901-2 ISBN 978-3-031-70899-2 (eBook)
https://doi.org/10.1007/978-3-031-70899-2

This Springer imprint is published by the registered company Springer Nature Switzerland AG
The registered company address is: Gewerbestrasse 11, 6330 Cham, Switzerland

Preface

In the field of cardiac surgery, the need for efficient, patient-centered approaches has never been more critical than it is at this moment, given the rapidly evolving landscape.

Fast Track in Cardiac Surgery in the Era of Eras aims to highlight some important strategies that have emerged and been formalized from enhanced recovery after surgery (ERAS) recommendations in Cardiac surgery. The "fast track" concept in cardiac surgery gained significant momentum since 2019, when the ERAS Cardiac Society was established and its well-known guidelines were published. These protocols are revolutionizing perioperative surgical care, improving not only clinical outcomes and the overall patient experience but also reducing hospital costs.

This book is designed for anesthesiologists, as well as cardiac surgeons and nurses specializing in adult cardiac surgery setting. It serves as a comprehensive guide, providing insights into the implementation of ERAS protocols, minimally invasive cardiac surgery, principles of fast-track extubation, and recent and emerging locoregional anesthesia practices that promote rapid recovery and improved outcomes in this setting.

We hope that this volume will reach a wide readership.

It is our hope and objective that this book will inspire a commitment to excellence and innovation in our practices, redefining the standards of care for our patients.

The editors are very grateful to the many experts and colleagues who cooperated with us. We are deeply grateful to all these colleagues for their invaluable support.

Maddaloni, Caserta, Italy — Giuseppe Sepolvere
Genova, Italy — Simona Silvetti

Contents

Contributors

Alfonso Agnino Heart-Surgery Department, Humanitas Gavazzeni, Bergamo, Italy

Valentina Ajello Department of Cardiac Anesthesia, Tor Vergata University Hospital, Rome, Italy

Giovanni Albano Anesthesiology Department, Humanitas Gavazzeni, Bergamo, Italy

Ottavio Alfieri Alfieri Heart Foundation, Milan, Italy

Cardiac Surgery Department, San Raffaele University Hospital, Milan, Italy

Tommaso Aloisio Department of Cardiothoracic and Vascular Anesthesia and Intensive Care Unit (ICU), Istituto di Ricovero e Cura a Carattere Scientifico (IRCCS) Policlinico San Donato, San Donato Milanese, Milan, Italy

Pietro Bertini Department of Anesthesia and Intensive Care, Casa di Cura San Rossore, Pisa, Italy

Giacomo Bianchi Division of Cardiac Surgery, Ospedale del Cuore, Fondazione Toscana Gabriele Monasterio, Massa, Italy

Cesare Biuzzi Department of Emergency-Urgency, Anesthesia and Intensive Care Unit, University Hospital of Siena, Siena, Italy

Rafael Blanco Corniche Hospital, Abu Dhabi, UAE

Alessandro Caldarola Alfieri Heart Foundation, Milan, Italy

Danilo Canzio Department of Anesthesia and Intensive Care Unit and Pain Therapy, Mater Dei Hospital, Bari, Italy

Paolo Capuano Department of Anesthesia and Intensive Care, Istituto Mediterraneo per i Trapianti e Terapie ad alta Specializzazione (IRCCS-ISMETT), UPMCI (University of Pittsburgh Medical Center Italy), Palermo, Italy

Giulio Carinci Department of Medical Science, Surgery and Neurosciences, Anesthesia and Intensive Care Unit, University Hospital of Siena, Siena, Italy

Guohao Chang Department of Cardiac, Thoracic and Vascular Surgery, National University Heart Center, Singapore (NUHCS), Singapore, Singapore

Loredana Cristiano Department of Anesthesia and Cardiac Surgery Intensive Care Unit, San Michele Hospital, Maddaloni, Caserta, Italy

Mauro D'Amora Department of Cardiac, Thoracic and Vascular Anesthesia, University Hospital "San Giovanni di Dio e Ruggi D'Aragona", Salerno, Italy

Cristiano D'Errico Intensive Care Unit, Department of Anesthesia, AORN Cardarelli, Naples, Italy

Blanca Martinez Lopez De Arroyabe Cardiothoracic and Vascular Anesthesia and Intensive Care Unit, University Hospital of Verona, Verona, Italy

Antonio De Bellis Department of Cardiac Surgery, San Michele Hospital, Maddaloni, Caserta, Italy

Andrea De Martino Cardiac Surgery Division, Ospedale Policlinico San Martino, Genoa, Italy

Francesca De Sanctis Unit of Anesthesia and Intensive Care, S. MAria Hospital, Terni, Italy

Fabrizio Di Zazzo Department of Anesthesia and Cardiac Surgery Intensive Care Unit, San Michele Hospital, Maddaloni, Caserta, Italy

Rapetti Francesca Department of Cardiac Anesthesia and Intensive Care, Cardiovascular Network, IRCCS Ospedale Policlinico San Martino, Genoa, Italy

Maisano Francesco Valve Center, Cardiac Surgery Department, San Raffaele University Hospital, Milana, Italy

Federico Franchi Department of Medical Science, Surgery and Neurosciences, Cardiothoracic and Vascular Anesthesia and Intensive Care Unit, University Hospital of Siena, Siena, Italy

Pierfrancesco Fusco Unit of Anesthesia and Intensive Care, SS Filippo e Nicola Hospital, Avezzano, L'Aquila, Italy

Luca Gentili Department of Anesthesia and Intensive Care Unit, Santa Maria Goretti Hospital, Latina, Italy

Azzola Nicolò Guicciardi Valve Center, Cardiac Surgery Department, San Raffaele University Hospital, Milano, Italy

Dorela Haxhiademi Department of Anesthesia and Intensive Care Unit, Heart Hospital "G. Pasquinucci", National Research Council-Tuscany Foundation "G. Monasterio", Massa, Italy

Daniele Marianello Department of Medical Science, Surgery and Neurosciences, Cardiothoracic and Vascular Anesthesia and Intensive Care Unit, University Hospital of Siena, Siena, Italy

Michele Martinelli Department of Surgical Sciences and Integrated Diagnostics, School of Medical and Pharmaceutic Sciences, University of Genoa, Genoa, Italy

Ciprian Nita Cardiothoracic Anaesthesia and Intensive Care, Royal Papworth Hospital, Cambridge, UK

Denti Paolo Valve Center, Cardiac Surgery Department, San Raffaele University Hospital, Milano, Italy

Matteo Parrinello Anesthesiology Department, Humanitas Gavazzeni, Bergamo, Italy

Gianluca Paternoster Department of Health Science Cardiovascular Anesthesia and ICU School of Medicine, San Carlo Hospital University of Basilicata, Potenza, Italy

Department of Health Science Anaesthesia and ICU School of Medicine, University of Basilicata San Carlo Hospital, Potenza, Italy

Gian Marco Petroni Unit of Anesthesia and Intensive Care, S. MAria Hospital, Terni, Italy

Marco Ranucci Department of Cardiac Anesthesia and Intensive Care, IRCCS Policlinico San Donato, Milan, Italy

Davide Ricci Department of Integrated Surgical and Diagnostic Sciences, University of Genova, Genoa, Italy

Division of Cardiac Surgery, IRCCS University Hospital San Martino-IST, Genoa, Italy

Antonio Rubino Cardiothoracic Anaesthesia and Intensive Care, Royal Papworth Hospital, Cambridge, UK

Antonio Salsano Cardiac Surgery Division, Ospedale Policlinico San Martino, Genoa, Italy

Disc Department, University of Genoa, Genoa, Italy

Filippo Sanfilippo University Hospital Policlinico G. Rodolico-San Marco, Catania, Italy

Department of Surgery and Medical-Surgical Specialties, University of Catania, Catania, Italy

Fabio Sangalli Anaesthesia and Intensive Care, ASST Valtellina e Alto Lario, Milan, Italy

Francesco Santini Division of Cardiac Surgery, Ospedale Policlinico San Martino, Genoa, Italy

Department of Integrated Surgical and Diagnostic Sciences, University of Genova, Genoa, Italy

Valeria Rita Scialdone Department of Anesthesia and Cardiac Surgery Intensive Care Unit, San Michele Hospital, Maddaloni, Caserta, Italy

Paolo Scimia Department of Anesthesia and Intensive Care Unit, Giuseppe Mazzini Hospital, Teramo, Italy

Unit of Anesthesia and Intensive Care, Mazzini Hospital, Teramo, Italy

Sabino Scolletta Department of Medical Science, Surgery and Neurosciences, Anesthesia and Intensive Care Unit, University Hospital of Siena, Siena, Italy

Tarek Senussi Department of Cardiac Anesthesia and Intensive Care, Cardiovascular Network, IRCCS Ospedale Policlinico San Martino, Genoa, Italy

Giuseppe Sepolvere Department of Anesthesia and Cardiac Surgery Intensive Care Unit, San Michele Hospital, Maddaloni, Caserta, Italy

Simona Silvetti Department of Cardiac Anesthesia and Intensive Care, Cardiovascular Network, IRCCS Ospedale Policlinico San Martino, Genoa, Italy

Mario Tedesco Department of Anesthesia and Intensive Care Unit and Pain Therapy, Mater Dei Hospital, Bari, Italy

Andrea Tognù Department of Anesthesia, Intensive Care and Pain Therapy, Orthopedic University Hospital Rizzoli, Bologna, Italy

Antonio Toscano Department of Anesthesia and Critical Care, Città della Salute e della Scienza di Torino, University of Turin, Turin, Italy

Valentina Trinchero Department of Surgical Sciences and Integrated Diagnostics School of Medical and Pharmaceutic Sciences, University of Genoa, Genoa, Italy

Part I

Introduction

Society for Enhanced Recovery After Cardiac Surgery

1

Simona Silvetti and Marco Ranucci

1.1 Introduction

The ERAS® Study Group was established in 2001, and since its beginning, it spearheaded the developments made in different surgical care and recovery. Since its inception, the ERAS® Society has expanded to include several subspecialtics, emphasizing the benefits of standardized best practices in the perioperative period. In 2005, the Study Group developed and published the first consensus program for patients undergoing colon-rectal surgery. In the following years, the specialty subgroups moved forward, and at the beginning of 2017, a team including cardiac surgeons, anesthesiologists, and intensivists established the Enhanced Recovery After Cardiac Surgery (ERACS) Society to obtain these goals for patients undergoing cardiac surgery.

In this chapter, we would summarize the Society history and give some tips focused on ERAS program.

S. Silvetti (✉)
Department of Cardiac Anesthesia and Intensive Care, Cardiovascular Network, IRCCS Ospedale Policlinico San Martino, Genoa, Italy

M. Ranucci
Department of Cardiac Anesthesia and Intensive Care, IRCCS Policlinico San Donato, Milan, Italy

1.2 ERAS Cardiac Surgery Society

The ERACS was established in 2017 by a group of cardiac surgeons, anesthesiologists, and intensivists, with the purpose of improving the quality of care of patients undergoing heart surgery. Basically, the main pillars of this Society are research, education, and implementation of evidence-based techniques leading to an enhanced post-procedural recovery. Within this context, ERACS is a direct derivate of the ERAS Society, which started as a Study Group in 2001.

ERAS is a concept inclusive of many different surgical subspecialties, and it is not surprising that cardiac surgery gained the relevance to establish its own Society. Cardiac surgery is a peculiar type of surgery that includes many unique characteristics. The most relevant is certainly the need for cardiopulmonary bypass (CPB) in the majority of the procedures, but other specific aspects include the use of hypothermia in selected procedures, the coagulopathy associated with CPB, the need for systemic anticoagulation, the coagulation factor consumption, the inflammatory reaction due to the release of cytokines and other mediators, and others. The combination of these factors creates the perfect environment for the development of post-surgery complications. Depending on the severity of the procedure, major morbidity (defined as acute kidney injury, stroke, prolonged mechanical ventila-

G. Sepolvere, S. Silvetti (eds.), *Fast-Track in Cardiac Anesthesia*,
https://doi.org/10.1007/978-3-031-70899-2_1

tion, surgical reoperation for any cause, and deep sternal infection) ranges from 10 to 30% in the USA [1]. About 30% of the cardiac surgery patients are anemic [2], and cardiac surgery is one of the specialties with the highest rate of allogeneic blood transfusion.

Many attempts have been done to contain the risk of postoperative complications. They include the use of specific drugs and products to contain bleeding [3]; the CPB modification toward a minimally invasive technique [4]; the surgical access minimization (mini-thoracotomy, mini-sternotomy) [5]; the application of robotic surgery [5]; and others.

Given this very specific scenario, the need for a specific approach to ERAS in cardiac surgery appears clear and requires adequate steps. In particular, the multidisciplinary nature of the team ("the heart team") is warranted, because the interventions to contain the postoperative complications and speed up the recovery process, fulfilling the ERAS philosophy, can be applied at different levels by different players. The preoperative optimization is usually managed by cardiologists, internists, cardiac surgeons, and cardiac anesthesiologists; the choice of the surgical technique is up to the cardiac surgeon, and the application of mini-invasive CPB should be decided and controlled by the combined efforts of the perfusionist, the cardiac surgeon, and the anesthesiologist; finally, anesthesiologists-intensivists are responsible for the application of programs enabling a fast discharge from the intensive care unit, like early extubation programs.

The ERACS Society provided a comprehensive attempt to cover all these topics composing an ERACS program. The first Consensus Document dates back to 2017, when a multidisciplinary group of 16 individuals was ultimately selected that included cardiac surgeons, anesthesiologists, and intensivists demonstrating expertise in subjects related to recovery, as well as specifically those who had experience with ERAS. The group identified a list of 22 potential interventions divided into preoperative, intraoperative, and postoperative phases. After following a process of mutual agreement on each proposed statement, a Consensus Document was finalized and presented at the American Association for Thoracic Surgery (AATS) meeting on April 28, 2018, and May 2, 2018. Following this important step, in 2019, the ERACS published the complete guidelines and a list of 22 recommendations [6]. The most important anesthesiologic items emphasized by the ERACS Society are multimodal analgesia and early extubation. These two points are analyzed in this book, while all the ERACS recommendations are treated in the next chapter.

After this cornerstone published from ERACS in JAMA in 2019, other important scientific contributions were provided by this Society. A consensus statement published in 2023 [7] emphasizes the two previously discussed points: within the multimodal analgesia, for the first time officializing the importance of chest wall block in cardiac surgery patients, defining this as "effective component of multimodal approach in perioperative pain management"; within the early extubation (6 postoperative hours), this is defined as a safe practice in elective patients. In this consensus statement, for the first time, and despite a low level of evidence, also the ultrafast-track extubation was included. The ultrafast-track extubation is defined as intraoperative or immediately postoperative (within 1 h), a practice founding a place only in highly selected patients who have undergone low-risk cardiac surgery. A specific chapter on ultrafast-track extubation is included in this book.

To validate the pain management as a hinge in cardiac surgery patients, another consensus statement focused only on pain management was released by ERACS in 2023 [8]. The process resulted in the promulgation of six recommendations regarding pain management and opioid stewardship in cardiac surgery, focused on avoiding the use of high-dose opioids, as well as encouraging more widespread application of foundational aspects of ERAS, such as the use of multimodal nonopioid medications and regional anesthesia techniques, formal patient and provider education, and structured system-level opioid prescription practices.

In recent years, the interest in the application of ERAS to cardiac surgery has grown significantly. It must however be recognized that the application of ERAS protocol to cardiac surgery is difficult because it involves a methodical shift more in the culture than in clinical practice, meeting the challenges of initiating and sustaining meaningful organizational change, and pivoting to a patient-centered system of care to optimize speed and completeness of recovery.

1.3 ERACS Program

1.3.1 Why Start an ERACS Program

Despite the evident and known difficulties in organizing an ERACS program, in this book, we will emphasize the importance of adhesion to this culture.

High compliance with these protocols is shown to reduce surgical insult, promote recovery, and prevent postoperative complications, thereby improving the value of delivered care without compromising patient safety. The ERAS protocol is safe and feasible in an elective setting, and reducing patient complications leads to a quicker ICU and hospital discharge.

1.3.2 How to Start an ERACS Program

Initiating an ERACS program is a long path; it is a huge change in mentality and practice not only for the physicians but also for the hospital organization. To follow this way, many objectives should be aimed, and many collaborations must work well. Here, we suggest some fundamental points to start an adequate ERACS program (Fig. 1.1) [9].

The first step is organizing a dedicated multidisciplinary ERACS team that includes all figures, surgeons, anesthesiologist, intensivists, nurses, and other consultants. The team will be tasked to developing their own center-specific ERAS protocol, promote education initiatives, and check and evaluate the evolution of the program constantly applying the needed changes.

The second step is to draw up and follow this ERACS protocol. In addition to using the ERACS guideline [6], each hospital should base its program on the local expertise. Obviously, each program should include in their protocol some fundamental goals of ERAS as multimodal analgesia and early extubation (these two points are the main topic of this book), but a standard proto-

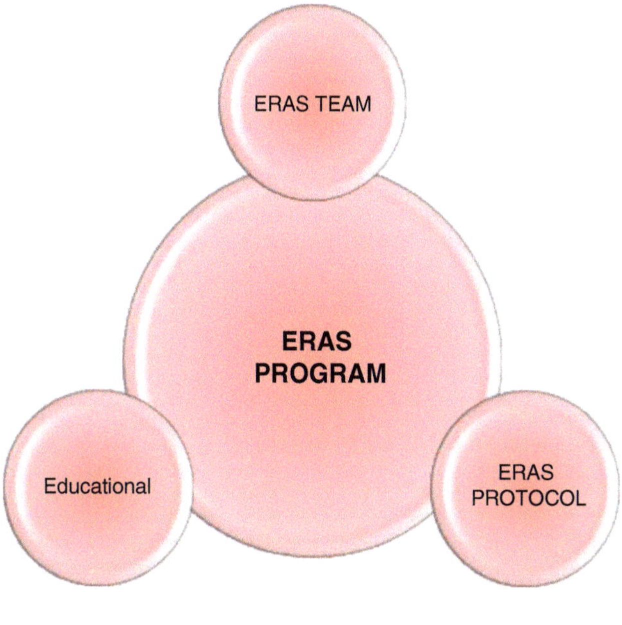

Fig. 1.1 Component of ERAS program

col suitable for every center cannot be proposed. For example, some centers usually and routinely perform peripheral blocks but other centers do not.

Each protocol should have a multidisciplinary approach and includes three moments: careful preoperative planning, intraoperative management, and comprehensive postoperative care.

Third and probably the most important point is the educational planning for anyone who takes care of the patients and for patients themselves. Patient education is crucial for understanding and cooperation to the postoperative care protocols. Educating patients about the goals of care, including the benefits and processes of early extubation, helps them understand the importance of participating in the recovery phase. Effective education can reduce anxiety, improve compliance with rehabilitation protocols, and enhance patient outcomes. Furthermore, nursing team must be involved and prepared. As a matter of fact, nursing care adjustments are essential for supporting the complex needs of postoperative patients and achieving the goal of early extubation. Nurses frequently assess pain, respiratory distress, and signs of neurological changes to early detect any complications. They closely collaborate with respiratory therapists to wean patients from the ventilator according to established criteria. Proper management of surgical wounds, including appropriate dressings and monitoring for signs of infection, is also an essential aspect of nursing care.

ERACS program, as all new initiatives, must overcome some barriers, economic, organizational, and interpersonal. A good ERAS program will start only with hospital authorization and will operate only when all healthcare personnel involved agree and apply the aforementioned protocol.

1.3.3 Who Is a Candidate to an ERACS Program?

At the moment, there are no standardized criteria for fast-track extubation, and each institution has eventually developed its own internal procedure. The matter of understanding the most appropriate clinical criteria and the best approach for patient selection in terms of pursuing a fast-track extubation is a difficult matter and currently relies on a low quality of evidence, mainly because it is influenced by local factors that cannot be fully accounted for in the research produced by single centers. Indeed, most of the evidence and literature available remain related to single-center experience reported with retrospective analyses. Further, in order to increase the sample size, the authors usually pool together data collected during long time periods, where several local factors such as change of policies, staffing, and processes are likely to influence the results.

A score for patient selection should be developed because it would be really useful for our work and for the safety of patient himself. Furthermore, this score should have a "two-stage" structure, with a first selection based on patient and procedure characteristics, and a second selection based on intraoperative and early postoperative factors.

1.4 Conclusion

ERAS program represents a paradigm shift towards a more efficient, patient-centered model of care, optimizing surgical outcomes and resource utilization in cardiac surgery. However, personalized care plans and continuous quality improvement are mandatory to maintain the effectiveness of these protocols and obtain all benefits.

References

1. STS Public Reporting. Adult Cardiac Surgery Public Reporting I STS Public Reporting. Accessed 10 June 2024.
2. Muñoz M, Gómez-Ramírez S, Campos A, Ruiz J, Liumbruno GM. Pre-operative anaemia: prevalence, consequences and approaches to management. Blood Transfus. 2015;13(3):370–9.
3. Task Force on Patient Blood Management for Adult Cardiac Surgery of the European Association for Cardio-Thoracic Surgery (EACTS) and the European Association of Cardiothoracic Anaesthesiology

(EACTA), Boer C, Meesters MI, Milojevic M, Benedetto U, Bolliger D, von Heymann C, Jeppsson A, Koster A, Osnabrugge RL, Ranucci M, Ravn HB, Vonk ABA, Wahba A, Pagano D. 2017 EACTS/EACTA guidelines on patient blood management for adult cardiac surgery. J Cardiothorac Vasc Anesth. 2018;32(1):88–120.

4. Anastasiadis K, Antonitsis P, Murkin J, Serrick C, Gunaydin S, El-Essawi A, Bennett M, Erdoes G, Liebold A, Punjabi P, Theodoropoulos KC, Kiaii B, Wahba A, de Somer F, Bauer A, Kadner A, van Boven W, Argiriadou H, Deliopoulos A, Baker RA, Breitenbach I, Ince C, Starinieri P, Jenni H, Popov V, Moorjani N, Moscarelli M, Di Eusanio M, Cale A, Shapira O, Baufreton C, Condello I, Merkle F, Stehouwer M, Schmid C, Ranucci M, Angelini G, Carrel T. 2021 MiECTiS focused update on the 2016 position paper for the use of minimal invasive extracorporeal circulation in cardiac surgery. Perfusion. 2023;38(7):1360–83.
5. Faerber G, Mukharyamov M, Doenst T. Is there a future for minimal access and robots in cardiac surgery? J Cardiovasc Dev Dis. 2023;10(9):380.
6. Engelman DT, Ben Ali W, Williams JB, Perrault LP, Reddy VS, Arora RC, Roselli EE, Khoynczhad A, Gerdisch M, Levy JH, Lobdell K, Fletcher N, Kirsch M, Nelson G, Engelman RM, Gregory AJ, Boyle EM. Guidelines for perioperative care in cardiac surgery: enhanced recovery after surgery society recommendations. JAMA Surg. 2019;154(8):755–66.
7. Grant MC, Crisafi C, Alvarez A, Arora RC, Brindle ME, Chatterjee S, et al. Perioperative care in cardiac surgery: a joint consensus statement by the enhanced recovery after surgery (ERAS) cardiac society, ERAS International Society, and the Society of Thoracic Surgeons (STS). Ann Thorac Surg. 117:669. https://doi.org/10.1016/j.athoracsur.2023.12.006.
8. Grant MC, Chappell D, Gan TJ, Miller TE, Brodt JL, On Behalf of the PeriOperative Quality Initiative (POQI) and the Enhanced Recovery After Surgery (ERAS) Cardiac Society Workgroup. Pain management and opioid stewardship in adult cardiac surgery: joint consensus report of the PeriOperative Quality Initiative and the Enhanced Recovery After Surgery Cardiac Society. J Thorac Cardiovasc Surg. 2023;166(6):1695–1706.e2. https://doi.org/10.1016/j.jtcvs.2023.01.020.
9. Jawitz OK, Bradford WT, McConnel G, Engel J, Allender JE, Williams JB. How to start an enhanced recovery after cardiac surgery program. Crit Care Clin. 2020;36(4):571–9.

2 Enhanced Recovery After Surgery (ERAS) Recommendations

Mauro D'Amora,
Blanca Martinez Lopez De Arroyabe,
and Gianluca Paternoster

2.1 Perioperative Care and Outcomes

A surgery fast track, often referred to as fast-track surgery program or enhanced recovery after surgery (ERAS), consists of perioperative protocols designed to improve the recovery process for surgical patients [1]. The need for multimodal surgical care converged towards the ERAS® Society, officially registered as a no-profit medical society based in Stockholm, Sweden. The mission of the Society is to develop perioperative care and improve recovery through research, education, audit, and implementation of evidence-based practice. High-quality perioperative care has been shown to minimize postoperative complications and decrease postoperative length of hospital stay.

ERAS is a multidisciplinary approach aimed at providing bundled best practice interventions and therapies in the perioperative period. ERAS adopts evidence-based protocols that are published and regularly updated across various surgical specialties. Registry-based observational studies indicate that high compliance with these protocols reduces surgical insult, promotes recovery, and prevents postoperative complications [2].

In the setting of cardiac surgery, the main objectives of a fast-track cardiac approach include the reduction in hospital length of stay, the enhancement of the quality of care, and then the improvement in patient satisfaction. To achieve these objectives, the optimization of the various phases of hospitalization (preoperative, intraoperative, and postoperative) is necessary (Table 2.1) [3].

This chapter was conceived with the contribution of Blanca Martinez, a brilliant anesthesiologist and a sincere friend who prematurely passed away. This chapter is dedicated to Blanca.

M. D'Amora
Department of Cardiac, Thoracic and Vascular Anesthesia, University Hospital "San Giovanni di Dio e Ruggi D'Aragona", Salerno, Italy

B. M. L. De Arroyabe
Cardiothoracic and Vascular Anesthesia and Intensive Care Unit, University Hospital of Verona, Verona, Italy

G. Paternoster (✉)
Department of Health Science Cardiovascular Anesthesia and ICU School of Medicine, San Carlo Hospital University of Basilicata, Potenza, Italy

G. Sepolvere, S. Silvetti (eds.), *Fast-Track in Cardiac Anesthesia*,
https://doi.org/10.1007/978-3-031-70899-2_2

Table 2.1 Essential elements of ERAS protocol

Preoperative	Intraoperative	Postoperative
Risk assessment	Bleeding management	Active tube drainage clearance
Prehabilitation program with patient education	Sternotomy closure with rigid plate fixation	Glycemic control
Screening for undiagnosed diabetes	Temperature management	Hypothermia prevention
Serum albumin control	Intraoperative lung-protective ventilation	Postoperative nausea and vomiting prevention
Nutritional supplementation	Hemodynamic management	Early extubation
Oral carbohydrate drink loading		Vascular thrombotic event prevention
Antibiotic therapy		Acute kidney injury prevention
		Early postoperative rehabilitation
		Goal-directed fluid therapy
		Postoperative atrial fibrillation prevention
		Delirium screening and prevention
		Pain control and locoregional analgesia
		Blood management protocol

2.2 Preoperative Strategies

The preoperative strategies include the following:

Risk assessment is an important tool to analyze the basic characteristics to recognize the aspects used for an optimization strategy and actions to reduce the surgical risk. The European Heart Surgery Risk Assessment System 2011 revision (EuroSCORE II) calculator is the most widely used tool to determine in-hospital and early postoperative mortality and morbidity [4, 5] (Table 2.2).

Prehabilitation program with patient education, nutritional optimization, exercise training, social support, and anxiety management should

Table 2.2 EuroSCORE risk assessment: set of risk factors to assess the Euro-SCORE mortality score

Risk factor	Definition and explanation
Renal dysfunction	This is assessed by CC, estimated using the Cockcroft–Gault formula, and falls into three categories: CC 51–85, on dialysis (regardless of serum creatinine), and CC ≤50
NYHA	Classification for dyspnea
CCS 4 class angina	The inability to perform any activity without angina, or experiencing angina at rest
IDDM	Insulin-dependent diabetes mellitus
Extracardiac arteriopathy	Claudication; carotid occlusion or >50% stenosis (according to north American symptomatic carotid endarterectomy trial criteria); amputation due to arterial disease; previous or planned intervention on the abdominal aorta, limb arteries, or carotids
Poor mobility	Severe mobility impairment due to musculoskeletal or neurological dysfunction
Previous cardiac surgery	One or more previous major cardiac operations
Active endocarditis	Patients undergoing surgery while still receiving antibiotic treatment for endocarditis
Critical preoperative state	One or more of the following occurring preoperatively during the same hospital admission as the operation: ventricular tachycardia or fibrillation, aborted sudden death, cardiac massage, ventilation before arrival in the anesthetic room, use of inotropes, intra-aortic balloon counterpulsation or ventricular-assist device before arrival in the anesthetic room, or acute renal failure (anuria or oliguria <10 mL/h)
LVEF	Good (LVEF better than 51%); moderate (LVEF 31–50%); poor (LVEF 21–30%); very poor (LVEF 20% or less)

(continued)

Table 2.2 (continued)

Risk factor	Definition and explanation
Urgency of procedure	– Elective: routine admission for operation – Urgent: patients not electively admitted for operation but who require surgery during the current admission for medical reasons and cannot be discharged without a definitive procedure – Emergency: operation before the beginning of the next working day after the decision to operate – Salvage: patients requiring cardiopulmonary resuscitation (external cardiac massage) en route to the operating theatre or before induction of anesthesia. This does not include cardiopulmonary resuscitation after induction of anesthesia
Recent myocardial infarction	Within 90 days before operation
Weight of procedure	This evaluates the complexity or scale of the procedure. The baseline is isolated CABG. Procedures considered more complex than the baseline fall into three categories: (1) Isolated non-CABG major procedure (e.g., single-valve procedure, replacement of ascending aorta, correction of septal defect). (2) Two major procedures (e.g., CABG + AVR, CABG + MVR, AVR + replacement of ascending aorta, CABG + maze procedure, AVR + MVR). (3) Three or more major procedures (e.g., AVR + MVR + CABG, MVR + CABG + tricuspid annuloplasty), or aortic root replacement when it includes AVR or repair + coronary reimplantation + root and ascending replacement

CC creatinine clearance, *NYHA* New York Heart Association, *LVEF* left ventricular ejection fraction, *CABG* coronary artery bypass graft, *AVR* aortic valve replacement, *MVR* mitral valve repair

be considered. Prehabilitation helps patients to support the stress of surgery by enhancing functional ability. Approximately 50% of patients scheduled for cardiac surgery are considered fragile patients. Smoking cessation and abstinence from alcohol for 1 month should be incorporated into a prehabilitation program because they reduce the risk of respiratory failure, wound infections, bleeding, and metabolic derangement.

Screening for undiagnosed diabetes, assessed by hemoglobin A1c, is necessary to analyze the glucose control in the previous 3 months. Optimal preoperative glycemic control, defined as a hemoglobin A1c level below 6%, has been associated with significant reductions in deep sternal wound infections, ischemic events, and other complications [6]. Despite this recommendation, approximately 25% of patients undergoing cardiac surgery have hemoglobin A1c levels above 7%, and 10% have undiagnosed diabetes [6].

Serum albumin control: Low serum albumin (<4.0 g/L) is associated with an increased risk of morbidity and mortality despite the body mass index (BMI) [7]. Hypoalbuminemia is an important predictor of perioperative risk; it is related to prolonged mechanical ventilation, acute kidney injury (AKI), infections, extended hospital length of stay, and mortality [8, 9].

Nutritional supplementation: It improves nutritional support from 7 to 10 days before surgery has been associated with a reduction in infections [10]. For example, an oral carbohydrate drink 2 h before surgery may reduce insulin resistance and tissue glycosylation, improve postoperative glycemic control, and enhance return of gut function [11].

Antibiotics: Antibiotics administered intravenously 30–60 min before surgery, and skin antiseptic cleaning treatments can help in reducing surgical site infections [12]. The Society of Thoracic Surgeons' practice guidelines state that a beta-lactam antibiotic is indicated as a single antibiotic of choice for standard cardiac surgical prophylaxis in populations that do not have a high incidence of methicillin-resistant Staphylococcus aureus. Prophylactic antibiotic therapy needs 24–48h of administration.

2.3 Intraoperative Strategies

The intraoperative strategies include the following:

Bleeding management: Bleeding is a common complication after cardiac surgery and is related to increased mortality and morbidity [13]. The strategies proposed to reduce the risk of bleeding include treatment of preoperative anemia, definition of a safe transfusion threshold value, implementation of intraoperative blood scavenging, dynamic monitoring of the coagulation cascade, and use of data-driven algorithms.

Sternotomy closure with rigid plate fixation: If compared with traditional wire cerclage, this technique seems to be superior, in particular in patients with high body max index (BMI), in previous chest wall radiation, in severe chronic obstructive pulmonary disorders, or in patients under steroid therapies [14].

Temperature management is different from many other surgical procedures, because intentional mild or deep hypothermia is often used during cardiopulmonary bypass (CPB) as a neuroprotective and cardioprotective strategy. However, normothermia (>36 °C) should be maintained before and after CPB. Hypothermia after weaning off CPB may lead to platelet dysfunction, coagulopathy, increased bleeding and need for transfusion [15]. Furthemore, hypothermia has multiple additional systemic adverse effects including myocardial depression, arrhythmias, pulmonary hypertension, altered drug metabolism, increased surgical site infections, and increased mortality. All of these complications increase length of stay and healthcare costs [16, 17]. Use of forced-air warming blankets, fluid warmers, and increased room temperature helps to prevent hypothermia.

Intraoperative lung-protective ventilation: In patients undergoing cardiac surgery, it is common (up to 25%) to observe derangements in pulmonary function [18]. A recent observational study investigating the effects of intraoperative mechanical ventilation on postoperative pulmonary complications after cardiac surgery demonstrated that the application of an intraoperative lung-protective ventilation bundle, consisting of low tidal volume ventilation (<8 mL/kg predicted body weight), modified driving pressure (peak inspiratory pressure, PEEP) <16 cm H_2O, and PEEP ≥5 cm H_2O, was independently associated with reduced pulmonary complications after cardiac surgery [19]. At this time, during CPB, there is no strong evidence on the type of ventilation to reduce the postoperative complications.

Hemodynamic management: In patients with hemodynamic instability, there are multiple cardioactive and vasoactive drugs to select, in order to maintain relatively stable hemodynamic parameters (≤20% deviation from the baseline). In this clinical situation, it is crucial to know how inotropes and vasoactive drugs work in terms of selective actions (receptors) and side effects. This is critical for the success of ERAS protocol and patients' clinical outcomes.

2.4 Postoperative Strategies

The postoperative strategies include the following:

Active tube clearance aims at increasing chest tube drainage efficiency [12]. Immediately after surgery, most patients have some bleeding from surgical drains. Retained blood can cause tamponade or hemothorax. It also causes hemolysis and promotes oxidative inflammatory process, potentially causing pleural and pericardial effusions and triggering postoperative atrial fibrillation [20]. While there are no standard criteria for the timing of mediastinal drain removal, evidence suggests that they can be safely removed once the drainage becomes macroscopically serous. Maintaining chest tube patency without breaking the sterile field is recommended to prevent complications from retained blood. Stripping or breaking the sterile field of chest tubes to remove clots is not recommended.

Glycemic control: is associated with improved outcomes [21]. After cardiac surgery, hyperglycemia (glucose >160/180 mg/dL) is common and multifactorial and can increase oxidative stress, prothrombotic effects, and hyperinflammation. Postoperative hypoglycemia should be avoided [22].

Temperature control: Hypothermia is defined as the inability to achieve or maintain normothermia (>36 °C) within 2–5 h after admission to the intensive care unit (ICU) following cardiac surgery and is associated with increased bleeding, prolonged ICU stay, and death [15]. This condition should be prevented by using convection heating methods, as forced-air warming blankets, raising the room temperature, and using fluid warmers for intravenous fluids.

Postoperative nausea and vomiting (PONV): Reported incidence of PONV after cardiac surgery varies from 10 to 70%. This delays recovery, creates electrolyte imbalances, and delays early extubation [23, 24]. Identifying risk factors and providing prophylactic medications decrease the incidence of postoperative nausea and vomiting [25]. The main risk factors are perioperative opioid use, being nonsmoker, being female, and history of motion sickness or postoperative nausea and vomiting. Treatment options include 5-HT3 antagonists, dexamethasone, scopolamine, perphenazine, diphenhydramine, propofol, droperidol, NK-1 antagonists, and acupuncture techniques.

Early extubation: Prolonged mechanical ventilation is associated with longer hospitalization, high morbidity and mortality, and increased costs. Early extubation is recommended **within 6 h** after ICU arrival. ERAS recommends the implementation of a structured extubation protocol as it can reduce time to extubation [26]. There are studies comparing ultrafast-track extubation (within 1 h) versus fast-track extubation [27, 28]; however, at this time, we do not recommend this practice, at least not routinely, but only in selected patients and in certain institute with a greater experience.

Prophylactic anticoagulation: Vascular thrombotic events, including deep venous thrombosis and pulmonary embolism, are potentially preventable complications after cardiac surgery [29]. Prophylactic anticoagulation should be considered on the first postoperative day and daily thereafter. All patients benefit from mechanical thromboprophylaxis achieved with compression stockings and/or intermittent pneumatic compression during hospitalization to reduce the incidence of deep-vein thrombosis.

Acute kidney injury (AKI) prevention: The incidence of AKI ranges from 5 to 20% of cardiac surgery procedures is associated with an increased risk of chronic kidney failure as well as increased mortality and costs [30]. In patients at risk of AKI, it is recommended avoiding nephrotoxic agents and discontinuing angiotensin-converting enzyme inhibitors and angiotensin II antagonists for 48 h. A close monitoring of creatinine and urine output is also recommended, along with strict glycemic control to optimize volume status and hemodynamic parameters [31, 32].

Early postoperative rehabilitation: Early mobilization after cardiac surgery is crucial to the success of ERAS. Early mobilization can significantly reduce the incidence of complications, improve functional capacity, and decrease hospital length of stay [33]. It is a safe procedure as long as it is done under close hemodynamic and clinical monitoring in the ICU setting [33]. In mechanically ventilated patients, there is a high risk of immobilization. In particular, in these patients, early mobilization helps functional recovery and improves outcomes [33]. It also prevents thrombotic events as stroke and pulmonary embolism.

Goal-directed fluid therapy: This approach uses hemodynamic monitoring techniques to guide the appropriate administration of fluids and drugs; this helps preventing low cardiac output, hypotension, and hypertension throughout the perioperative period [34].

Postoperative atrial fibrillation prevention and management (POAF): POAF is a frequent complication with an incidence from 15 to 40%. It is associated with an increased risk of perioperative stroke, hospital length of stay, and costs [35]. Identification of patients with a higher risk of POAF allows the initiation of preventive methods. The CHA_2DS_2-VASc score (Table 2.3) has relatively good performance in predicting POAF after cardiac surgery and may help identify the patients at high risk of POAF [36]. The use of prophylactic β-blockers administered both preoperatively and postoperatively has been shown to

Table 2.3 CHA_2DS_2-VASc score: a score to predict postoperative atrial fibrillation

		Score
C	Congestive heart failure	1
H	Hypertension (>150/90 mmHg)	1
A	Age ≥75	2
D	Diabetes mellitus	1
S_2	Prior TIA or stroke	2
V	Vascular disease	1
A	Age 65–74	1
Sc	Sex (female = 1)	1

0 = low risk; 1 = moderate risk; ≥2 = high risk
TIA transitory ischemic attack

be effective in reducing the incidence of POAF. Posterior pericardial drainage, defined as posterior pericardiotomy incision, chest tube to posterior pericardium, or both, is a safe and straightforward technique that significantly decreases not only the occurrence of early pericardial effusion and POAF but also late pericardial effusion and cardiac tamponade. These advantages contribute to improved survival after cardiac surgery [37].

Delirium: It affects approximately 20–50% of patients following cardiac surgery and is related to decreased in-hospital and long-term survival and impaired cognitive and functional recovery [38]. Early detection of delirium is crucial for its management and should start in the preoperative phase by identifying key risk factors for its development. Due to the complexity of delirium pathogenesis, it is unlikely that a single drug will reduce its incidence after cardiac surgery; non-pharmacologic strategies are the first-line component of management, and there is no evidence that prophylactic antipsychotic use, or other drugs, can reduce delirium. Clinicians should consider the implementation of "ABCDEF liberation bundle" that includes assess, prevent, and manage pain; both spontaneous awakening and spontaneous breathing trials; choice of analgesia and sedation; delirium: assess, prevent, and manage; early mobility and exercise; and family engagement [39].

Pain control is likely the most critical aspect to achieve fast track in cardiac surgery. Inadequate pain management during the early postoperative phase can lead to adverse effects on pulmonary (atelectasis, pneumonia, and stagnation of bronchial secretions), cardiovascular (increased oxygen consumption and tachycardia), and musculoskeletal (muscle weakness and disuse) systems, potentially necessitating reintubation [40].

Poorly controlled pain can lead to clinical syndromes such as chronic postoperative pain or contribute to psychiatric disorders like post-traumatic stress disorder.

ERAS recommends a multimodal analgesia approach as well as opioid sparing and the inclusion of locoregional analgesia protocols in the management of all patients undergoing cardiac surgery procedures. This approach is characterized by the additive or synergistic effects of different medications, thereby reducing total dosages and consequently minimizing adverse effects. In addition to reducing opioid-related adverse events, this approach also appears to result in lower pain scores at all assessment points within the first 72 h and shortened hospital stays [41].

Different medications are used in pain control in ICU as well as in operating room.

Tramadol reduces postoperative morphine consumption by approximately 25%, enhances patient comfort, and decreases pain scores [42]. However, it is associated with an increased incidence of delirium.

Nonsteroidal anti-inflammatory drugs, such as ibuprofen, appear to be associated with an increased risk of renal dysfunction.

Selective COX-2 inhibitors, such as parecoxib and valdecoxib, following CABG surgery are associated with a higher incidence of cardiovascular events, raising significant concerns regarding their use [43].

Paracetamol appears to be a safe choice when administered at a dose of 1 g every 8 h. When combined with opioids, it enhances pain control and reduces the need for opioids. Paracetamol also appears to have an independent antiemetic effect [44].

Dexmedetomidine, an intravenous α-2 agonist, decreases opioid requirements and may reduce postoperative delirium. It also appears to shorten intubation times, but it may increase bradycardia in cardiac surgery patients compared to propofol [45].

Locoregional analgesia strategies, as part of a multimodal analgesic approach in cardiac surgery, enhance patient satisfaction and functional recovery.

Fascial blocks, as a part of locoregional anesthesia in cardiac surgery, reduce opioid use and promote early recovery after surgery [46]. The most common and effective fascial blocks for cardiac surgery procedures are superficial parasternal intercostal plane block, serratus anterior plane block, and rectus sheath nerve block. All these are easy approaches to be applied with a very short learning curve and a lower risk of periprocedural complications; it is important to standardize techniques and protocols along with patient selection. All these techniques are fully described in this book.

Blood management protocol: It is essential to use a patient blood management program that involves local protocols for the reduction of transfusion rate. Any protocol must take into consideration these major points: (1) preoperative screening and optimization of anemia and iron deficiency, (2) minimization of intraoperative blood loss and hemodilution, and (3) permissive anemia during and after surgery [47] (Table 2.4).

Table 2.4 Essential elements for a blood management program

Preoperative assessment	Intraoperative	Postoperative
It is advisable to perform laboratory measurements of antiplatelet drug effect in patients receiving preoperative dual-antiplatelet therapy to determine the optimal timing of surgery	Minimizing the priming volume in the cardiopulmonary bypass circuit decreases hemodilution and the need for blood transfusion	A standardized and conservative perioperative red blood cell transfusion protocol is preferred over a liberal approach to minimize transfusion requirements
Administering intravenous iron and/or erythropoietin-stimulating agents before surgery to boost red blood cell volume	It is recommended to routinely utilize intraoperative red blood cell salvage through centrifugation for blood conservation purposes	Goal-directed transfusion algorithms that integrate point-of-care testing, such as viscoelastic devices, have been demonstrated to decrease bleeding and the need for transfusion
Assessing and treating anemia and iron deficiency with B12, folate, and intravenous iron preparations, as appropriate	The administration of synthetic antifibrinolytic agents such as epsilon-aminocaproic acid (EACA) or tranexamic acid has been demonstrated to decrease the need for blood transfusion	Any blood management program should be optimized according to hospital resources and adapted to local protocols

2.5 ERAS Limitations

In developing an ERAS program in cardiac surgery, we have to consider the potential barriers. Usually, they are represented by patient-related factors, poor health literacy, poor patient engagement, and comorbidities. Important limitations may also come from staff-related factors, lack of information, and poor communication and cooperation; also, lack of leadership and financial problems can represent a brake in the development of an Enhanced Recovery After Cardiac Surgery (ERACS) program.

2.6 Conclusion

ERACS includes interventions with the aim to decrease complications and improve patient outcomes after cardiac surgery. The ERACS approach is focused on optimizing preoperative patient assessment, decrease surgical injury, and minimize postoperative stress. If compared to non-ERACS approach, it has been demonstrated to lower the rates of complications and speed the patient's return to ordinary daily life. To achieve an excellent outcome and optimize the fast track for cardiac surgery patients, a multidisciplinary approach is necessary, including cardiac surgeons, cardiologists, anesthetists, perfusionists, nurses, pharmacists, dietitians, and cardiac rehabilitation specialists. A team should choose the best therapeutic path for each patient, highlighting potential complications on a case-by-case basis. The main challenge in implementing such pathways is the lack of communication between the various disciplines, which also limits the implementation of ERAS protocols. Selecting an ERAS coordinator is recommended to create a point of reference between all the actors, as well as overseeing data collection and protocol implementation.

Anesthesiologists play a pivotal role in the ERACS approach. In this chapter, we gave an outline of the ERACS program from the anesthesiologist perspective.

References

1. Wall J, Dhesi J, Snowden C, Swart M. Perioperative medicine. Future Healthc J. 2022;9(2):138–43.
2. Grant MC, Crisafi C, Alvarez A, Arora RC, Brindle ME, Chatterjee S, et al. Perioperative Care in Cardiac Surgery: a joint consensus statement by the Enhanced Recovery After Surgery (ERAS) Cardiac Society, ERAS International Society, and the Society of Thoracic Surgeons (STS). Ann Thorac Surg. 2024;117(4):P669–89.
3. Hirji SA, Salenger R, Boyle EM, Williams J, Reddy VS, Grant MC, et al. Expert consensus of data elements for collection for enhanced recovery after cardiac surgery. World J Surg. 2021;45(4):917–25.
4. Engelman DT, Ben Ali W, Williams JB, Perrault LP, Reddy VS, Arora RC, et al. Guidelines for perioperative care in cardiac surgery. JAMA Surg. 2019;154(8):755.
5. Nashef SAM, Roques F, Sharples LD, Nilsson J, Smith C, Goldstone AR, et al. EuroSCORE II†. Eur J Cardiothorac Surg. 2012;41(4):734–45.
6. Robich MP, Iribarne A, Leavitt BJ, Malenka DJ, Quinn RD, Olmstead EM, et al. Intensity of glycemic control affects long-term survival after coronary artery bypass graft surgery. Ann Thorac Surg. 2019;107(2):477–84.
7. Engelman DT, Adams DH, Byrne JG, Aranki SF, Collins JJ, Couper GS, et al. Impact of body mass index and albumin on morbidity and mortality after cardiac surgery. J Thorac Cardiovasc Surg. 1999;118(5):866–73.
8. Li N, Qiao H, Guo JF, Yang HY, Li XY, Li SL, et al. Preoperative hypoalbuminemia was associated with acute kidney injury in high-risk patients following non-cardiac surgery: a retrospective cohort study. BMC Anesthesiol. 2019;19(1):171.
9. Karas PL, Goh SL, Dhital K. Is low serum albumin associated with postoperative complications in patients undergoing cardiac surgery? Interact Cardiovasc Thorac Surg. 2015;21(6):ivv247.
10. Waitzberg DL, Saito H, Plank LD, Jamieson GG, Jagannath P, Hwang TL, et al. Postsurgical infections are reduced with specialized nutrition support. World J Surg. 2006;30(8):1592–604.
11. Ljungqvist O. Modulating postoperative insulin resistance by preoperative carbohydrate loading. Best Pract Res Clin Anaesthesiol. 2009;23(4):401–9.
12. Grieshaber P, Heim N, Herzberg M, Niemann B, Roth P, Boening A. Active chest tube clearance after cardiac surgery is associated with reduced reexploration rates. Ann Thorac Surg. 2018;105(6):1771–7.
13. Dyke C, Aronson S, Dietrich W, Hofmann A, Karkouti K, Levi M, et al. Universal definition of perioperative bleeding in adult cardiac surgery. J Thorac Cardiovasc Surg. 2014;147(5):1458–1463.e1.
14. Allen KB, Thourani VH, Naka Y, Grubb KJ, Grehan J, Patel N, et al. Randomized, multicenter trial comparing sternotomy closure with rigid plate fixation to wire cerclage. J Thorac Cardiovasc Surg. 2017;153(4):888–896.e1.
15. Karalapillai D, Story D, Hart GK, Bailey M, Pilcher D, Cooper DJ, et al. Postoperative hypothermia and patient outcomes after elective cardiac surgery. Anaesthesia. 2011;66(9):780–4.
16. Campbell G, Alderson P, Smith AF, Warttig S. Warming of intravenous and irrigation fluids for preventing inadvertent perioperative hypothermia. Cochrane Database Syst Rev. 2015;4(4):CD009891.
17. Grocott HP, Mathew JP, Carver EH, Phillips-Bute B, Landolfo KP, Newman MF. A randomized controlled trial of the Arctic Sun Temperature Management System versus conventional methods for preventing hypothermia during off-pump cardiac surgery. Anesth Analg. 2004;98:298–302.
18. Brown P, Kugelmass AD, Cohen D, Reynolds MR, Culler SD, Dee AD, et al. The frequency and cost of complications associated with coronary artery bypass grafting surgery: results from the United States Medicare Program. Ann Thorac Surg. 2008;85(6):1980–6.
19. Mathis MR, Duggal NM, Likosky DS, Haft JW, Douville NJ, Vaughn MT, et al. Intraoperative mechanical ventilation and postoperative pulmonary

complications after cardiac surgery. Anesthesiology. 2019;131(5):1046–62.
20. Boyle EM, Gillinov AM, Cohn WE, Ley SJ, Fischlein T, Perrault LP. Retained blood syndrome after cardiac surgery: a new look at an old problem. Innovations: technology and techniques in cardiothoracic and vascular surgery. Innovations (Phila). 2015;10(5):296–303.
21. MacIsaac RJ, Jerums G. Intensive glucose control and cardiovascular outcomes in type 2 diabetes. Heart Lung Circ. 2011;20(10):647–54.
22. Lazar HL, Chipkin SR, Fitzgerald CA, Bao Y, Cabral H, Apstein CS. Tight glycemic control in diabetic coronary artery bypass graft patients improves perioperative outcomes and decreases recurrent ischemic events. Circulation. 2004;109(12):1497–502.
23. Hijazi EM, Edwan H, Al-Zoubi N, Radaideh H. Incidence of nausea and vomiting after fast-track anaesthesia for heart surgery. Braz J Cardiovasc Surg. 2018;33(4):371.
24. Sawatzky JAV, Rivet M, Ariano RE, Hiebert B, Arora RC. Post-operative nausea and vomiting in the cardiac surgery population: who is at risk? Heart Lung. 2014;43(6):550–4.
25. Champion S, Zieger L, Hemery C. Prophylaxis of postoperative nausea and vomiting after cardiac surgery in high-risk patients: a randomized controlled study. Ann Card Anaesth. 2018;21(1):8–14.
26. Flynn BC, He J, Richey M, Wirtz K, Daon E. Early extubation without increased adverse events in high-risk cardiac surgical patients. Ann Thorac Surg. 2019;107(2):453–9.
27. Dorsa AG, Rossi AI, Thierer J, Lupiañez B, Vrancic JM, Vaccarino GN, et al. Immediate extubation after off-pump coronary artery bypass graft surgery in 1196 consecutive patients: feasibility, safety and predictors of when not to attempt it. J Cardiothorac Vasc Anesth. 2011;25(3):431–6.
28. Dawn S, Gangopadhyay S, Acharjee A, Nayak S, Piplai G, Gupta K. Immediate extubation versus standard postoperative ventilation: our experience in on pump open heart surgery. Indian J Anaesth. 2010;54(6):525.
29. Parolari A, Mussoni L, Frigerio M, Naliato M, Alamanni F, Galanti A, et al. Increased prothrombotic state lasting as long as one month after on-pump and off-pump coronary surgery. J Thorac Cardiovasc Surg. 2005;130(2):303–8.
30. Hu J, Chen R, Liu S, Yu X, Zou J, Ding X. Global incidence and outcomes of adult patients with acute kidney injury after cardiac surgery: a systematic review and meta-analysis. J Cardiothorac Vasc Anesth. 2016;30(1):82–9.
31. Göcze I, Jauch D, Götz M, Kennedy P, Jung B, Zeman F, et al. Biomarker-guided intervention to prevent acute kidney injury after major surgery. Ann Surg. 2018;267(6):1013–20.
32. Zarbock A, Küllmar M, Ostermann M, Lucchese G, Baig K, Cennamo A, et al. Prevention of cardiac surgery-associated acute kidney injury by implementing the KDIGO guidelines in high-risk patients identified by biomarkers: the PrevAKI-multicenter randomized controlled trial. Anesth Analg. 2021;133(2):292–302.
33. Ljungqvist O, Scott M, Fearon KC. Enhanced recovery after surgery. JAMA Surg. 2017;152(3):292.
34. Osawa EA, Rhodes A, Landoni G, Galas FRBG, Fukushima JT, Park CHL, et al. Effect of perioperative goal-directed hemodynamic resuscitation therapy on outcomes following cardiac surgery: a randomized clinical trial and systematic review. Crit Care Med. 2015;44(4):724–33.
35. Eikelboom R, Sanjanwala R, Le ML, Yamashita MH, Arora RC. Post-operative atrial fibrillation after cardiac surgery: a systematic review and meta-analysis. Ann Thorac Surg. 2020;111:544.
36. Chen YL, Zeng M, Liu Y, Xu Y, Bai Y, Cao L, et al. CHA2DS2-VASc score for identifying patients at high risk of postoperative atrial fibrillation after cardiac surgery: a meta-analysis. Ann Thorac Surg. 2020;109(4):1210–6.
37. Gozdek M, Pawliszak W, Hagner W, Zalewski P, Kowalewski J, Paparella D, et al. Systematic review and meta-analysis of randomized controlled trials assessing safety and efficacy of posterior pericardial drainage in patients undergoing heart surgery. J Thorac Cardiovasc Surg. 2017;153(4):865–875.e12.
38. Arenson BG, MacDonald LA, Grocott HP, Hiebert BM, Arora RC. Effect of intensive care unit environment on in-hospital delirium after cardiac surgery. J Thorac Cardiovasc Surg. 2013;146(1):172–8.
39. Devlin JW, Skrobik Y, Gélinas C, Needham DM, Slooter AJC, Pandharipande PP, et al. Clinical practice guidelines for the prevention and management of pain, agitation/sedation, delirium, immobility, and sleep disruption in adult patients in the ICU. Crit Care Med. 2018;46(9):825–73.
40. Barr LF, Boss MJ, Mazzeffi MA, Taylor BS, Salenger R. Postoperative multimodal analgesia in cardiac surgery. Crit Care Clin. 2020;36(4):631–51.
41. Li M, Zhang J, Gan TJ, Qin G, Wang L, Zhu M, et al. Enhanced recovery after surgery pathway for patients undergoing cardiac surgery: a randomized clinical trial. Eur J Cardiothorac Surg. 2018;54(3):491–7.
42. But AK, Erdil F, Yucel A, Gedik E, Durmus M, Ersoy MO. The effects of single-dose tramadol on post-operative pain and morphine requirements after coronary artery bypass surgery. Acta Anaesthesiol Scand. 2007;51(5):601–6.
43. Nussmeier NA, Whelton AA, Brown MT, Langford RM, Hoeft A, Parlow JL, et al. Complications of the COX-2 inhibitors parecoxib and valdecoxib after cardiac surgery. N Engl J Med. 2005;352(11):1081–91.
44. Jelacic S, Bollag L, Bowdle A, Rivat C, Cain KC, Richebe P. Intravenous acetaminophen as an adjunct analgesic in cardiac surgery reduces opioid consumption but not opioid-related adverse effects: a randomized controlled trial. J Cardiothorac Vasc Anesth. 2016;30(4):997–1004.

45. Liu X, Xie G, Zhang K, Song S, Song F, Jin Y, et al. Dexmedetomidine vs propofol sedation reduces delirium in patients after cardiac surgery: a meta-analysis with trial sequential analysis of randomized controlled trials. J Crit Care. 2017;38(38):190–6.
46. Capuano P, Sepolvere G, Toscano A, Scimia P, Silvetti S, Tedesco M, et al. Fascial plane blocks for cardiothoracic surgery: a narrative review. J Anesth Analg Crit Care. 2024;4(1):20.
47. Boer C, Meesters MI, Milojevic M, Benedetto U, Bolliger D, von Heymann C, et al. 2017 EACTS/EACTA guidelines on patient blood management for adult cardiac surgery. J Cardiothorac Vasc Anesth. 2018;32(1):88–120.

Part II

Loco-regional Anesthesia in Cardiac Procedures

3 Assessment and Pathophysiology of Pain in Cardiac Surgery

Giuseppe Sepolvere and Rafael Blanco

3.1 Introduction

Cardiac surgery represents one of the main surgeries burdened by the highest and most severe rates of perioperative pain leading to impairment of pulmonary function, increased hospital length of stay, and increased mortality and morbidity [1]. The intensity of pain perceived by the patient is significantly influenced by several factors including the use of extracorporeal circulation (ECC), the position during surgery, the anatomical extension of the surgical cut, the tissue damage, the level of preoperative anxiety negatively affecting the patient's psyche, and the analgesic drugs and techniques used in the perioperative period [2, 3]. The etiology of pain comes from different types of insults: damage to tissues, organs, and peripheral nerves; smooth and striated muscle spasm compression of visceral structures; from costal cartilage tissue trauma to ribs and sternum fractures; and inflammatory injuries determining both superficial and deep somatic and visceral pain. If pain is not addressed, it can cause impaired respiratory mechanics, and this will be accompanied by reduced mobility, leading to pulmonary complications or muscle atrophy. Patients feeling pain will breathe more rapidly and less deeply, with cough inhibition and mucus expectoration. There will also be an increased risk of mechanical ventilation, pneumonia, atelectasis, and antibiotic administration. Uncontrolled pain may increase the neurovegetative and metabolic activity inducing dangerous hemodynamic alterations. These conditions may develop hypoxemia, myocardial ischemia or infarction, cerebrovascular accidents, thromboembolism, and delayed wound healing [4, 5] (Fig. 3.1a, b). An important concept is that the cardiac surgery pain is self-limiting. This is particularly severe in the first 24 postoperative hours, decreasing its intensity over the next days. The highest intensity of this pain occurs during the first 6–12 h [6, 7]. Extracorporeal circulation plays a primary role. When used, it activates a systemic inflammatory response syndrome up to organ failure so that patients report more pain than those in whom ECC is not used. Several factors are involved in the inflammatory syndrome such as blood contact with ECC device's surface, blood loss, and ischemic reperfusion injury. Moreover, myocardial reperfusion may activate leukocytes, which in turn may induce atrial fibrillation or several arrhythmias. It is noteworthy that ECC generates coagulopathy, active oxygen, and consequent oxidative stress [8]. Pain intensity depends on the sex and age of patients. It is perceived higher in women than men and less intense in the elderly population due to the higher

G. Sepolvere (✉)
Department of Anesthesia and Cardiac Surgery Intensive Care Unit, San Michele Hospital, Maddaloni, Caserta, Italy

R. Blanco
Corniche Hospital, Abu Dhabi, UAE

G. Sepolvere, S. Silvetti (eds.), *Fast-Track in Cardiac Anesthesia*,
https://doi.org/10.1007/978-3-031-70899-2_3

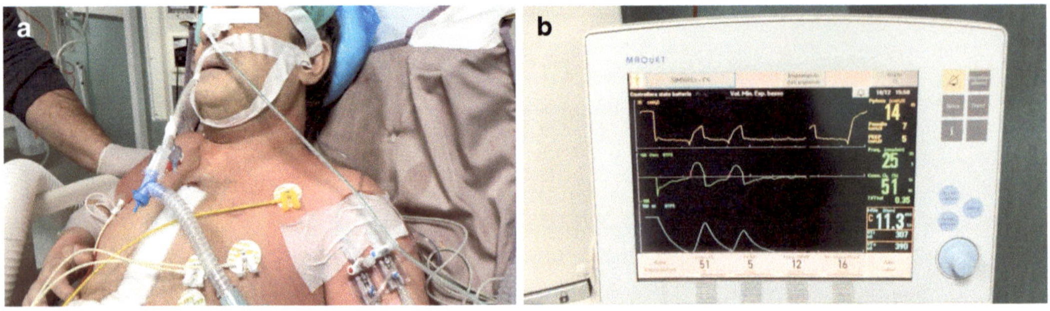

Fig. 3.1 Patient suffering from postoperative cardiac surgery pain. (**a**) Patient experiencing postoperative pain, clearly evident from facial expression. He is showing the location of chest pain in the subxiphoid region. (**b**) Impaired ventilation with high breathing frequency and low tidal volume

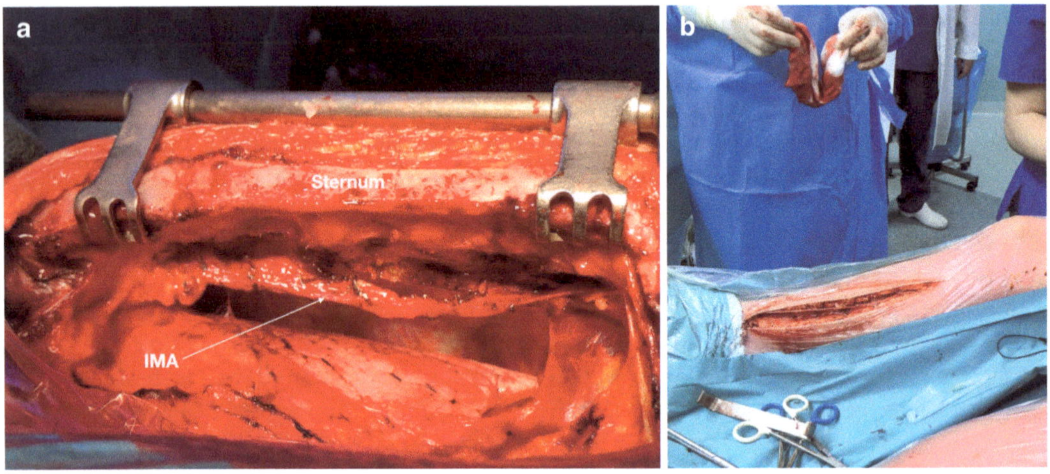

Fig. 3.2 Pain anatomical locations. (**a**) Internal mammary artery region. (**b**) Leg after right vein harvesting. *IMA* internal mammary artery, *Sternum* sternum

pain threshold. Different painful locations have been identified after cardiac surgery: median sternotomy and internal mammary artery harvesting area, leg after vein harvesting (Fig. 3.2a, b), subxiphoid region, oropharynx due to prolonged intubation, and back and shoulders from intraoperative surgery position [9–11]. Minithoracotomy determines a higher postoperative intensity pain compared to the one deriving from median sternotomy leading to potential respiratory complications if not adequately treated (Fig. 3.3b). In addition to that, drainage tubes insertion sites are maximal painful locations after cardiac surgery. The pain caused by subxiphoid drainage tube can be from skin incision, rubbing during the tube insertion, continuing irritation between adjacent tissue and the tube, and direct injury to the rectus abdominis muscles. Their positioning is burdened by a high incidence of severe postoperative pain reported in epigastric region often compromising patient's respiratory dynamics and increasing the risk of respiratory complications especially in severe chronic obstructive pulmonary disease patients (COPD) and delayed extubation [12] (Fig. 3.3a). Moreover, the presence of postoperative drainages may represent a direct nociceptive impulse on parietal pleura innervated by the intercostal and phrenic nerves. Despite continuous advances in the field of cardiac surgery, perioperative pain assessment and relief are still inappropriate. A correct protocol of pain management, in order to avoid complications related to the side effects of opioid administration and delayed extubation or

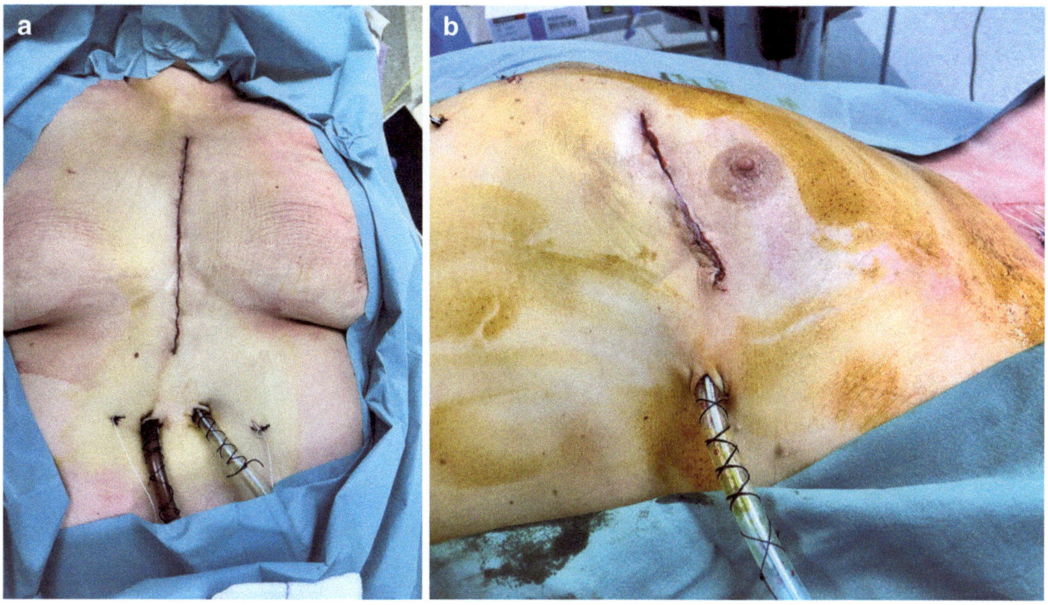

Fig. 3.3 Pain anatomical locations. (**a**) Anterior chest wall and median sternotomy, subxiphoid region, and drainage insertion. (**b**) Lateral chest wall and left or right minithoracotomy

rehabilitation, should be standardized and adopted in the era of fast track and multimodal opioid sparing to improve the patient's quality of life. On this basis, it is mandatory to understand the pathomechanism of postoperative pain exploring the conditions affecting the intensity and perception of pain in patients undergoing cardiac surgery [13, 14].

3.2 Patient Typology and Surgical and Anesthetic Techniques

Coronary artery bypass grafting (CABG) and heart valve surgery (replacement or annuloplasty) are the most common procedures performed in cardiac surgery worldwide. The continuous improving of surgical and anesthetic techniques allows complex surgery in elderly population affected by several comorbidities or low left ventricular contraction (Fig. 3.4a, b). To minimize as far as possible pain experienced by cardiac surgery patients, minimally invasive surgical techniques and ultrasound chest fascial blocks should be adopted as a standardized approach by the heart team. Minimally invasive procedures are well standardized for mitral or aortic valve surgery (Fig. 3.5), atrioventricular surgery and atrial septal defect decreasing postoperative bleeding, reducing incidence of sternal wound infections, and shortening length of stay. Chest wall blocks ensure an optimal and effective postoperative pain relief, decreasing the incidence of pulmonary complications through an early and fast-track extubation and reducing the administration of opioids. Both minimally invasive direct CABG and totally endoscopic CABG could be performed through minithoracotomy without sternum opening (Fig. 3.6). The limitation of both procedures is that only one or two vessels can be achieved on the anterior wall surface of the heart. The further procedure evolution is represented by the transcutaneous approaches. Transcatheter aortic valve implantation (TAVI) or transcatheter mitral valve repair system is considered an effective alternative to surgical treatment for patients at high risk or not eligible for open-heart surgery (Fig. 3.7). An alternative technique useful in avoiding the use of extracorporeal circulation and reducing the inflammatory systemic response is the off-pump CABG where the grafts are sewn on

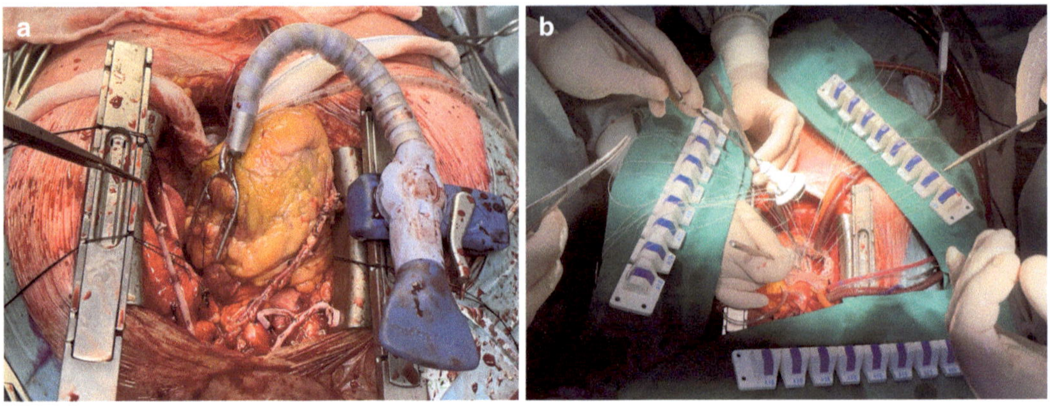

Fig. 3.4 Most common cardiac surgery procedures. (**a**) Off-pump beating heart coronary artery bypass grafting. (**b**) Mitral valve replacement through median sternotomy

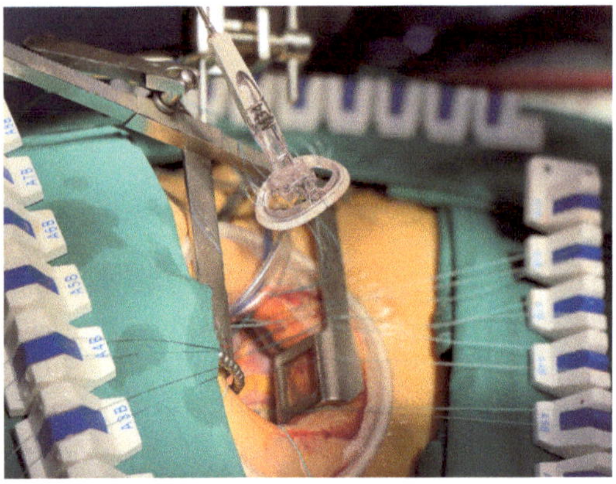

Fig. 3.5 Minimally invasive mitral valve replacement through right minithoracotomy

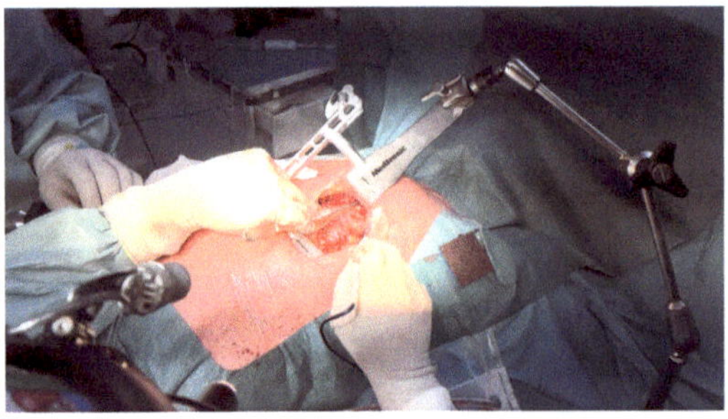

Fig. 3.6 Internal mammary artery harvesting through left minithoracotomy for minimally invasive coronary artery bypass grafting

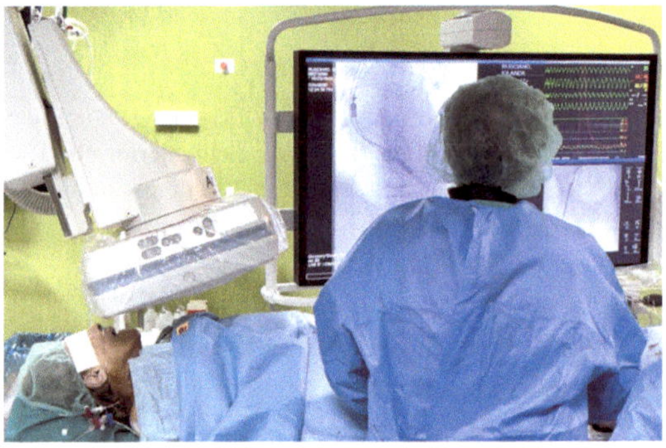

Fig. 3.7 Sedation and spontaneous breathing during pacing phase in a patient undergoing transcatheter aortic valve implantation (TAVI)

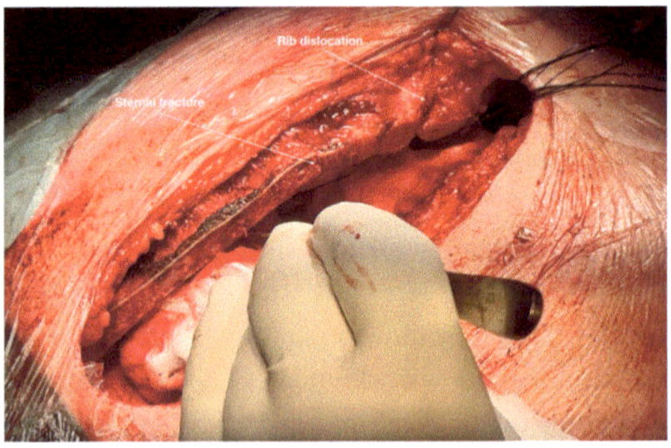

Fig. 3.8 Sternal fracture and costosternal rib dislocation after median sternotomy

a beating heart (Fig. 3.4a). The anterior and posterior chest wall blocks, described in Chap. 8, should be an integral part of multimodal opioid-sparing and ERAS protocols also in emergency conditions. Parasternal block is used to manage pain deriving from median sternotomy, sternal fractures (Fig. 3.8), and anatomical sternal region after the internal mammary artery harvesting. Rectus sheath block can be performed to relieve pain from subxiphoid drainages. Serratus plane block is performed to manage pain deriving from lateral chest minithoracotomy or rib fractures and pneumothorax tube insertion. Pecs I and Pecs II are useful in case of pacemaker or subcutaneous implantable cardioverter defibrillator (S-ICD) implantation combined with serratus plane block. Erector spinae plane block (ESP) is performed to manage lateral and anterior cardiac surgery chest pain. It is noteworthy to underline that through a systematic review and meta-analysis in cardiac surgery patients, King et al. stated that ESP block was not associated with reduced postoperative pain, intraoperative opioid consumption, time extubation, and ICU length of stay [15–17].

3.3 Acute Postoperative Pain

Duration and type of surgery, extent of incision, and analgesic procedures are the main factors influencing the postoperative pain. On this basis, both surgeons and anesthesiologists modify the traditional approaches finding new minimally invasive techniques. Even if pain in cardiac surgery is the secondary effect of a planned surgery, its incidence is linked to direct trauma to tissues and organs and develops after the cessation of intraoperative analgesic drug action. This type of pain gradually reduces its intensity in the first 24 h, disappearing in the following days up to a maximum of about 10 days. Tissue damage leads to the release of several inflammatory mediators such as substance P, cytokines, serotonin, and histamine resulting in peripheral sensitization and activation of sleeping nociceptors so that it can also last up to 3 months and above, becoming chronic pain [18, 19]. Through a mechanism of central sensitization, the patients report excessive response to painful stimulations deriving from the surgical wound or from the site surrounding it (hyperalgesia) even after a light stimulus (allodynia). Often, it is difficult to locate and lasts longer than expected. In the era of minimally invasive procedures, rib fractures or dislocation of costosternal joints from minithoracotomy or sternal retractors may promote the development of acute and very intense postoperative pain (Fig. 3.8). The immediate postoperative period is crucial for early patient extubation, which represents the anesthetic goal for the fast track in cardiac surgery. In case of severe acute postoperative pain, the respiratory system results impaired, and the patients may lie immobilized in bed with breath shortness, reduced tidal volume and vital capacity, reduced pulmonary compliance, atelectasis, pulmonary infections, and subsequent delayed extubation and increased risk of length of stay or further postoperative complications [20]. Due to the general hemodynamic instability of cardiac patients, the activation of the sympathetic nervous system on the cardiovascular system and gastrointestinal and urinary tracts has a relevant aspect. Acute postoperative pain may induce heart rate acceleration, increase contractility and tone of the heart walls, and elevate arterial blood pressure. The latter may result to be particularly dangerous in patients in the postoperative period due to the increased potential incidence of blood loss, heart valve failure, or primary heart failure deriving from the increased vascular resistances. This way, peripheral blood flow is reduced with consequent venous stasis (increased by immobilization) and development of deep-vein thrombosis. The postoperative inflammatory condition makes platelets more susceptible to aggregate with increased risk of cerebrovascular thrombosis or bypass grafting dysfunction. Activation of the sympathetic system also impairs the motility of the gastrointestinal tract (spasm of the sphincters), the urinary bladder, and the urethra and activates the catabolic phase with reduced insulin level and increased level of cortisol, catecholamine, antidiuretic hormone, corticotropic hormone, renin, angiotensin, and aldosterone. A prolonged pain stimulation may induce a suppression of immune system leading to a delayed wound healing and increased incidence of systemic infections [21, 22]. Perception of pain is a subjective sensation influenced not only by the surgical trauma and anesthetic procedures but also by biological, psychological, and sociological factors. Uncovered acute pain causes fear, sleep disorders, anxiety,

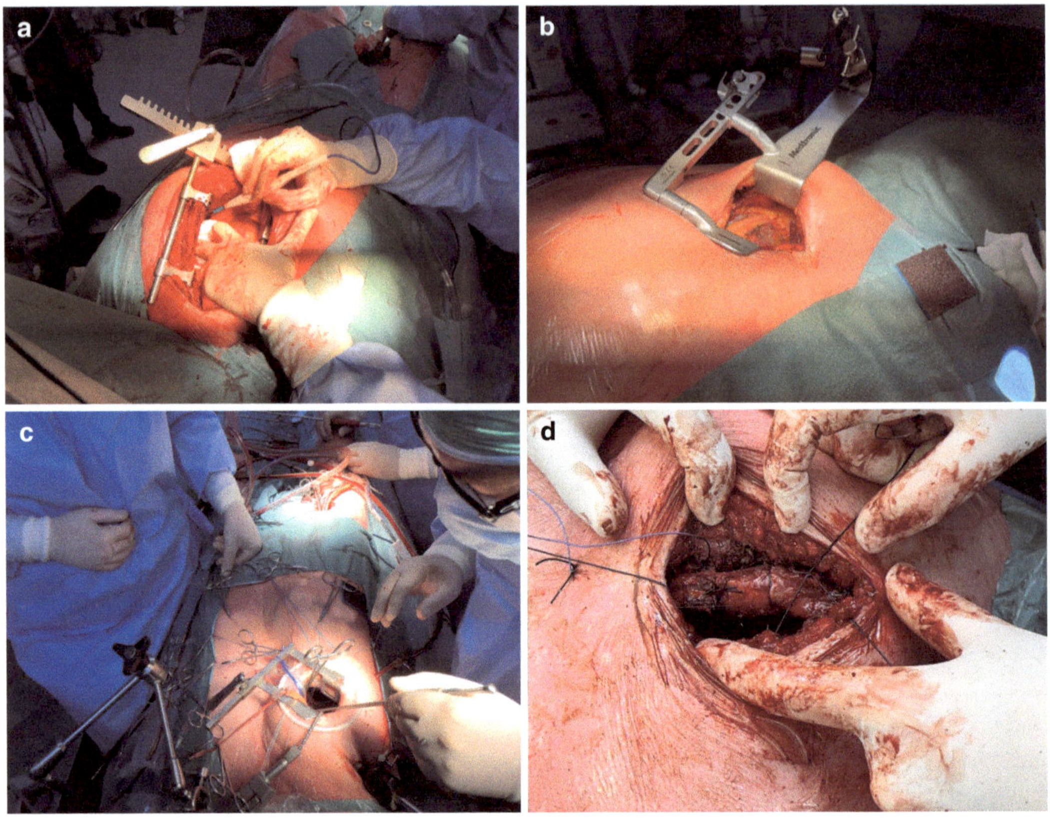

Fig. 3.9 Intercostal nerve trauma caused by surgical dilator compression or rib and sternal fractures. (**a**) Sternal dilator. (**b**) Left minithoracotomy retractor for minimally invasive coronary artery bypass grafting. (**c**) Right minithoracotomy dilator for minimally invasive mitral valve replacement. (**d**) Rib fracture caused by left minithoracotomy dilator for minimally invasive coronary artery bypass grafting

and depression. It should not be forgotten that psychological components, such as high levels of anxiety, emotional lability, and pessimistic attitude, can increase pain sensations. In addition, the intensive care unit could be perceived as the place in which the patients are thirsty and have tube and probes in mouth or nose but much more importantly when they are not able to sleep [23]. In addition to the subxiphoid region, postoperative drainages generate pain from parietal pleura innervated by intercostal and phrenic nerves. When the intercostal space is opened as for minithoracotomy, the intercostal nerves are exposed to injury or trauma due to a potential rib fractures or by the surgery dilator compression leading to demyelination and both acute and chronic pain [24] (Fig. 3.9). The most intense pain is associated with coughing or deep breathing during respiratory physiotherapy, movements, or getting up from bed. The pain anatomical areas vary from day to day. In the first 24 h, the thoracotomy region, the chest and mediastinal and pleural drain placement sites, the sternal and subxiphoid regions, and the back, shoulders, and buttocks related to the intubation and intraoperative surgery position are predominant. On the following days, pain in these areas gradually decreases, probably due to the removal of drains and the possibility to move within the bed.

3.4 Chronic Postoperative Pain

If it persists longer than the patient's recovery, it may take the characteristics of chronic pain. Patients undergoing cardiac surgery are exposed to several nociceptive stimulations that can lead to chronic postoperative pain (CPOP) and related persistent postoperative pain (PPP), thus losing their protective action and becoming a serious and disabling condition itself. In some patients, CPOP lasts for many years or suddenly reappears a long time after surgery. It is stated that 37% of cardiac surgery patients suffer from PPP in the first six postoperative months, while in 17%, it remains for more than 2 years after surgery. Steegers et al. demonstrated that among patients with chronic pain, only in 53% the neuropathic pain component was present, while in 47% of patients, pain was not neuropathic. The etiology of CPOP is multifactorial, but intercostal nerve damage, prolonged chest tube placement, or inadequate perioperative pain management can be associated with continuous stimulation, hypersensitivity, and reorganization of central nervous system, generating an important neuropathic component suggested by the presence of allodynia and/or hyperalgesia. Stecco et al. demonstrated the presence of free nerve endings, corpuscles, and autonomic nerve fibers inside the deep fascia, such as if it were a very "fascial system" participating in the regulation of force transmission, sensory functions, wound regulation, dynamic proprioception, and pain control. Based on these studies, Fusco et al. demonstrated through elastography that the injection of local anesthetic (LA) in the fascial plane may involve the free nerve endings reducing pain and fascial densification and stiffness and increasing homogeneity and elasticity of muscles. As suggested by Werner and Kongsgaard, it could be defined chronic pain if it has the following specific criteria: pain develops or increases its intensity after surgical procedure, it is of at least 3–6 months' duration and significantly affects the quality of life, it is a continuation of acute postoperative surgery or develops after a silent and asymptomatic period, and it directly derives from the surgical site or refers to a dermatome or to a wider anatomical area innervated by the nerves of the surgical site [25–28]. Even if it can manifest as visceral or somatic or mixed pain simulating a myocardial ischemia, sternal instability or mediastinitis after cardiac surgery and CPOP should be differentiated from these acute conditions. Pain after sternotomy could have from mild to moderate intensity mostly located over the anterior chest wall and internal mammary artery harvesting regions. Other factors may influence the development of CPOP such as allergy or intolerance to the wires used for sternal closure or previous cardiac surgery. The main clinical predictive condition of CPOP which should alert the anesthesiologists is the continuous and constant presence of severe postoperative acute pain during the first 24 h. For every 10% increasing time with severe pain, the risk and incidence of CPOP go up to 30% [29]. It is noteworthy that a significant and correct preventive and perioperative analgesia is associated with decreased incidence of CPOP and PPP. Current literature suggests prevention and treatment of PPP through multimodal pharmacology, regional anesthesia, and multidisciplinary involvement. Although opioids have been historically the primary analgesic approach to cardiac surgery, an opioid-sparing and multimodal protocol should be taken into consideration in reducing side effects and avoiding secondary opioid hyperalgesia as happens for ultrashort-acting remifentanil. Multimodal analgesic protocols are often combined with ultrasound fascial blocks able to reduce opioid requirements and their side effects including delirium, hypotension, bradycardia, bleeding, ileus, respiratory depression, and sedation. For refractory neuropathic pain, antiepileptic agents (carbamazepine, lamotrigine, topiramate, etc.), NMDA receptor antagonists such as memantine, and infusions including ketamine or lidocaine are options to take into consideration. In patients with muscle spasms or myofascial pain, muscle relaxants can provide some symptom relief [30]. Adverse effects of CPOP and PPP manifesting as sleep disturbances can be observed even a year after the procedure.

3.5 Assessment of Cardiac Surgery Pain

Pain assessment is the first and most important step for an effective acute and chronic pain treatment. The most commonly used scales include the verbal rating scale (VRS), numeric pain rating scale (NRS), visual analogue scale (VAS), and picture scales based on facial expressions. The VRS includes a sequential digit representing the pain intensity: 0 = no pain, 1 = low pain, 2 = moderate pain, 3 = severe pain, and 4 = very severe pain. NRS is an evaluating pain scale based on 0–10 point scores, where 0 means no pain and 10 means maximum pain. VAS rates the pain intensity on a horizontal line where no pain is located on the left and unbearable pain on the right. While VRS is well understood, the VAS is difficult to be easily comprised by neurological and cognitive disorder patients. The NRS has a sensitivity similar to the VAS, is easy to use, and is recommended for pain assessment by many authors (Fig. 3.10). A facial pain scale (FPS) can be used for both patients unable to communicate verbally and patients with tracheostomy where the smiling face means no pain and the crying one means severe pain (Fig. 3.11). In addition, a correct pain assessment should consider that some physiological behaviors during recovery are not necessarily pain indicators. Pain reported by patients may not be reflected in increased pulse rate or blood pressure or pain facial expressions but as a discomfortable emotional condition. Pain should be estimated at rest but also under dynamic conditions to get correct information when different analgesic protocols are compared. The Prince Henry Hospital Pain Score represents a scale evaluating painful symptoms during basic and physical activity. 0 = no pain on cough, 1 = pain on cough and no pain while taking deep breaths, 2 = pain on deep breathing and no pain at rest, 3 = slight pain at rest, and 4 = severe pain at rest (Fig. 3.12). A new concept of pain assessment is based on the ability of the patient to make movements as well as change position in bed to get comfortable. A patient able to change position on his own or make movements in bed during the very first postoperative hours will also be able to cough or deeply breathe stating a good pulmonary performance (Fig. 3.13a, b). Further pain assessment methods are represented by the graphic representation of location and perception of pain or by questionnaires for acute and chronic pain. The most used questionnaire is the McGill Pain Questionnaire consisting of a diagram of pain with NRS and 74 adjectives concerning location, character, frequency, and intensity of pain. The patients select the words that better describe the felt sensation. Effective treatment of postoperative pain should be based on the administration of analgesics, multimodal analgesia, and regional anesthesia techniques. Pharmacological therapy is based on the nonopioids, nonsteroidal anti-inflammatory drugs (NSAIDs), and paracetamol administrations. Their use is limited by the side

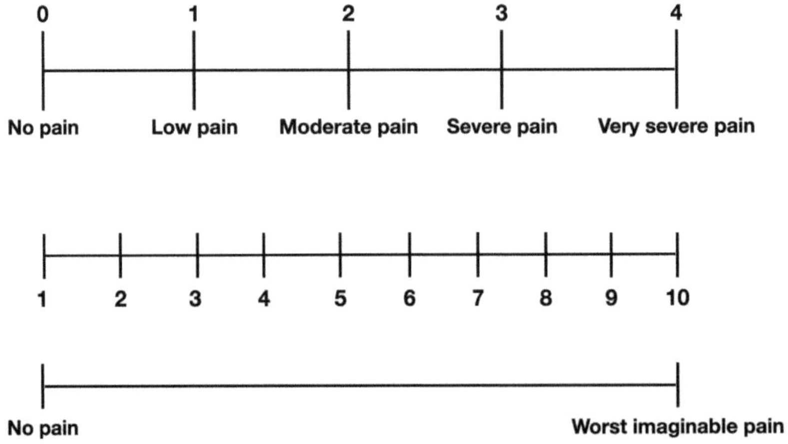

Fig. 3.10 Verbal rating scale, numeric pain rating scale, and visual analogue scale

Fig. 3.11 Facial pain scale

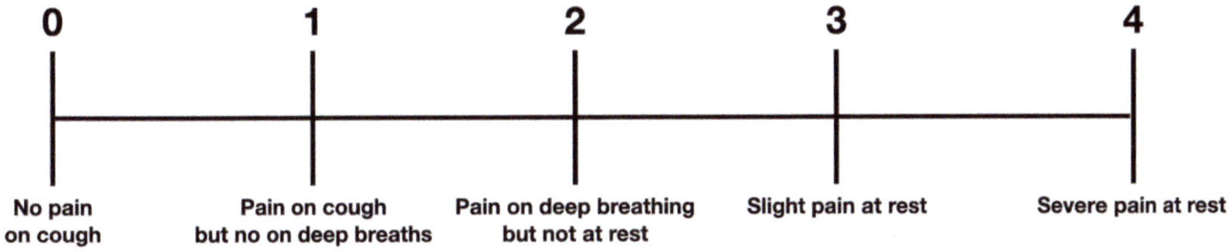

Fig. 3.12 The Prince Henry Hospital Pain Score

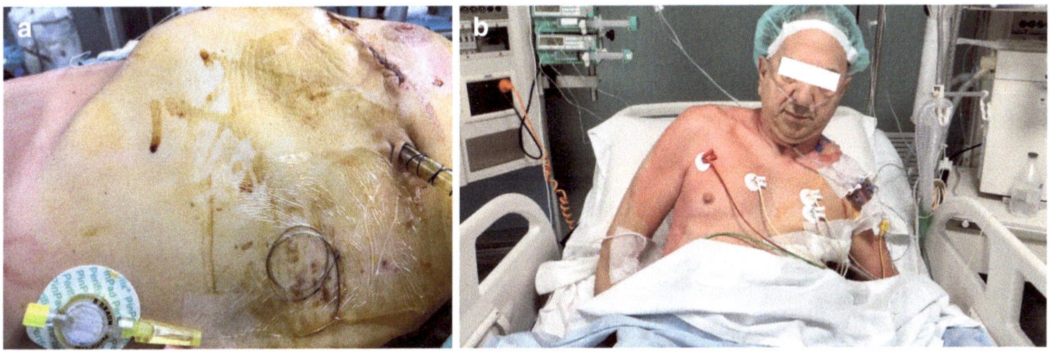

Fig. 3.13 Pain assessment under dynamic condition. (**a**) Continuous deep serratus plane block for left minithoracotomy. (**b**) Patient able to change position in bed during the very first postoperative hours certifying a good pulmonary performance

effects of opioids (ileus, vomiting, sedation, respiratory depression, and delayed extubation leading to prolonged intensive care unit stay) and by the risk of renal dysfunction and bleeding after NSAID administration. Multimodal analgesia is based on the analgesic drug administration together with regional analgesia techniques. In the era of fast-track, ERAS, and multimodal opioid-sparing protocols, the chest wall blocks represent a safe, effective, and valid procedure to be well integrated inside the multidimensional treatments.

3.6 Conclusion and Considerations

Pain management in cardiac and thoracic surgery is actually not well standardized and represents a challenge mostly depending on individual skills, experience, and protocols. It is due to the fact that the pathophysiological mechanisms are unknown or underestimated. Perioperative patient's quality of life is seriously compromised if pain is not well treated, while complications related to an inappropriate analgesia or drug administration side effects could increase the risk of length of stay in intensive care unit, morbidity, and mortality. In 2012, the American Society of Anesthesiologists published guidelines based on the World Health Organization's analgesic ladder with the scope of increasing the efficacy of acute perioperative pain management, improving the patient's quality of life, and decreasing the incidence of complications and chronic pain. Every cardiac anesthesiologist or surgeon should understand and better know the physiological disorders deriving from surgical trauma or extracorporeal circulation and the newest analgesic procedures adopted to reduce the perioperative pain as well as the development of protocols following the entire pathway of cardiac surgery patients. In the era of fast-track extubation, multimodal opioid-sparing, and ERAS approaches, the use of chest wall blocks represents the best choice to reduce acute and chronic perioperative pain and give patients life before the surgery.

References

1. Nachiyunde B, Lam L. The efficacy of different modes of analgesia in postoperative pain management and early mobilization in postoperative cardiac surgical patients: a systematic review. Ann Card Anaesth. 2018;21(4):363–70. https://doi.org/10.4103/aca.ACA_186_17. PMID: 30333328; PMCID: PMC6206788.
2. Apfelbaum JL, Chen C, Mehta SS, Gan TJ. Postoperative pain experience: results from a national survey suggest postoperative pain continues to be undermanaged. Anesth Analg. 2003;97(2):534–40.
3. Cogan J. Pain management after cardiac surgery. Semin Cardiothorac Vasc Anesth. 2010;14(3):201–4.
4. Kaplan JA. In: Kaplan JA, Cronin B, Maus T, editors. Essentials of cardiac anesthesia for cardiac surgery. 2nd ed. Elsevier; 2018.
5. Sasseron AB, Figueiredo LC, Trova K, et al. Does the pain disturb respiratory function after heart surgeries? Rev Bras Cir Cardiovasc. 2009;24(4):490–6.
6. Gerbershagen HJ, Aduckathil S, van Wijck AJ, Peelen LM, Kalkman CJ, Meissner W. Pain intensity on the first day after surgery: a prospective cohort study comparing 179 surgical procedures. Anesthesiology. 2013;118(4):934–44.
7. Bjørnnes AK, Rustøen T, Lie I, Watt-Watson J, Leegaard M. Pain characteristics and analgesic intake before and following cardiac surgery. Eur J Cardiovasc Nurs. 2016;15(1):47–54.
8. Fujii Y. Evaluation of inflammation caused by cardiopulmonary bypass in a small animal model. Biology (Basel). 2020;9(4):81. https://doi.org/10.3390/biology9040081. PMID: 32326072; PMCID: PMC7236599.
9. Mueller XM, Tinguely F, Tevaearai HT, Revelly JP, Chioléro R, von Segesser LK. Pain location, distribution, and intensity after cardiac surgery. Chest. 2000;118(2):391–6.
10. Piraccini E, Biondi G, Byrne H, Calli M, Bellantonio D, Musetti G, Maitan S. Ultrasound guided transversus thoracic plane block, parasternal block and fascial planes hydrodissection for internal mammary post thoracotomy pain syndrome. Eur J Pain. 2018;22(9):1673–7. https://doi.org/10.1002/ejp.1249. Epub 2018 May 31.
11. Roca J, Valero R, Gomar C. Pain locations in the postoperative period after cardiac surgery: chronology of pain and response to treatment. Rev Esp Anestesiol Reanim. 2017;64(7):391–400. https://doi.org/10.1016/j.redar.2017.01.002. Epub 2017 Feb 22.
12. Sepolvere G, Tedesco M, Fusco P, Scimia P, Donatiello V, Cristiano L. Subxiphoid cardiac drainage pain management: could ultrasound rectus sheath block be the answer? Minerva Anestesiol. 2020;86(9):994–6. https://doi.org/10.23736/S0375-9393.20.14576-0. Epub 2020 May 18.
13. Hendrix H, Kamlak V, Prisadov G, Welcker K. Pain treatment after thoracic surgery. Zentralbl Chir. 2017;142(3):337–47.
14. Rothaug J, Zaslansky R, Schwenkglenks M, et al. Patients' perception of postoperative pain management: validation of the international pain outcomes (IPO) questionnaire. J Pain. 2013;14(11):1361–70.
15. Melidi E, Latsios G, Toutouzas K, et al. Cardio-anesthesiology considerations for the trans-catheter aortic valve implantation (TAVI) procedure. Hell J Cardiol. 2016;57(6):401–6.
16. Soylu E, Harling L, Ashrafian H, et al. A systematic review of the safety and efficacy of distal coronary artery anastomotic devices in MIDCAB and TECAB surgery. Perfusion. 2016;31(7):537–43.
17. Easterwood RM, Bostock IC, Nammalwar S, Mccullough JN, Iribarne A. The evolution of minimally invasive cardiac surgery: from minimal access to transcatheter approaches. Future Cardiol. 2018;14(1):75–87.
18. Chapman CR, Tuckett RP, Song CW. Pain and stress in a systems perspective: reciprocal neural, endocrine, and immune interactions. J Pain. 2008;9(2):122–45.
19. Yaksh T, Woller S, Ramachandran R, Sorkin L. The search for novel analgesics: targets and mechanisms. F1000Prime Rep. 2015;7:56.
20. Shenkman Z, Shir Y, Weiss YG, Bleiberg B, Gross D. The effects of cardiac surgery on early and late pulmonary functions. Acta Anaesthesiol Scand. 1997;41(9):1193–9.
21. Bartoloni A, Polati E, Finco G, Facchin S, Rigo V, Gottin L. The neuroendocrine and metabolic responses to surgical stress. Chir Ital. 1995;47(6):3–11.

22. Schultz CH, Rivers EP, Feldkamp CS, et al. A characterization of hypothalamic–pituitary–adrenal axis function during and after human cardiac arrest. Crit Care Med. 1993;21(9):1339–47.
23. Uymaz B, Sezer G, Coskun PK, Tarcan O, Ozleme S, Aybek T. Clinical outcome, pain perception and activities of daily life after minimally invasive coronary artery bypass grafting. Anadolu Kardiyol Derg. 2014;14(2):172–7.
24. Gerner P. Postthoracotomy pain management problems. Anesthesiol Clin. 2008;26(2):355–67.
25. Sepolvere G, Scialdone VR. Chronic pain in cardiac surgery. Minerva Anestesiol. 2023;89(3):230–1. https://doi.org/10.23736/S0375-9393.22.16881-1.
26. Bignami E, Castella A, Pota V, Saglietti F, Scognamiglio A, Trumello C, Pace MC, Allegri M. Perioperative pain management in cardiac surgery: a systematic review. Minerva Anestesiol. 2018;84(4):488–503.
27. Gjeilo KH, Stenseth R, Klepstad P. Risk factors and early pharmacological interventions to prevent chronic postsurgical pain following cardiac surgery. Am J Cardiovasc Drugs. 2014;14(5):335–42.
28. Fusco P, Stecco C, Petroni GM, Ciaschi W, Marinangeli F. ESP block and chronic pain: the dark side of the moon. Minerva Anestesiol. 2022;88(6):528–9.
29. Fine PG, Karwande SV. Sternal wire-induced persistent chest pain: a possible hypersensitivity reaction. Ann Thorac Surg. 1990;49(1):135–6.
30. Krakowski JC, Hallman MJ, Smeltz AM. Persistent pain after cardiac surgery: prevention and management. Semin Cardiothorac Vasc Anesth. 2021;25(4):289–300. https://doi.org/10.1177/10892532211041320. Epub 2021 Aug 20. PMID: 34416847; PMCID: PMC8669213.

Multimodal Opioid Sparing

4

Antonio Toscano, Paolo Scimia,
and Pierfrancesco Fusco

4.1 Introduction

Perioperative pain management is a critical area where anesthesiologists play a key role. Effective postoperative pain relief is essential to prevent both immediate and long-term complications from unmanaged pain. Many anesthesiologists have adopted multimodal techniques to address these factors and optimize patient satisfaction. In addition to traditional opioid-based regimens, various agents can help reduce opioid requirements. Key agents include nonsteroidal anti-inflammatory drugs (NSAIDs), acetaminophen, ketamine, alpha-2 agonists, glucocorticoids, gabapentinoids, and fascial plane blocks. Multimodal analgesia employs a combination of these drugs, each with a different mechanism of action. This approach can potentially mitigate undesirable effects of opioids, such as nausea, vomiting, and respiratory depression, thereby reducing the risk of more serious complications.

A. Toscano (✉)
Department of Anesthesia and Critical Care, Città della Salute e della Scienza di Torino, University of Turin, Turin, Italy

P. Scimia
Department of Anesthesia and Intensive Care Unit, Giuseppe Mazzini Hospital, Teramo, Italy

P. Fusco
Unit of Anesthesia and Intensive Care, SS Filippo e Nicola Hospital, Avezzano, L'Aquila, Italy

4.2 Pain Following Cardiac Surgery

Cardiac surgery, compared to other major surgical procedures, is associated with significant postoperative pain [1], which complicates recovery. Pain is most intense on the first and second postoperative days (PODs 1 and 2); although pain gradually decreases as the postoperative period progresses, almost half of the patients still experience severe pain at rest by POD 4 [2]. Moreover, the location of pain shifts during the postoperative period. In the early stages after surgery, sources of pain include those directly related to surgery such as incisional pain, sternotomy, chest retraction, and intercostal nerve pain; after the second postoperative day (POD 2), significant pain also occurs in other areas such as the lower extremities, due to vein graft harvesting, and the shoulders caused by operative positioning, which is worse for patients with preexisting back or limb issues [2]. Postoperative sources of pain also include pain from the invasion of chest tubes, endotracheal tube, tracheal suctioning, urinary catheter, intravascular lines, nasogastric tube, and possibly postoperative pericarditis and pleuritis. Activities like coughing, moving, turning, deep breathing, and using incentive spirometry are associated with pain through the fourth to sixth postoperative days (POD 4–POD 6). Effective analgesia in cardiac surgery involves a multimodal approach to pain

G. Sepolvere, S. Silvetti (eds.), *Fast-Track in Cardiac Anesthesia*,
https://doi.org/10.1007/978-3-031-70899-2_4

management using two or more analgesics or techniques that target different mechanisms or pathways in the nociceptive system. This approach allows for the use of lower doses of each drug, reducing individual side effects while maintaining overall effectiveness. This theoretically results in better pain relief, improved functional recovery, and fewer opioid-related side effects.

4.3 Opioids

Opioids are the cornerstone of analgesic therapy in cardiac surgery.

The opioid-based cardiac anesthetic/analgesic technique, initiated in the late 1960s, used high-dose IV morphine as a stable primary anesthetic for open-heart surgery, leading to widespread acceptance and continued promotion in anesthesiology literature. Opioids, such as morphine, fentanyl, sufentanil, and remifentanil, became key components due to their hemodynamic stability and lack of negative inotropic effects. These agents act on the central nervous system to provide potent pain relief. However, their use must be carefully balanced to avoid side effects. In fact, opioids are associated with a multitude of undesirable side effects, including somnolence, ICU-associated delirium [3], prolonged mechanical ventilation [4], urinary retention, and delayed intestinal recovery after surgery [5]. Opioid use is also associated with the development of tolerance, hyperalgesia, and withdrawal [6], and there is a significant concern from a public health perspective as opioid abuse has become a global public health crisis, with increases in associated morbidity, mortality, and addiction worldwide [7].

High-dose opioids, associated with prolonged mechanical ventilation, contribute to protracted postoperative recovery, including the potential for lengthy intensive care. Two meta-analyses compared high-dose opioids (defined as fentanyl >20 μg/kg, sufentanil >2 μg/kg, remifentanil >1.7 mg, and morphine >2 mg/kg) versus low-dose opioids in cardiac surgery. Low-dose opioids are associated with shorter postoperative intubation time, while there is no significant difference in the risk of myocardial infarction, stroke, or reintubation between the two regimens [8, 9]. Opioid-related adverse drug events (ORADEs) are often highlighted in noncardiac surgeries, particularly among outpatient and colorectal surgery patients, impacting their overall recovery rates significantly. However, in cardiac surgery patients, ORADEs are typically overlooked. A study on Medicare patients undergoing cardiac surgery indicated that while ORADEs were officially documented in 0.7% of patients, approximately one-third (32.4%) likely experienced at least one of these events during their hospital stay [10]. Despite the theoretical benefits of high-dose opioids for cardiac surgery, low-dose opioid regimens have demonstrated similar hemodynamic profiles in addition to improving certain recovery milestones [9]. This has led to the adoption of ERAS pathways aiming to reduce opioid consumption by utilizing standardized multimodal analgesic regimens that include nonopioid alternatives. This helps minimize perioperative opioid use and promotes faster recovery [11, 12]. Enhanced recovery programs, designed to improve postoperative recovery through evidence-based interventions, have been adapted for cardiac surgery to optimize pain management and reduce opioid reliance. However, existing guidelines often lack specificity for cardiac surgery pain management. To address these issues, the PeriOperative Quality Initiative (POQI) and ERAS Cardiac Society held a joint conference to review the literature focusing on pain management and opioid stewardship in cardiac surgery patients. They aimed to identify strategies to minimize opioid use while optimizing pain management for cardiac surgery patients [13]. A team of experts in various fields including anesthesiology, surgery, critical care, pain medicine, and nursing came together to address key questions regarding the use of opioids in this patient population. The process involved a consensus-building initiative using the modified Delphi method, where participants engaged in discussions and reviewed literature to develop recommendations. The strength of evidence and recommendations were determined using the GRADE methodology. *The experts recommend against the routine use of high-dose opioid anesthesia or analgesia for patients undergoing cardiac surgery* and recommend *implementation of perioperative opioid stewardship (grade: strong; level of evidence B).*

4.4 Multimodal Opioid Sparing

Multimodal analgesia is the combination of different analgesic regimens or techniques to achieve an effective analgesic effect and reduce the consumption of opioids and their related adverse reactions. Decreased opioids have been shown to decrease hospital length of stay, long-term opioid use, and chronic pain. An important element of multimodal pain management is preemptive analgesic dosing rather than reactive medication use. Analgesics are started preoperatively and intraoperatively, and some agents are dosed around-the-clock. Preemptive analgesia has been identified as an approach to mitigate the phenomenon of central sensitization, which plays an important role in the development of chronic pain after surgery. Medications are titrated based on effects, mainly altered level of consciousness. Minimal supplemental opioids are added as needed. Regional anesthesia also has a central role. Here is an overview of some commonly used nonopioid analgesics in this context (Table 4.1).

4.4.1 Acetaminophen (Paracetamol)

Acetaminophen, thanks to its favorable safety profile, is the commonest ingredient in the multimodal analgesia protocols. Even if paracetamol has been used in medical practice for more than half the century, its mechanism of action is still not fully understood. It has analgesic and antipyretic properties similarly to nonsteroidal anti-inflammatory drugs (NSAIDs), but it does not possess any anti-inflammatory activity. Acetaminophen suppresses prostaglandin production and may also act through the potentiation of cannabinoid/vanilloid receptors in the central nervous system. Widely used for its analgesic and antipyretic properties, it reduces opioid requirements postoperatively, has a good safety profile, and is well tolerated [14, 15]. Acetaminophen is

Table 4.1 Nonopioid medications, dosing, and cardiac surgery considerations

Nonopioid medications, dosing, and cardiac surgery considerations			
Medication	Mechanism	Dosing	Side effects/limitations to use
Acetaminophen	Inhibits the synthesis of prostaglandins in the central nervous system	650–1000 mg PO/IV every 6–8 h; maximum 3–4 g/day; duration of 7–14 days	Liver toxicity
Gabapentin	Voltage-gated calcium channel modulator	300–600 mg once, 100–300 mg every 8 h; duration 5–7 days	Sedation and respiratory depression, renal excretion, age-based dose adjustment; questionable efficacy
Pregabalin	Voltage-gated calcium channel modulator	Pregabalin: 50–150 mg (preoperative); 50–150 mg every 8 h; duration 7–14 days	Altered vision, renal excretion, age-based dose adjustment
Ketamine	*N*-methyl-D-aspartate antagonist	0.1–1.0 mg/kg bolus; 0.1–0.2 mg/kg/h	Tachycardia and questionable efficacy with bolus, hallucinations
Dexmedetomidine	Alpha-2 agonist	0.5–1.5 μg/kg/h	Hypotension, bradycardia
NSAID	Cyclooxygenase inhibitor	Ketorolac: 15–30 mg IV every 6–8 h Ibuprofen: 400–800 PO mg every 6–8 h	Platelet dysfunction, gastrointestinal irritation, renal dysfunction; FDA “black-box warning” for CABG
Lidocaine	Voltage-gated sodium channel inhibitor	1 mg/kg bolus; 0.5–2.0 mg/kg/h	Optimal dosage uncertain, local anesthetic toxicity

mostly unexplored in the context of cardiac surgery, except for its intravenous form. Randomized studies have demonstrated that IV acetaminophen can lower opioid use, maintain comparable pain levels, and possibly decrease delirium (which can result from inadequate pain management or opioid side effects) when administered routinely [16].

4.4.2 Gabapentinoids

Modulated calcium channels to reduce excitatory neurotransmitter release seem to be effective for neuropathic pain as part of a multimodal regimen. Unfortunately, they are associated with a multitude of undesirable side effects, including sedation, dizziness, and respiratory depression; therefore, they require dosing adjustments according to kidney function. In one trial, a single preoperative dose of gabapentin 600 mg reduced opioid consumption and improved pain scores compared with placebo, but also increased sedation and was associated with a modest increase in postoperative mechanical ventilation [17]. On the contrary, another trial that used a larger preoperative dose of 1200 mg, followed by scheduled gabapentin at 600 mg twice daily, showed similar opioid consumption and pain scores without any significant difference in overall side effects [18]. Gabapentin has been extensively researched in noncardiac surgery patients. A recent meta-analysis indicated its minimal effectiveness in the acute postoperative setting and found it to be associated with somnolence and respiratory depression, especially when used alongside opioids [19]. Pregabalin also, by modulating voltage-gated calcium channels, diminishes opioid consumption, enhances pain relief, and potentially expedites extubation following cardiac surgery. This effect has been observed with a lone preoperative administration of 150 mg, followed by scheduled doses of 75 mg twice daily [20]. Despite initially being considered very promising, their routine use was discontinued due to their side effects.

4.4.3 Nonsteroidal Anti-inflammatory Drugs (NSAIDs)

These inhibit cyclooxygenase (COX) enzymes, reducing the synthesis of prostaglandins which mediate inflammation and pain. NSAIDs, widely used in noncardiac surgery, are reasonably well represented in cardiac surgery literature, and several small prospective studies generally support their utility in postoperative multimodal protocols of pain control. A 2006 meta-analysis [21] analyzed 20 randomized trials with 1065 patients showing that NSAIDs significantly reduced 24-h VAS pain scores and decreased morphine-equivalent consumption in the first 24 h without increasing mortality, myocardial infarction, renal dysfunction, or gastrointestinal bleeding. Potential kidney injury and gastrointestinal complications limit their widespread use. NSAIDs cause a clinically unimportant transient reduction in renal function in the early postoperative period in patients with normal preoperative renal function [22]; moreover, they are associated with gastrointestinal toxicity, affecting both upper gastrointestinal tract (peptic ulcer disease) and lower gastrointestinal tract (NSAID-induced enteropathy), and, in 2019, the Food and Drug Administration issued a formal warning regarding NSAIDs in patients undergoing coronary revascularization owing to an association with thrombotic cardiovascular complications [23]. For all these reasons, NSAIDs should be carefully managed in cardiac surgery patients.

4.4.4 Selective Cyclooxygenase-2 (COX-2) Inhibitors

Selectively inhibit the COX-2 enzyme, reducing prostaglandin production. COX-2 inhibitors provide analgesia with fewer gastrointestinal side effects compared to traditional NSAIDs. The selective cyclooxygenase-2 (COX-2) inhibitor valdecoxib (Bextra, Pfizer) and its intravenous prodrug parecoxib (Dynastat, Pfizer) demonstrated notable opioid-sparing benefits following dental, gynecologic, orthopedic, and various other noncardiac surgeries, seemingly without leading to severe side effects [24]. In a randomized double-blind study by Nussmeier et al. [25], the use of parecoxib and valdecoxib after CABG was associated with an increased incidence of cardiovascular events (including myocardial infarction, cardiac arrest, stroke, and pulmonary embolism), arousing serious concern about the use of these drugs in such circumstances.

4.4.5 *N*-methyl-D-aspartate (NMDA) Receptor Antagonists

Ketamine is a unique anesthetic drug that provides analgesia, hypnosis, and amnesia with minimal respiratory and cardiovascular depression. It essentially acts on glutamate-binding sites, *N*-methyl-D-aspartate (NMDA), and non-NMDA receptors [26]. The antagonism of NMDA receptor is responsible for the specific ketamine properties (amnesic and psychosensory effects, analgesia, and neuroprotection). There are also other glutamate-independent mechanisms: Ketamine interacts with many binding sites such as opioid, monoaminergic, cholinergic, nicotinic, and muscarinic receptors, and, in particular, it binds to opioid receptors including mu (μ), delta (∂), and kappa (K). It is a potentially useful anesthetic drug in patients with impaired ventricular function because it has sympathomimetic properties that may augment cardiac output. While early data suggested that ketamine might help prevent postoperative delirium, a recent study found that a single dose of ketamine (0.5–1.0 mg/kg) before incision did not affect delirium, opioid consumption, or pain scores but was linked to an increased incidence of hallucinations and nightmares [27]. Ketamine infusions (0.1–0.5 mg/kg/h) have shown modest results, with one trial indicating reduced opioid use and lower pain scores [28], although other trials did not replicate these findings [29]. This contrasts with noncardiac surgery patients, where subanesthetic ketamine has been found to reduce the need for rescue analgesics and pain intensity [30]. It has several significant side effects that have restricted its widespread use in cardiac surgery. Firstly, it reliably causes tachycardia, which can be detrimental for patients with stenotic heart lesions or coronary artery disease. In an animal model, ketamine increased myocardial oxygen consumption by as much as 50% [31]. Additionally, it may enhance the arrhythmogenic potential of epinephrine, a medication frequently used for hemodynamic support during cardiac surgery [32]. Perhaps the most significant concern preventing the wider adoption of ketamine as an anesthetic and sedative agent is emergence delirium and the potentially unpleasant psychotropic effects of the drug [33].

Magnesium exists as the second most common intracellular cation and the fourth most common plasma cation. It has a wide range of effects on the regulation of transmembrane ion exchange and enzymatic reactions. In the clinical setting, magnesium is typically used as an antiarrhythmic and tocolytic agent. Although not commonly considered as an analgesic agent, magnesium has also been shown to act as an NMDA receptor antagonist. This property, in addition to its role as a calcium channel blocker, leads to its potential as an analgesic adjunct. It can be administered in the perioperative period as an infusion, and pooled data from studies indicate that perioperative magnesium infusion is associated with a decrease in postoperative pain and opioid consumption without clinical toxic effects caused by toxic serum levels of magnesium [34]. Preoperative magnesium loading appears to be an effective prophylactic measure for preventing atrial fibrillation following cardiac surgery. It is an affordable and accessible option that can positively impact patient outcomes [34].

4.4.6 Dexmedetomidine

Dexmedetomidine is an alpha agonist having sedative, anxiolytic, hypnotic, analgesic, and sympatholytic properties. It produces these effects by inhibiting central sympathetic outflow by blocking the alpha receptors in the brainstem, thereby inhibiting the release of norepinephrine. IV dexmedetomidine has been extensively studied in randomized clinical trials and meta-analyses focused on cardiac surgery. These studies have highlighted various benefits, such as quicker extubation, fewer arrhythmias, decreased delirium, and shorter hospital stays [35]. Additionally, dexmedetomidine has shown promise as an analgesic, significantly reducing opioid needs and improving pain management for up to 24 h after cardiac surgery [36]. However, its use as a primary analgesic is potentially limited by side effects like hypotension and bradycardia, which can occur with bolus or rapidly increasing doses.

4.4.7 Lidocaine

Lidocaine is a sodium channel blocker that stabilizes neuronal membranes and inhibits nerve impulse conduction. It provides analgesia, reduces opioid requirements, and has anti-inflammatory properties.

Multimodal pain management after cardiac surgery frequently incorporates local anesthetics administered intravenously, infiltrated perineurally, or infused into the epidural space. Lidocaine is commonly employed during the perioperative phase. Unlike some other local anesthetic medications, lidocaine is easily accessible in topical formulations and can be safely administered intravenously, broadening its therapeutic applications. A systematic review by Boswell et al. [37] on the use of lidocaine for postoperative pain after cardiac surgery suggests that applying 2% lidocaine topically to chest tubes before their intraoperative insertion resulted in significantly reduced pain scores and lower total doses of fentanyl (low certainty of evidence). Additionally, administering 2% lidocaine intrapleurally was linked to significantly lower pain scores and notable improvements in FEV1 (very low certainty of evidence). However, lidocaine infusions, in contrast to noncardiac surgery, did not lead to significant changes in pain scores, and no significant associations were found between postoperative lidocaine use and overall mortality, hospital stay duration, or ICU stay length (very low certainty of evidence); moreover, it requires careful dosing to avoid toxicity.

4.4.8 Dexamethasone

Dexamethasone, a synthetic adrenocortical steroid with high glucocorticoid activity, has been used to reduce PONV and postoperative inflammation for years. However, it has also shown potential in improving postoperative pain and reducing discharge times from day surgery units. A meta-analysis examining the effects of perioperative dexamethasone on postoperative analgesia showed significantly lowered pain scores, an opioid-sparing effect at 2 and 24 h, and reduced PACU stays [38]. Study doses of dexamethasone ranged from 4 to 20 mg, with the most common dosage being 8 mg. There was no evidence of a dose-dependent effect on opioid requirements and a small but significant dose-dependent effect on 24-h pain scores. Comparable results were found in patients receiving dexamethasone during laparoscopic cholecystectomy. Despite its many benefits, dexamethasone has also potential significant side effects, such as perioperative hyperglycemia, postoperative infection, impaired wound healing, and adverse neuropsychiatric effects.

4.5 Fascial Plane Blocks

Fascial plane blocks, which have been extensively covered in other chapters, involve the injection of local anesthetic between the muscles through which the peripheral nerve travels. In these procedures, the focus is not on targeting the nerve itself, nor is the needle directed towards the neural axis. Consequently, the potential risks of severe complications such as neural injury and neuraxial hematoma can be mitigated or even avoided. This aspect is particularly advantageous for cardiac surgery patients who commonly receive heparin, making the avoidance of neuraxial needling highly appealing. Moreover, the added advantage of the relative simplicity of performing these blocks has contributed to their widespread adoption. The extensive utilization of chest wall blocks in cardiac surgery has generated a wealth of scientific literature on the subject. These blocks are now regarded as safe even within the challenging context of cardiac surgery [39]. Some blocks, originally designed for analgesic purposes and incorporated into multimodal analgesia protocols, have proven so effective that they are now used as anesthetic techniques for awake cardiac surgery. Consider, for instance, sternal wound revision, often performed with a parasternal or pectoralis-intercostal rectus sheath block in combination with light sedation [40]. A further consideration in opioid-free and opioid-sparing modalities is pain control after patients leave the hospital setting. Chronic pain lasting months after surgery can become a significant burden. A meta-analysis examined the effect of regional anesthetic techniques on the incidence of persistent postoperative pain, defined as pain persisting beyond 3 months after surgery. It was hypothesized that by preventing central sensitization, regional anesthetic techniques could possibly improve long-term pain outcomes. The authors found that regional anesthesia used in thoracotomy, breast surgery, and cesarean section showed significant reductions in patient risk of developing persistent postoperative pain compared with standard analgesia [41].

4.6 Adjunctive Therapies

Non-pharmacological interventions such as physical therapy, cognitive behavioral therapy, and acupuncture [42] may also play a role in comprehensive pain management, but the scientific literature on the subject is still limited.

4.7 Conclusion

A multimodal opioid-sparing approach to postoperative pain management uses several nonopioid medications and techniques to target different pain pathways. This approach is preemptive, and although the Enhanced Recovery After Surgery Cardiac Society recommends using multimodal analgesia for postoperative pain, evidence-based guidelines have yet to be established [43].

Preliminary studies suggest that this multimodal approach for cardiac surgery patients improves pain management and ameliorates side effects to improve functional recovery [44].

References

1. Gerbershagen HJ, Aduckathil S, van Wijck AJ, Peelen LM, Kalkman CJ, Meissner W. Pain intensity on the first day after surgery: a prospective cohort study comparing 179 surgical procedures. Anesthesiology. 2013;118(4):934–44. https://doi.org/10.1097/ALN.0b013e31828866b3.
2. Lahtinen P, Kokki H, Hynynen M. Pain after cardiac surgery: a prospective cohort study of 1-year incidence and intensity. Anesthesiology. 2006;105(4):794–800. https://doi.org/10.1097/00000542-200610000-00026.
3. Pisani MA, Murphy TE, Araujo KL, Slattum P, Van Ness PH, Inouye SK. Benzodiazepine and opioid use and the duration of intensive care unit delirium in an older population. Crit Care Med. 2009;37(1):177–83. https://doi.org/10.1097/CCM.0b013e318192fcf9. PMID: 19050611; PMCID: PMC2700732.
4. Wanzuita R, Poli-de-Figueiredo LF, Pfuetzenreiter F, Cavalcanti AB, Westphal GA. Replacement of fentanyl infusion by enteral methadone decreases the weaning time from mechanical ventilation: a randomized controlled trial. Crit Care. 2012;16(2):R49. https://doi.org/10.1186/cc11250. PMID: 22420584; PMCID: PMC3681375.
5. Beard TL, Leslie JB, Nemeth J. The opioid component of delayed gastrointestinal recovery after bowel resection. J Gastrointest Surg. 2011;15(7):1259–68. https://doi.org/10.1007/s11605-011-1500-3. Epub 2011 Apr 15.
6. Wang PP, Huang E, Feng X, Bray CA, Perreault MM, Rico P, Bellemare P, Murgoi P, Gélinas C, Lecavalier A, Jayaraman D, Frenette AJ, Williamson D. Opioid-associated iatrogenic withdrawal in critically ill adult patients: a multicenter prospective observational study. Ann Intensive Care. 2017;7(1):88. https://doi.org/10.1186/s13613-017-0310-5. PMID: 28866754; PMCID: PMC5581799.
7. Kim B, Nolan S, Ti L. Addressing the prescription opioid crisis: potential for hospital-based interventions? Drug Alcohol Rev. 2017;36(2):149–52. https://doi.org/10.1111/dar.12541. PMID: 28326630; PMCID: PMC5802354.
8. Wong WT, Lai VK, Chee YE, Lee A. Fast-track cardiac care for adult cardiac surgical patients. Cochrane Database Syst Rev. 2016;9(9):CD003587. https://doi.org/10.1002/14651858.CD003587.pub3. PMID: 27616189; PMCID: PMC6457798.
9. Rong LQ, Kamel MK, Rahouma M, Naik A, Mehta K, Abouarab AA, Di Franco A, Demetres M, Mustapich TL, Fitzgerald MM, Pryor KO, Gaudino M. High-dose versus low-dose opioid anesthesia in adult cardiac surgery: a meta-analysis. J Clin

Anesth. 2019;57:57–62. https://doi.org/10.1016/j.jclinane.2019.03.009. Epub 2019 Mar 11.
10. Allen KB, Brovman EY, Chhatriwalla AK, Greco KJ, Rao N, Kumar A, Urman RD. Opioid-related adverse events: incidence and impact in patients undergoing cardiac surgery. Semin Cardiothorac Vasc Anesth. 2020;24(3):219–26. https://doi.org/10.1177/1089253219888658. Epub 2019 Nov 27.
11. Shafi S, Collinsworth AW, Copeland LA, Ogola GO, Qiu T, Kouznetsova M, Liao IC, Mears N, Pham AT, Wan GJ, Masica AL. Association of opioid-related adverse drug events with clinical and cost outcomes among surgical patients in a large integrated health care delivery system. JAMA Surg. 2018;153(8):757–63. https://doi.org/10.1001/jamasurg.2018.1039. PMID: 29799927; PMCID: PMC6142954.
12. Urman RD, Seger DL, Fiskio JM, Neville BA, Harry EM, Weiner SG, Lovelace B, Fain R, Cirillo J, Schnipper JL. The burden of opioid-related adverse drug events on hospitalized previously opioid-free surgical patients. J Patient Saf. 2021;17(2):e76–83. https://doi.org/10.1097/PTS.0000000000000566.
13. Grant MC, Chappell D, Gan TJ, Manning MW, Miller TE, Brodt JL, PeriOperative Quality Initiative (POQI) and the Enhanced Recovery After Surgery (ERAS) Cardiac Society Workgroup. Pain management and opioid stewardship in adult cardiac surgery: joint consensus report of the PeriOperative quality initiative and the enhanced recovery after surgery cardiac society. J Thorac Cardiovasc Surg. 2023;166(6):1695–1706.e2. https://doi.org/10.1016/j.jtcvs.2023.01.020. Epub 2023 Jan 28.
14. Macario A, Royal MA. A literature review of randomized clinical trials of intravenous acetaminophen (paracetamol) for acute postoperative pain. Pain Pract. 2011;11(3):290–6.
15. Mamoun NF, Lin P, Zimmerman NM, Mascha EJ, Mick SL, Insler SR, Sessler DI, Duncan AE. Intravenous acetaminophen analgesia after cardiac surgery: a randomized, blinded, controlled superiority trial. J Thorac Cardiovasc Surg. 2016;152(3):881–889.e1. https://doi.org/10.1016/j.jtcvs.2016.04.078. Epub 2016 May 5.
16. Subramaniam B, Shankar P, Shaefi S, Mueller A, O'Gara B, Banner-Goodspeed V, Gallagher J, Gasangwa D, Patxot M, Packiasabapathy S, Mathur P, Eikermann M, Talmor D, Marcantonio ER. Effect of intravenous acetaminophen vs placebo combined with propofol or dexmedetomidine on postoperative delirium among older patients following cardiac surgery: the DEXACET randomized clinical trial. JAMA. 2019;321(7):686–96. https://doi.org/10.1001/jama.2019.0234. PMID: 30778597; PMCID: PMC6439609.
17. Menda F, Köner O, Sayın M, Ergenoğlu M, Küçükaksu S, Aykaç B. Effects of single-dose gabapentin on postoperative pain and morphine consumption after cardiac surgery. J Cardiothorac Vasc Anesth. 2010;24(5):808–13. https://doi.org/10.1053/j.jvca.2009.10.023. Epub 2010 Jan 6.
18. Rapchuk IL, O'Connell L, Liessmann CD, Cornelissen HR, Fraser JF. Effect of gabapentin on pain after cardiac surgery: a randomised, double-blind, placebo-controlled trial. Anaesth Intensive Care. 2010;38(3):445–51. https://doi.org/10.1177/0310057X1003800306.
19. Verret M, Lauzier F, Zarychanski R, Perron C, Savard X, Pinard AM, Leblanc G, Cossi MJ, Neveu X, Turgeon AF, Canadian Perioperative Anesthesia Clinical Trials (PACT) Group. Perioperative use of gabapentinoids for the management of postoperative acute pain: a systematic review and meta-analysis [Erratum in: Anesthesiology 2020 Aug 21;:null]. Anesthesiology. 2020;133(2):265–79. https://doi.org/10.1097/ALN.0000000000003428.
20. Joshi SS, Jagadeesh AM. Efficacy of perioperative pregabalin in acute and chronic post-operative pain after off-pump coronary artery bypass surgery: a randomized, double-blind placebo controlled trial. Ann Card Anaesth. 2013;16(3):180–5. https://doi.org/10.4103/0971-9784.114239.
21. Bainbridge D, Cheng DC, Martin JE, Novick R, Evidence-Based Perioperative Clinical Outcomes Research (EPiCOR) Group. NSAID-analgesia, pain control and morbidity in cardiothoracic surgery. Can J Anaesth. 2006;53(1):46–59. https://doi.org/10.1007/BF03021527.
22. Lee A, Cooper MG, Craig JC, Knight JF, Keneally JP. Effects of nonsteroidal anti-inflammatory drugs on postoperative renal function in adults with normal renal function. Cochrane Database Syst Rev. 2007;2007(2):CD002765. https://doi.org/10.1002/14651858.CD002765.pub3. PMID: 17443518; PMCID: PMC6516878.
23. Food and Drug Administration Drug Safety Communication. FDA strengthens warning that non-aspirin nonsteroidal anti-inflammatory drugs (NSAIDs) can cause heart attacks or strokes. FDA. https://www.fda.gov/drugs/drug-safety-and-availability/fda-drug-safety-communication-fda-strengthens-warning-non-aspirin-nonsteroidal-anti-inflammatory.
24. Ng A, Smith G, Davidson AC. Analgesic effects of parecoxib following total abdominal hysterectomy. Br J Anaesth. 2003;90(6):746–9. https://doi.org/10.1093/bja/aeg139. PMID: 12765890.
25. Nussmeier NA, Whelton AA, Brown MT, Langford RM, Hoeft A, Parlow JL, Boyce SW, Verburg KM. Complications of the COX-2 inhibitors parecoxib and valdecoxib after cardiac surgery. N Engl J Med. 2005;352(11):1081–91. https://doi.org/10.1056/NEJMoa050330. Epub 2005 Feb 15.
26. Kohrs R, Durieux ME. Ketamine: teaching an old drug new tricks. Anesth Analg. 1998;87(5):1186–93. https://doi.org/10.1097/00000539-199811000-00039.
27. Avidan MS, Maybrier HR, Abdallah AB, Jacobsohn E, Vlisides PE, Pryor KO, Veselis RA, Grocott HP, Emmert DA, Rogers EM, Downey RJ, Yulico H, Noh GJ, Lee YH, Waszynski CM, Arya VK, Pagel

PS, Hudetz JA, Muench MR, Fritz BA, Waberski W, Inouye SK, Mashour GA, PODCAST Research Group. Intraoperative ketamine for prevention of postoperative delirium or pain after major surgery in older adults: an international, multicentre, double-blind, randomised clinical trial [Epub 2017 May 30. Erratum in: Lancet. 2017 Jul 15;390(10091):230]. Lancet. 2017;390(10091):267–75. https://doi.org/10.1016/S0140-6736(17)31467-8. PMID: 28576285; PMCID: PMC5644286.
28. Cogan J, Lalumière G, Vargas-Schaffer G, Deschamps A, Yegin Z. Low-dose intravenous ketamine for postcardiac surgery pain: effect on opioid consumption and the incidence of chronic pain. Ann Card Anaesth. 2017;20(4):395–8. https://doi.org/10.4103/aca.ACA_54_17. PMID: 28994672; PMCID: PMC5661306.
29. Cameron M, Tam K, Al Wahaibi K, Charghi R, Béïque F. Intraoperative ketamine for analgesia post-coronary artery bypass surgery: a randomized, controlled, double-blind clinical trial. J Cardiothorac Vasc Anesth. 2020;34(3):586–91. https://doi.org/10.1053/j.jvca.2019.10.010. Epub 2019 Oct 11.
30. Bell RF, Dahl JB, Moore RA, Kalso E. Peri-operative ketamine for acute post-operative pain: a quantitative and qualitative systematic review (Cochrane review). Acta Anaesthesiol Scand. 2005;49(10):1405–28. https://doi.org/10.1111/j.1399-6576.2005.00814.x.
31. Patschke D, Brückner JB, Gethmann JW, Tarnow J, Weymar A. Einfluss der Ketaminnarkose auf die Hämodynamik und den myokardialen Sauerstoffverbrauch narkotisierter Hunde [The effect of ketamine on haemodynamics and myocardial oxygen consumption in anaesthetized dogs (author's transl)]. Prakt Anaesth. 1975;10(6):325–34. German.
32. Koehntop DE, Liao JC, Van Bergen FH. Effects of pharmacologic alterations of adrenergic mechanisms by cocaine, tropolone, aminophylline, and ketamine on epinephrine-induced arrhythmias during halothane-nitrous oxide anesthesia. Anesthesiology. 1977;46(2):83–93. https://doi.org/10.1097/00000542-197702000-00001.
33. Mazzeffi M, Johnson K, Paciullo C. Ketamine in adult cardiac surgery and the cardiac surgery intensive care unit: an evidence-based clinical review. Ann Card Anaesth. 2015;18(2):202–9. https://doi.org/10.4103/0971-9784.154478. PMID: 25849690; PMCID: PMC4881646.
34. Fairley JL, Zhang L, Glassford NJ, Bellomo R. Magnesium status and magnesium therapy in cardiac surgery: a systematic review and meta-analysis focusing on arrhythmia prevention. J Crit Care. 2017;42:69–77. https://doi.org/10.1016/j.jcrc.2017.05.038. Epub 2017 Jun 21.
35. Elgebaly AS, Sabry M. Sedation effects by dexmedetomidine versus propofol in decreasing duration of mechanical ventilation after open heart surgery. Ann Card Anaesth. 2018;21(3):235–42. https://doi.org/10.4103/aca.ACA_168_17. PMID: 30052208; PMCID: PMC6078043.
36. Habibi V, Kiabi FH, Sharifi H. The effect of dexmedetomidine on the acute pain after cardiothoracic surgeries: a systematic review. Braz J Cardiovasc Surg. 2018;33(4):404–17. https://doi.org/10.21470/1678-9741-2017-0253. PMID: 30184039; PMCID: PMC6122757.
37. Boswell MR, Moman RN, Burtoft M, Gerdes H, Martinez J, Gerberi DJ, Wittwer E, Murad MH, Hooten WM. Lidocaine for postoperative pain after cardiac surgery: a systematic review. J Cardiothorac Surg. 2021;16(1):157. https://doi.org/10.1186/s13019-021-01549-0. PMID: 34059093; PMCID: PMC8166031.
38. Luo J, Min S. Postoperative pain management in the postanesthesia care unit: an update. J Pain Res. 2017;10:2687–98. https://doi.org/10.2147/JPR.S142889. PMID: 29180895; PMCID: PMC5695271.
39. Toscano A, Capuano P, Galatà M, Tazzi I, Rinaldi M, Brazzi L. Safety of ultrasound-guided serratus anterior and erector spinae fascial plane blocks: a retrospective analysis in patients undergoing cardiac surgery while receiving anticoagulant and antiplatelet drugs. J Cardiothorac Vasc Anesth. 2022;36(2):483–8. https://doi.org/10.1053/j.jvca.2021.05.037. Epub 2021 May 24.
40. Toscano A, Balzani E, Capuano P, Vaninetti A, Perrucci C, Simonato E, Rinaldi M, Brazzi L. Awake cardiac surgery using the novel pectoralis-intercostal-rectus sheath (PIRS) plane block and subxiphoid approach. J Card Surg. 2022;37(9):2923–6. https://doi.org/10.1111/jocs.16658. Epub 2022 Jun 4.
41. Andreae MH, Andreae DA. Regional anaesthesia to prevent chronic pain after surgery: a Cochrane systematic review and meta-analysis. Br J Anaesth. 2013;111(5):711–20. https://doi.org/10.1093/bja/aet213. Epub 2013 Jun 28. PMID: 23811426; PMCID: PMC3793661.
42. Feingold KL, Moskowitz JT, Elenbaas C, Andrei AC, Victorson D, Kruse J, Grote V, Patil KD, Shafiro T, Grimone A, Lin F, Davidson CJ, Ring M, McCarthy PM. Acupuncture after valve surgery is feasible and shows promise in reducing postoperative atrial fibrillation: the ACU-heart pilot trial. JTCVS Open. 2023;16:321–32. https://doi.org/10.1016/j.xjon.2023.05.010. PMID: 38204624; PMCID: PMC10774881.
43. Ward CT, Moll V, Boorman DW, et al. The impact of a postoperative multimodal analgesia pathway on opioid use and outcomes after cardiothoracic surgery. J Cardiothorac Surg. 2022;17:342. https://doi.org/10.1186/s13019-022-02067-3.
44. Barr LF, Boss MJ, Mazzeffi MA, Taylor BS, Salenger R. Postoperative multimodal analgesia in cardiac surgery. Crit Care Clin. 2020;36(4):631–51. https://doi.org/10.1016/j.ccc.2020.06.003. Epub 2020 Aug 12.

Anatomy and Ultrasound: General Considerations

5

Paolo Scimia, Luca Gentili, Paolo Capuano, and Giuseppe Sepolvere

5.1 Anatomy and Ultrasound: General Considerations

In recent years, the advent and wide use of Enhanced Recovery After Surgery (ERAS) programs have led to the proliferation of minimally invasive surgical techniques, in order to reduce tissue trauma and postoperative pain compared to open techniques. At the same time, the need was felt to research less invasive analgesic strategies compared to canonical techniques such as systemic opioids, neuraxial analgesia, and paravertebral block. Despite their proven effectiveness, standard analgesic techniques are associated with a variety of side effects that limit their clinical utility. In particular, the use of opioid analgesics may determine sedation, respiratory depression, nausea and vomiting, itching, urinary retention, constipation, tolerance, hyperalgesia, decreased gastric motility, muscle rigidity, myoclonus, sleep-disordered breathing, hormonal dysfunction, and immune system suppression. For these reasons, recent evidences promote opioid-sparing strategies, recommending that opioid administration should be used in the lowest effective doses as part of multimodal analgesia. With this in mind, regional anesthetic (RA) techniques are candidates as the cornerstone of opioid-free anesthesia (OFA). Thoracic epidural analgesia (TEA) has always been considered the "queen" of analgesic techniques for major surgery, as it obtunds the stress of surgical response, provides better dynamic pain control compared to systemic opioids, reduces the incidence of postoperative complications, and enhances the quality of recovery shortening hospital stay. Thoracic paravertebral block (TPVB) represents a valid alternative to epidural for all surgery of the trunk, providing equivalent pain relief with fewer adverse effects. However, it has currently been questioned whether these techniques can still be the gold standard per postoperative analgesia, since their use requires proven practical skills and a careful risk-benefit assessment, especially in frail patients. Just think of the risk of epidural hematoma related to catheter in situ in patients taking antithrombotic therapies. Similarly, TPVB is not a technique for beginners as its target is very close to the pleura and posterior intercostal ves-

P. Scimia (✉)
Department of Anesthesia and Intensive Care Unit, Giuseppe Mazzini Hospital, Teramo, Italy

L. Gentili
Department of Anesthesia and Intensive Care Unit, Santa Maria Goretti Hospital, Latina, Italy

P. Capuano
Department of Anesthesia and Intensive Care, Istituto Mediterraneo per i Trapianti e Terapie ad alta Specializzazione (IRCCS-ISMETT), UPMCI (University of Pittsburgh Medical Center Italy), Palermo, Italy

G. Sepolvere
Department of Anesthesia and Cardiac Surgery Intensive Care Unit, San Michele Hospital, Maddaloni, Caserta, Italy

G. Sepolvere, S. Silvetti (eds.), *Fast-Track in Cardiac Anesthesia*,
https://doi.org/10.1007/978-3-031-70899-2_5

sels. For these reasons, it may be associated with the risk of potentially severe complications, such as pneumothorax, sympathetic blockade, and intravascular injection [1]. In light of these observations, researchers are focusing their efforts on developing equally effective but safer analgesic alternatives. In recent years, the advent of ultrasound and a better understanding of the human fascial system have led to the introduction of different fascial plane blocks (FPBs) [2]. These techniques have been increasingly utilized as part of a multimodal analgesia in various branches of surgery, providing in many cases a safer alternative to standard techniques. By virtue of these properties, FPBs currently represent the minimally invasive evolution of regional anesthesia for acute and chronic pain management [3, 4]. FPBs are traditionally considered a new class of RA techniques where a local anesthetic (LA) mixture is injected into a plane between two layers of fascia or between a fascia and a bone surface, aiming to spread along that anatomical plane and block the nerves lying inside or crossing through it [5]. In the last decade FPBs have become popular, and many techniques have been described and applied in clinical practice, providing a right balance between analgesic efficacy, safety profile, and fast acquisition of skills. Despite the FPBs' success, their mechanisms of action remain controversial [6]. To date, various mechanisms have been hypothesized to explain the analgesic effect of FPBs, such as a direct LA action on nerve fibers traveling inside the fascial plane or crossing through it, LA action on nerve fibers or sensory receptors within the fascia, LA reabsorption in bloodstream, a mechanical action on sensory receptors within the fascia, and a direct anti-inflammatory action when blocking close to target tissues [5, 6]. Although several clinical studies have shown the effectiveness of FPBs, patterns of injectate spread and dermatomal distribution of the sensory blockade are associated with significant interindividual variability. A recent experts' opinion by Fusco et al. has highlighted that the variability of FPBs outcome may depend on various factors that may be classified into three categories: operator related, patient related, and drug related (Table 5.1). All of these factors should be taken into consideration by anesthesiologists in order to perform successful FPBs [5].

Table 5.1 Factors to consider for fascial plane blocks

Parameters	Variables
Operator related/ technique related	Personal skill and experience Choice of technique Needle bevel contour and angle Needle insertion angle Fascia disruption with multiple passages Static or dynamic injection Injection pressure and speed Probe pressure
Patient related	Type of fascial plane: anatomical site Age BMI Anatomical variants and lines of fusion History of previous surgery, trauma, disease, irradiation and adhesions, or scar tissue Patient positioning Muscle contractions after the block Muscle stiffness Spontaneous or artificial ventilation Patient physical status
Drug related	Drug Volume Concentration Adjuvants pH, temperature

Integration of FPBs into clinical practice has undoubtedly revolutionized the individualized approach to anesthetic management in various surgical branches and pain therapy. However, the exponential growth of these techniques has led to the development of innumerable novel approaches described in the scientific literature. These approaches often target similar anatomical structures generating confusion particularly regarding their nomenclature.

The heterogeneity in the names and anatomical descriptions of FPBs may have adverse consequences on education, research, and implementation of these techniques into clinical practice. For this reason, there is a need of harmonization and standardization of nomenclature in order to improve education, research, and ultimately patient care. In 2021, El-Boghdadly et al.

presented the first international consensus on nomenclature and anatomical descriptions of blocks of the abdominal wall, chest wall, and paraspinal blocks, involving both the American Society of Regional Anesthesia (ASRA) Pain Medicine and European Society of Regional Anaesthesia and Pain Therapy (ESRA) [7]. In conclusion, the authors recommend using the consensus results in academic and clinical practice. However, while the recent ASRA-ESRA consensus has clarified many doubts related to the nomenclature of FPBs, the lack of specific sonoanatomical signs which are able to confirm the correct execution of FPBs has limited more widespread adoption of these RA techniques by practitioners who have not received advanced training with significant implications for improving patient perioperative care. Fortunately, in recent years, some researchers have introduced different signs as unequivocal markers of the correct execution of FPBs. For example, looking at the ultrasound-guided transversus abdominis plane block (US-TAP block), recent reviews suggested that this technique, when correctly executed as part of a multimodal analgesic regimen for abdominal surgery, may improve postoperative pain control reducing opioid consumption. However, current findings about the utility of US-TAP block in cesarean section are contradictory. The discrepancy between results could be attributed to the primary block failure due to a not correct execution of the technique rather than lack of its clinical efficacy. In 2019, Fusco et al. introduced a novel sonographic sign in order to confirm the correct execution of all FPBs defined as "double V" sign [8]. The rationale of this sign is that if the injection is correctly performed, the spread of LA within the target fascial plane determines the opening of this plane and the separation of the two fasciae of the compartment visible bilaterally as a "double V." This sign should be considered a marker of a correct execution of the technique allowing to exclude a peri-fascial injection in all FPBs in which the target fascial plane is located between two muscular structures, such as US-guided TAP block or interpectoral block. The same authors have recently described an evolution of this sign in order to guarantee reproducibility and efficacy in FPBs defining it as "dynamic double V" sign [9]. The rationale for performing a dynamic block is to favor the opening of the fascial plane promoting a more homogeneous diffusion of LA by the advancement of the needle inside this compartment. The visualization of this sign in fact is a marker of the correct spread of LA in the target fascial plane during the whole time of injection, thus ensuring that all the drug dose is positioned in the right compartment. This approach may determine stretching of the fascia resulting in LA active transport via a pumping mechanism in addition to passive movement along lower resistance planes. Moreover, the progression of the needle within the fascial plane can favor the rupture of fibrous septa often present in patients with chronic inflammatory stimuli. To clarify this concept, Scimia et al. in 2022 reported a case in which starting from the transversus abdominis plane (TAP), a quadratus lumborum block type 1 (QLB1) was dynamically performed as the sole anesthetic technique for a 55-year-old man, ASA2, who underwent open right inguinal hernia repair (Figs. 5.1 and 5.2) [10]. Because US-TAP block is limited to somatic analgesia of the abdominal wall and being highly dependent on interfascial spread, US-QLB1 has been proposed as a more consistent method. In fact, prospective studies between US-QLB and TAP block showed that the former provides higher and longer lasting analgesia than TAP block, which could be due to a more reli-

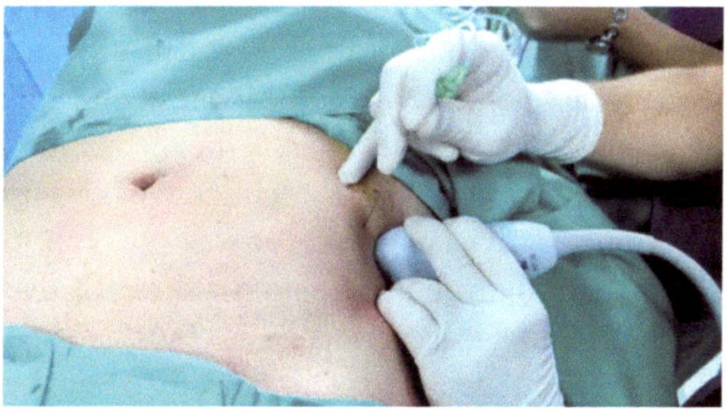

Fig. 5.1 Approach to perform lateral US-TAP block. A linear transducer was placed in the axial plane between the subcostal margin and the iliac crest. A 22 G-100 mm needle was inserted in plane in medial to lateral direction

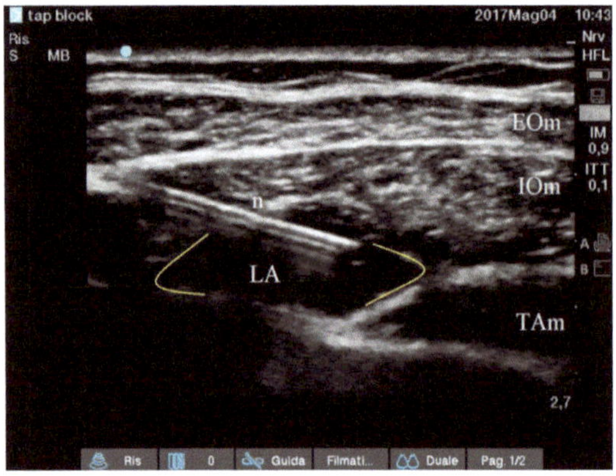

Fig. 5.2 The injection of local anesthetic in the fascial plane between oblique internal and transversus abdominis muscles describes the "double V sign." *EOm* external oblique muscle, *IOm* internal oblique muscle, *TAm* transversus abdominis muscle, *N* needle, *LA* local anesthetic. "Double V" sign highlighted in yellow

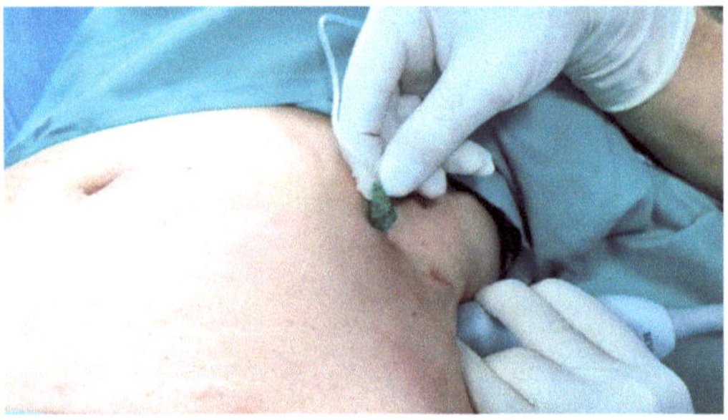

Fig. 5.3 The needle is progressively advanced within the target fascial plane in order to favor posterior spread of local anesthetic (dynamic fascial block)

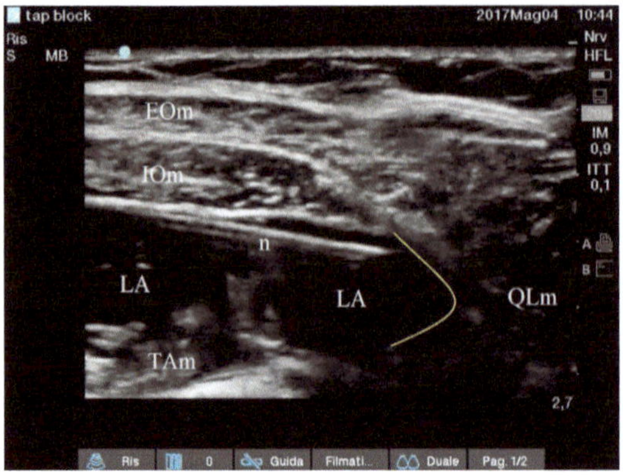

Fig. 5.4 The anterior surface of quadratus lumborum muscle is reached in a dynamic way advancing the needle within the target fascial plane. *EOm* external oblique muscle, *IOm* internal oblique muscle, *TAm* transversus abdominis muscle, *QLm* quadratus lumborum muscle, *N* needle, *LA* local anesthetic. Dynamic "double V" sign highlighted in yellow

able block of the iliohypogastric/ilioinguinal as well as genitofemoral nerves in the posterior pararenal space. Authors concluded that a dynamic way of injecting LA could represent the new approach to perform all FPBs in order to reach wider metamers, save local anesthetic volume, and improve the block efficacy. In this report, Scimia et al. have highlighted how by performing a dynamic block, it was possible to transform a somatic block into a more effective block obtaining visceral analgesia (Figs. 5.3 and 5.4). At least, Sepolvere et al. recently opened a discussion about potential ultrasound signs for FPBs in which the anesthetic solutions are injected into a plane between a deep fascia of a muscle and a bone surface [11], including the erector spinae plane (ESP) block, the deep serratus anterior plane (SAP) block, the superficial parasternal intercostal plane block with a modified approach [12], or the more recent serratus posterior superior intercostal plane (SPSIP) block described by Tulgar et al. [13]. Researchers have hypothesized characteristic ultrasound signs for these blocks, including the lifting of the muscle overlying the bone surface after injection and the homogeneous diffusion of LA along the bone surface (Figs. 5.5 and 5.6). For example, in a recent study, Forero et al. showed that the effectiveness of the US-ESP block depends on targeting the transverse process (TP) with needle tip and on ensuring distribution of the injectable below the deep fascia of the erector spinae muscle overlying the TP [14].

In conclusion, today, we should always keep in mind that the success of FPBs depends on several factors that may be summarized in three categories: operator related, patient related, and drug related.

Furthermore, we must never forget to check for the presence of characteristic sonoanatomical signs confirming correct execution of the FPBs, in order to best integrate these techniques into contemporary perioperative analgesia protocols.

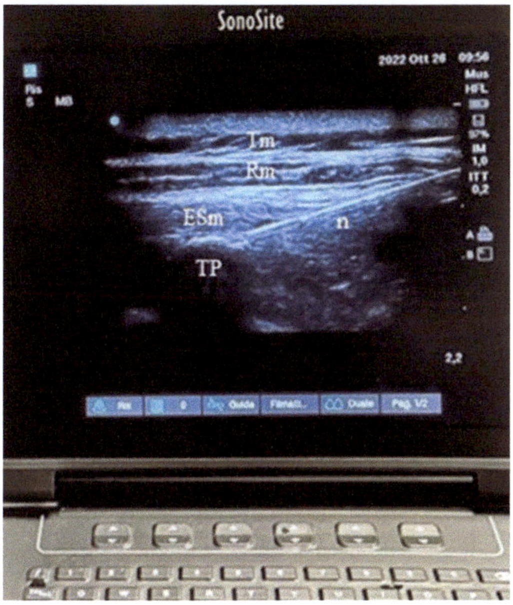

Fig. 5.5 Preinjection US-ESP block sonoanatomy. Needle contacting the tip of the transverse process below the deep fascia of the erector spinae muscle. *Tm* trapezius muscle, *Rm* rhomboid muscle, *ESm* erector spinae muscle, *n* needle, *TP* transverse process

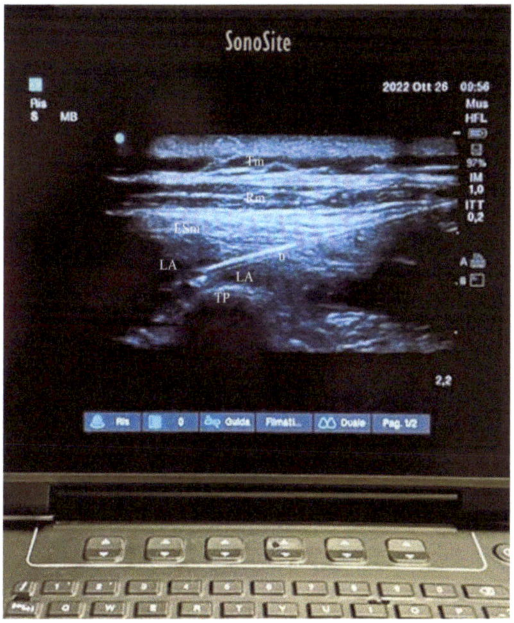

Fig. 5.6 Postinjection US-ESP block sonoanatomy. Local anesthetic is injected between the deep fascia of the erector spinae muscle deep fascia and the bone surface of the transverse process producing cranial to caudal spread. *Tm* trapezius muscle, *Rm* rhomboid muscle, *ESm* erector spinae muscle, *N* needle, *TP* transverse process, *n* needle

References

1. Kietaibl S, Ferrandis R, Godier A, et al. Regional anaesthesia in patients on antithrombotic drugs. Joint ESAIC/ESRA guidelines. Eur J Anaesthesiol. 2022;39:100–32.
2. Machi A, Joshi GP. Interfascial plane blocks. Best Pract Res Clin Anaesthesiol. 2019;33:303e315.
3. Fusco P, Pascarella G, Stecco C, et al. Factors to consider for fascial plane blocks' success in acute and chronic pain management. Minerva Anestesiol. 2024;90(1–2):87–97.
4. Chin KJ, Lirk P, Hollmann MW, et al. Mechanisms of action of fascial plane blocks: a narrative review. Reg Anesth Pain Med. 2021;46:618–28.
5. Fusco P, Stecco C, Petroni GM, et al. ESP block and chronic pain: the dark side of the moon. Minerva Anestesiol. 2022;88(6):528–9.
6. Fusco P, Nazzaro E, Petroni G, et al. Fascial plane blocks and chronic pain: another step towards the future. J Clin Anesth. 2023;84:111010.
7. El-Boghdadly K, Wolmarans M, Stengel AD, et al. Standardizing nomenclature in regional anesthesia: an ASRA-ESRA Delphi consensus study of abdominal wall, paraspinal, and chest wall blocks. Reg Anesth Pain Med. 2021;46:571–80.
8. Fusco P, Petrucci E, Marinangeli F, et al. Block failure or lack of efficacy? The "double V" sign: a novel sonographic sign for a successful interfascial plane block. Minerva Anestesiol. 2019;85:917–8.
9. Fusco P, Petroni GM, Walter C, et al. Dynamic double V sign: another step to the efficacy of fascial plane block. Minerva Anestesiol. 2022;88:1079–81.
10. Scimia P, Gentili L, Fusco P, et al. When a TAP becomes a QL block: a dynamic way to perform the fascial blocks. Minerva Anestesiol. 2022;88(11):976–8.
11. Sepolvere G, Stecco C, Gentili L, et al. Defining the fascial blocks: lights and shadows. Minerva Anestesiol. 2024;90(1–2):99–101.
12. Scimia P, Gentili L, Tedesco M, Fusco P, Sepolvere G. A modified approach to a parasternal block: a case report. A A Pract. 2023;17(1):e01644.
13. Tulgar S, Ciftci B, Ahiskalioglu A, et al. Serratus posterior superior intercostal plane block: a technical report on the description of a novel periparavertebral block for thoracic pain. Cureus. 2023;15(2):e34582. https://doi.org/10.7759/cureus.34582.
14. Forero M, Roqués V, Olejnik L. Erector spinae plane block technique: being thorough is crucial. Reg Anesth Pain Med. https://doi.org/10.1136/rapm-2024-105588. Epub ahead of print.

6 Anterior and Posterior Chest Wall Anatomy

Giuseppe Sepolvere, Danilo Canzio, and Cristiano D'Errico

6.1 Introduction

The anatomical knowledge represents a crucial condition for choosing the appropriate fascial block matching the surgical procedure. In the era of ultrasound imaging, the understanding of the sole ultrasound anatomy should be considered incomplete performing a fascial technique. It is mandatory to know competently the spinal roots from which the nerves arise, their pathway, the plexuses they constitute, the muscles they cross, the dermatomes and the anatomical structures they innerve, the fascial planes, and the bony and vascular structures. The innervation of the chest wall is essential for fascial blocks both for analgesia and anesthesia and plays a key role in the achievement of effective outcomes. It is not intended to be a detailed description of the whole anatomy, but the main anatomical structures involved in the fascial block techniques will be shortly described below [1].

G. Sepolvere (✉)
Department of Anesthesia and Cardiac Surgery Intensive Care Unit, San Michele Hospital, Maddaloni, Caserta, Italy

D. Canzio
Department of Anesthesia and Intensive Care Unit and Pain Therapy, Mater Dei Hospital, Bari, Italy

C. D'Errico
Intensive Care Unit, Department of Anesthesia, AORN Cardarelli, Naples, Italy

6.2 Anterior Chest Wall Anatomy

The anterior and lateral chest wall receive innervation from the intercostal nerves, the supraclavicular branches of the superficial cervical plexus, the pectoral nerves and the thoracic long nerve, the thoracodorsal nerve, and the intercostobrachial nerve in the axillary region. The anterolateral chest wall is composed of the skin, subcutaneous fat, muscles, ribs, and nerves [2, 3].

6.2.1 Muscles

The muscles involved in chest wall fascial blocks for cardiac surgery are:

- Pectoralis major muscle (PMM)
- Pectoralis minor muscle (pmm)
- Serratus anterior muscle (SAM)
- Intercostal muscle (IM)
- Latissimus dorsi muscle (LDM)
- Transversus thoracis muscle (TTM)

6.2.1.1 Pectoralis Major Muscle

The PMM is a fan-shaped triangular muscle that makes up most of the anterior chest wall. It is divided into two portions, the clavicular which originates from the medial half of the clavicle and the costosternal which arises from the anterior surface of the lateral border of the sternum, from the first seven costal cartilages and from the

G. Sepolvere, S. Silvetti (eds.), *Fast-Track in Cardiac Anesthesia*,
https://doi.org/10.1007/978-3-031-70899-2_6

aponeurosis of the external oblique muscle. Both muscle portions joint laterally originating a tendon with a flat structure inserting on the lateral lip of the bicipital groove (or intertubercular groove) of the humerus. It also represents the anterior fold of the armpit. The PMM receives its innervation from the lateral (LPN) and medial (MPN) pectoral nerves both arising from the brachial plexus (BP). The clavicular portion is innervated by the LPN, while the costosternal portion is innervated by both the LPN and the MPN. It is involved in flexion, adduction, and medial rotation of the humerus. It also allows the downward movement of the shoulder and upper limb and the lifting of the ribs [4]. The interfascial plane between the PMM and the pmm, together with the pectoral branch of the thoracoacromial artery, represents the ultrasound landmark for PECS I or interpectoral plane (IPP) block (Fig. 6.1).

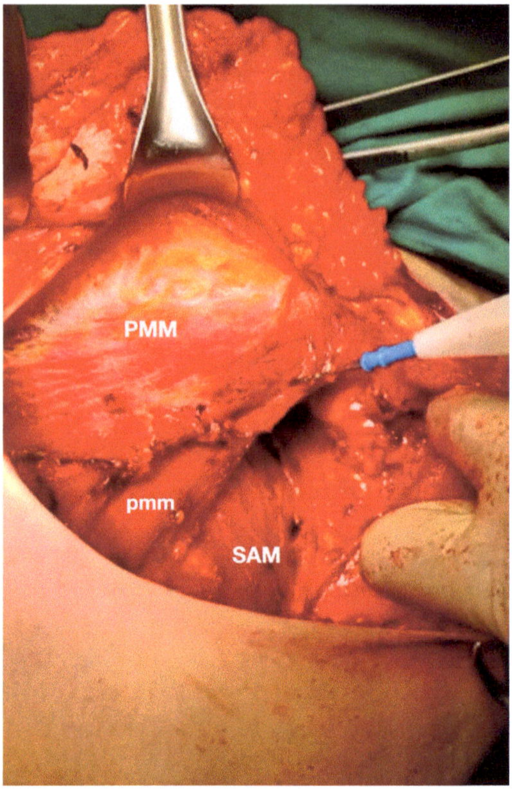

Fig. 6.1 The anatomical relationships between the pectoralis major, pectoralis minor, and serratus anterior muscles. *PMM* pectoralis major muscle, *pmm* pectoralis minor muscle, *SAM* serratus anterior muscle. (Courtesy of Dr. Giuseppe Sepolvere)

6.2.1.2 Pectoralis Minor Muscle

The pmm has a thinner and triangular structure located deeply under the PMM. It originates from the external surface of the third and fourth ribs converging superiorly and laterally to form a thin tendon that sticks to the coracoid process of the scapula. It also constitutes a portion of the anterior wall of the axillary cavity. The pmm receives its innervation from the LPN and the MPN. It allows the lowering and the rising of the shoulder and together with the SAM allows the anterior movement of the scapula. The interfascial plane between the pmm and the PMM, together with the thoracoacromial artery, represents the ultrasound landmark of the IPP (PECS I) block. The fascial plane between the pmm and the SAM represents the ultrasound landmark of PECS II or pectoserratus plane block. The anatomical relationships between PMM, pmm, and SAM are depicted in Fig. 6.1.

6.2.1.3 Serratus Anterior Muscle

The SAM, so named due to its morphology that resembles a wedge, covers most of the lateral chest wall and originates from the external surface of the first up to the eighth–ninth ribs. The muscle fibers then converge posteriorly inserting on the medial edge of the scapula. The SAM is part of the medial wall of the axilla and envelops the thorax like a wing participating in breathing and stabilizing the scapula (Fig. 6.2). Through its action, it elevates both the ribs participating in forced inspiration (accessory muscles) and the arm in the frontal and sagittal planes together with the trapezius muscle. It allows both the abduction and the external rotation of the scapula and its adherence to the chest. It is also called the “boxer’s muscle” as it allows the scapula to move forward and around the chest (typical punch movement). Furthermore, it is involved in the upward rotation of the scapula when a weight is lifted above the head. The SAM is innervated by the thoracic long nerve which runs caudally on its outer surface. The thoracic long nerve injury may lead to the detachment of the scapula from the chest producing a phenomenon known as

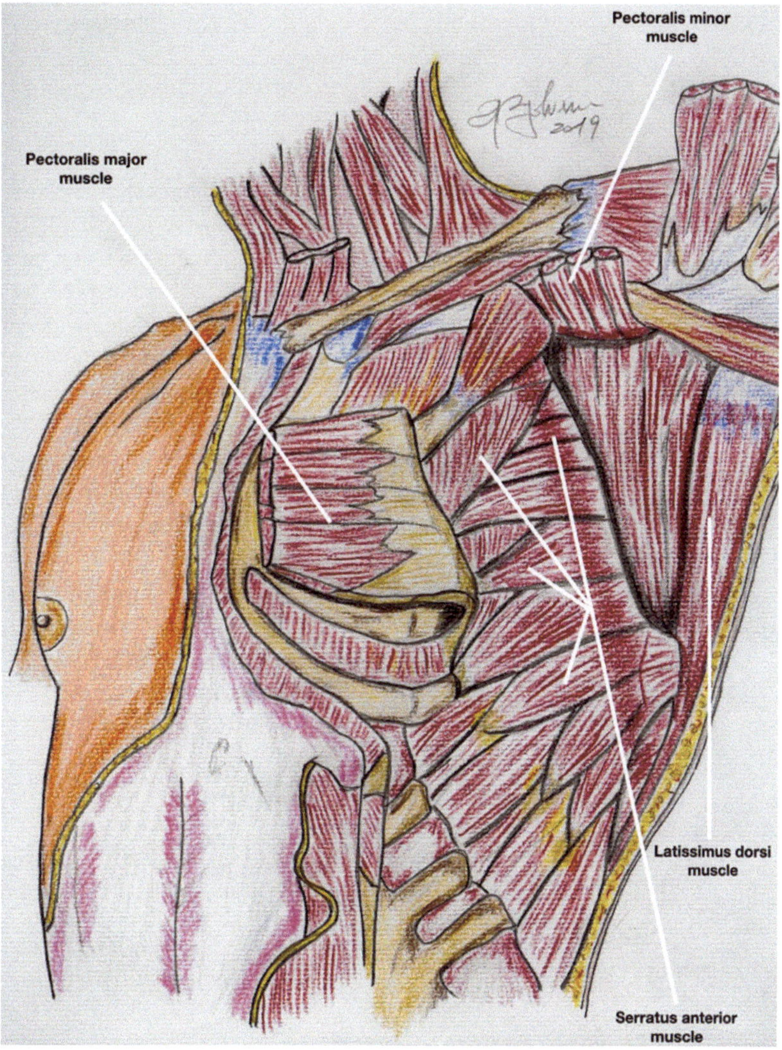

Fig. 6.2 The anatomical relationships between the serratus anterior muscle, the lateral chest wall, and the latissimus dorsi muscle. (Courtesy of Dr. Giuseppe Sepolvere)

"winged scapula." The fascial plane between pmm and SAM represents the ultrasound landmark for pectoserratus plane (PECS II) block (Fig. 6.3). Furthermore, the plane between SAM and LDM represents the ultrasound landmark of superficial serratus anterior plane block, while the plane between the SAM and the underlying costal plane is the ultrasound landmark of deep serratus anterior plane block [5].

6.2.1.4 Latissimus Dorsi Muscle

The LDM is a large, thin, and flat muscle which covers all back muscles of the posterior trunk. It arises from the spinous processes of the last six thoracic vertebrae (T7–T12), the thoracolumbar fascia, and the posterior third of the outer border of the iliac crest. It converges cranially to form a flattened tendon that inserts on the floor of the bicipital sulcus anteriorly to the junction of teres major muscle. It is involved in the adduction, extension, and internal rotation of the upper limb (Fig. 6.4). It is innervated by the thoracodorsal nerve which runs inferiorly together with the thoracodorsal artery, which represents a vascular landmark for the serratus anterior plane block. The fascial plane between the LDM and SAM, together with the thoracodorsal artery, represents the ultrasound landmark of superficial serratus anterior plane block.

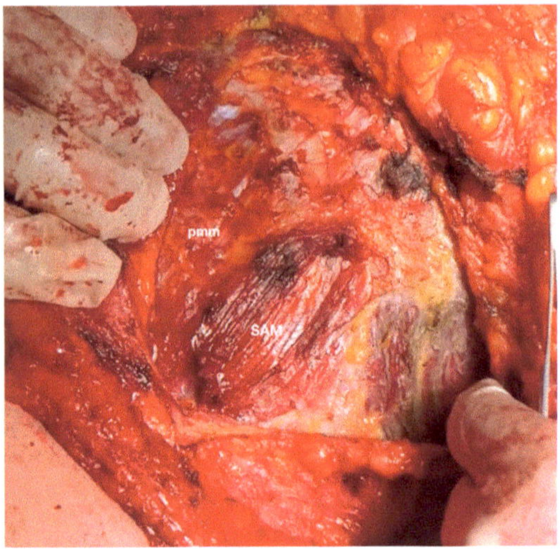

Fig. 6.3 The tooth structure of the serratus anterior muscle and its anatomical relationship with the pectoralis minor muscle. *SAM* serratus anterior muscle, *pmm* pectoralis minor muscle. (Courtesy of Dr. Giuseppe Sepolvere)

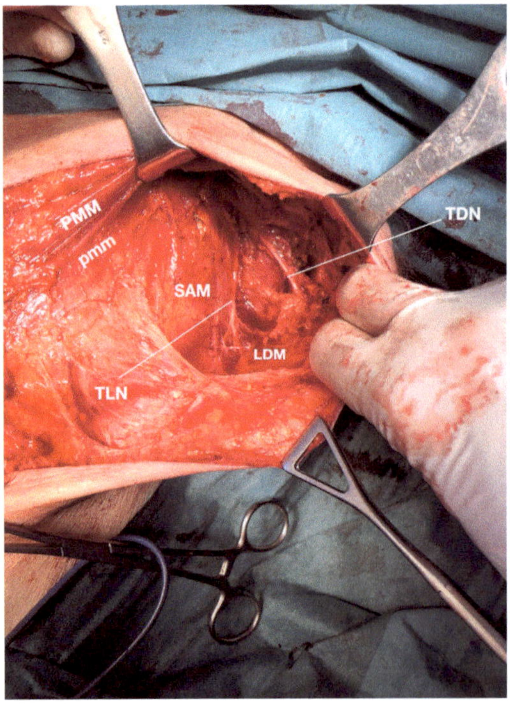

Fig. 6.4 The anatomical relationships between the pectoralis major, pectoralis minor, serratus anterior, and latissimus dorsi muscle. *PMM* pectoralis major muscle, *pmm* pectoralis minor muscle, *SAM* serratus anterior muscle, *LDM* latissimus dorsi muscle, *TLN* thoracic long nerve, *TDN* thoracodorsal nerve. (Courtesy of Dr. Giuseppe Sepolvere)

6.2.2 Nerves

The nervous structures involved in the chest wall blocks are:

- Intercostal nerves and intercostobrachial nerve (INs and ICBN)
- Supraclavicular nerves (SCNs)
- Pectoral nerves (PNs)–lateral pectoral nerve (LPN)–medial pectoral nerve (MPN)
- Thoracic long nerve (TLN)
- Thoracodorsal nerve (TDN)

The main nervous structures involved in fascia blocks and their anatomical origin are reported in Table 6.1.

6.2.2.1 Supraclavicular Nerves

A limited portion of the skin of the upper chest region and the clavicle is innervated by the SCNs originating from the superficial cervical plexus (SCP) reaching the anatomical border area

Table 6.1 Main nervous structures involved in fascia blocks and their anatomical origin

Nerves	Anatomical arise
Supraclavicular nerves	Superficial cervical plexus
Lateral intercostal nerves	From T2 to T6–T7
Anterior intercostal nerves	From T1 to T6
Intercostobrachial nerve	Lateral branch of second intercostal nerve (T2)
Lateral pectoral nerve	C5–C7 (50%) C6 and C7 (50%) Anterior divisions of the superior and middle trunks of the brachial plexus (33.8%) Lateral cord of the brachial plexus (23.4%)
Medial pectoral nerve	C8 to T1 (73.3%), C8 (23.4%), T1 (3.3%) Medial cord (49.3%) Anterior division of the lower trunk (43.8%), directly from the lower trunk (4.7%)
Long thoracic nerve	Ventral branches of C5, C6, and C7
Thoracodorsal nerve	Posterior cord of the brachial plexus with a spinal contribution from C6 to C8

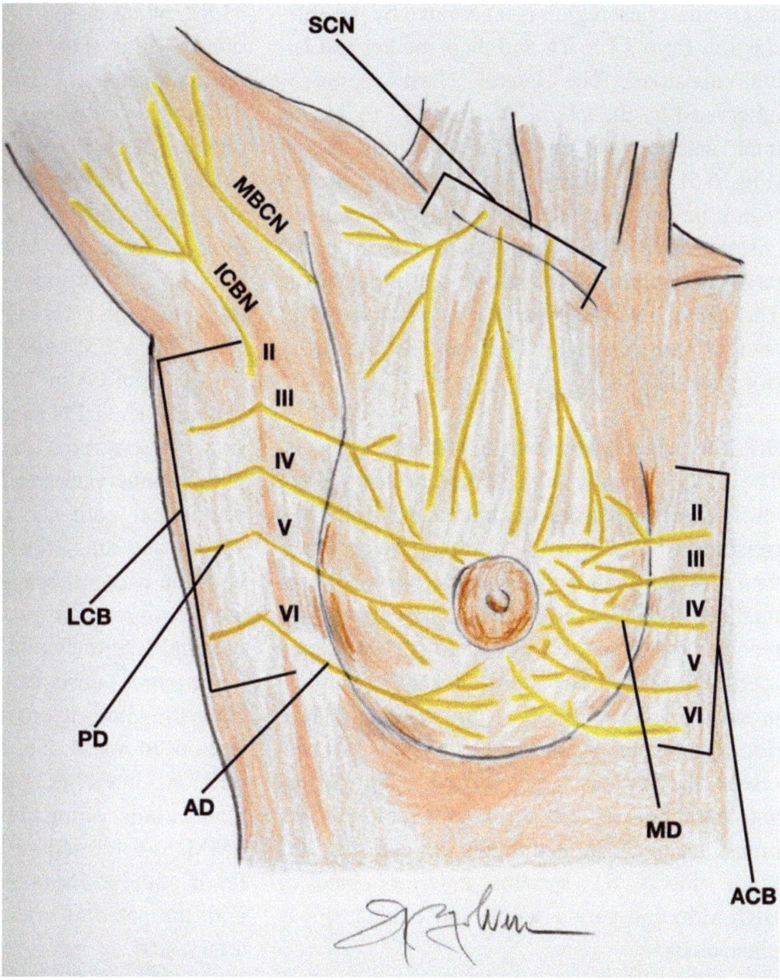

Fig. 6.5 Chest innervations. The anteromedial chest region is innervated by the anterior branches of T1–T2 to T6 intercostal nerves and their medial and lateral divisions. The lateral chest region is innervated by the lateral branches of T2–T6 intercostal nerves and their anterior and posterior divisions. The superior portion of the chest is innervated by supraclavicular nerves, which arise from the superficial cervical plexus. The lateral cutaneous branch of T2 represents the intercostobrachial nerve. *SCN* supraclavicular nerves, *ACB* anterior cutaneous branches, *LCB* lateral cutaneous branches, *MD* medial division, *PD* posterior divisions, *AD* anterior division, *ICBN* intercostobrachial nerve, *MBCN* medial brachial cutaneous nerve. (Courtesy of Dr. Giuseppe Sepolvere)

between the upper medial and lateral quadrants of the breast (Fig. 6.5). This anatomical area is involved in the pacemaker implantation [6].

6.2.2.2 Intercostal Nerves

The INs are primarily responsible for sensory innervation of the anterior and posterior chest wall and the mammary gland. Each spinal nerve exits the intervertebral foramen dividing into dorsal and ventral rami. The dorsal rami innervate the muscles, bones, joints, and skin. The ventral rami run initially close to the vessels between pleura and endothoracic fascia and then between the internal and innermost intercostal muscles, innervating the lateral and anterior chest walls. They are represented by the anterior branches of the thoracic spinal nerves from T1 to T11 and run in the intercostal spaces below the corresponding ribs having the same number, in close association with the vessels. The 12th IN is also called subcostal because it is not included between two ribs but runs under the 12th. At the level of sternal region, the anterior INs from T2 to T6 emit collateral branches that can be divided into lateral (LD) and medial (MD) cutaneous divisions, while the lateral INs, in the lateral chest region, emit lateral branches divided into anterior (AD) and posterior (PD) cutaneous divisions (Fig. 6.5). The lateral cutaneous branch of the second IN is called ICBN, which leaves the chest wall to anastomose with the medial brachial cutaneous nerve (MBCN) of the arm, and it is responsible of the armpit innervation together with TDN and TLN nerves [7] (Fig. 6.5). In summary, the anterior and medial chest region is innervated by the anterior INs from T1 to T6 and their medial and lateral divisions. The lateral chest region is innervated by the lateral INs from T2 to T6 and their anterior and posterior divisions [8, 9] (Fig. 6.5). The anterior INs in the parasternal region lie between the PMM and internal intercostal muscle (IIM) and represent the nervous target of superficial and deep parasternal block. The lateral INs represent the nervous target of pectoserratus plane (PECS II) and serratus anterior plane blocks.

6.2.2.3 Intercostobrachial Nerve

The ICBN, which is the lateral branch of the second IN, emerges from the intercostal space and runs laterally towards the limb supplying innervation to the axilla and the upper portion of the medial arm (Fig. 6.5). The ICBN may also receive contributions from the first, third, and fourth INs. The ICBN injury during the surgical procedure leads to the post-lymph node dissection chronic pain syndrome [10]. The ICBN represents the nervous target for the analgesic and anesthetic coverage of the lateral region of the breast and the armpit through the pectoserratus plane (PECS II), serratus anterior plane or BRILMA, and paravertebral and erector spinae plane blocks.

6.2.2.4 Pectoral Nerves

The PNs are commonly described as motor nerves; however, the increasing scientific evidences demonstrate their involvement in nociceptive and proprioceptive nervous afferents. Nociceptive afferents can be transferred to PNs directly from anatomical structures such as the acromioclavicular joint, coracoclavicular ligaments, subacromial bursa, shoulder joint capsule, clavicular periosteum, and pectoral muscles. Through the cutaneous branches, they innervate the anterior chest wall and the anterior border of the deltoid muscle. They are represented by the LPN and medial MPN. The LPN is anatomically more represented than MPN, and the communications between them is defined as "pectoral nerve loop." Recent studies demonstrate that in 33.8% of cases, the LPN emerges from the anterior divisions of the superior and middle trunks of the brachial plexus (BP), while in 23.4% of cases, it can also originate from the lateral cord of the plexus. The MPN has a variable origin and can emerge from the medial cord (49.3%), from the anterior division of the lower trunk (43.8%), or directly from the lower trunk (4.7%) of the BP. The LPN originates from C5–C7 in 50% of individuals and from C6 and C7 in the remaining 50%. The MPM can originate from C8 to T1 in 73.3%, from C8 in 23.4%, and from T1 in 3.3% of cases. The LPN runs anteriorly to the axillary vessels, crosses the clavipectoral fascia, and supplies its innervation to PMM. The LPN shares its anatomical pathway with the thoracoacromial vessels and runs under the PMM fascia together with the pectoral branch of the thoracoacromial artery. After its origin, the MPN courses inferiorly and anteriorly to the axillary artery and deep to the pmm. Subsequently, at the level of the midclavicular line, it crosses the pmm at the third intercostal space. The PNs can also have three different branches represented by a superior branch innervating the clavicular fibers of the PMM, an intermediate branch running below the fascia of the PMM taking anatomical relationship with the pectoral branch of the thoracoacromial artery, and an inferior branch which innervates the pmm and the costal portion of the PMM (Fig. 6.6). Due to the anatomical variability, we can describe a "subpectoral plexus" consisting of the roots of C5–T1, the two PNs, and the three terminal branches. Based on this anatomical arrangement, the superior and middle branches are divisions of the LPN, while the inferior branch is formed by the fusion of the MPN and the pectoral nerve loop arising from C7 (Fig. 6.7). The PNs, which travel in the fascial plane between PMM and pmm accompanied by the thoracoacromial artery, represent the nervous target of IPP (PECS I) block (Fig. 6.8).

6.2.2.5 Thoracic Long Nerve

The TLN, also known as the "nerve of Bell," originates from the ventral branches of C5, C6, and C7 and runs along the lateral region of the

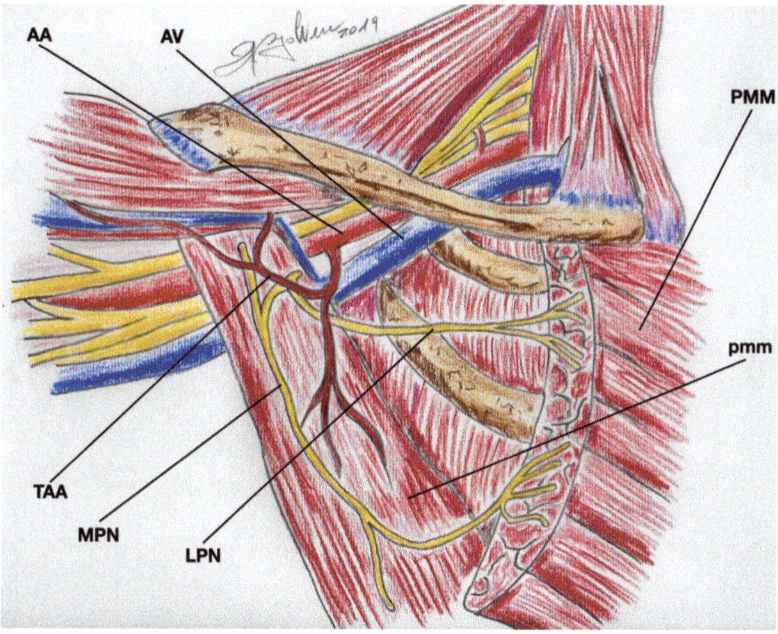

Fig. 6.6 Pectoral nerves and pectoral branch of the thoracoacromial artery. The lateral and medial pectoral nerves are included in the fascial plane between the pectoralis major and minor muscles near the pectoral branch of the thoracoacromial artery. *AA* axillary artery, *AV* axillary vein, *TAA* thoracoacromial artery, *LPN* lateral pectoral nerve, *MPN* medial pectoral nerve, *pmm* pectoralis minor muscle, *PMM* pectoralis major muscle. (Courtesy of Dr. Giuseppe Sepolvere)

thorax where it innervates SAM (Figs. 6.4 and 6.8). The TLN is the nervous target for pectoserratus plane (PECS II) block and the *block* of the lateral branches of the intercostal nerves in the middle axillary line (*BRILMA*).

6.2.2.6 Thoracodorsal Nerve

The TDN originates from the posterior cord of the BP with a spinal contribution from C6 to C8. It descends along the posterior wall of the axilla, and accompanied by the thoracodorsal artery, it innervates the LDM (Figs. 6.4 and 6.8). The TDN represents the nervous target for pectoserratus plane (PECS II) block and BRILMA.

6.2.3 Vascular Structures

The main arteries which supply the chest and breast are the internal thoracic artery, commonly known as the internal mammary artery, the lateral thoracic artery, the intercostal arteries, the thoracoacromial artery, and the thoracodorsal artery.

Specifically, the vascular structures used as peculiar landmarks for the fascial blocks in cardiac surgery are:

- Thoracoacromial artery (TAA)
- Thoracodorsal artery (TDA)
- Internal mammary artery (IMA)

6.2.3.1 Thoracoacromial Artery

The TAA is a short trunk that originates from the axillary artery and travels a short distance along the upper border of the pmm. Penetrating the clavipectoral fascia, it divides into its lateral branches: the clavicular, acromial, deltoid, and pectoralis (Figs. 6.6 and 6.9). The TAA represents an important vascular landmark for the interpectoral plane (PECS I) block, since the PNs and the pectoral nerve loop have an anatomical relationship with the artery. The LPN runs parallel to the pectoral branch of the TAA in the myofascial plane between PMM and pmm.

6.2.3.2 Thoracodorsal Artery

The TDA is a branch of the subscapularis artery and runs inferiorly along the lateral chest wall. It initially runs deep to the LDM and then moves to the outer surface of the SAM (Figs. 6.9 and 6.10). It is accompanied by the TDN and supplies innervation to the LDM. It represents a useful ultrasound landmark for the

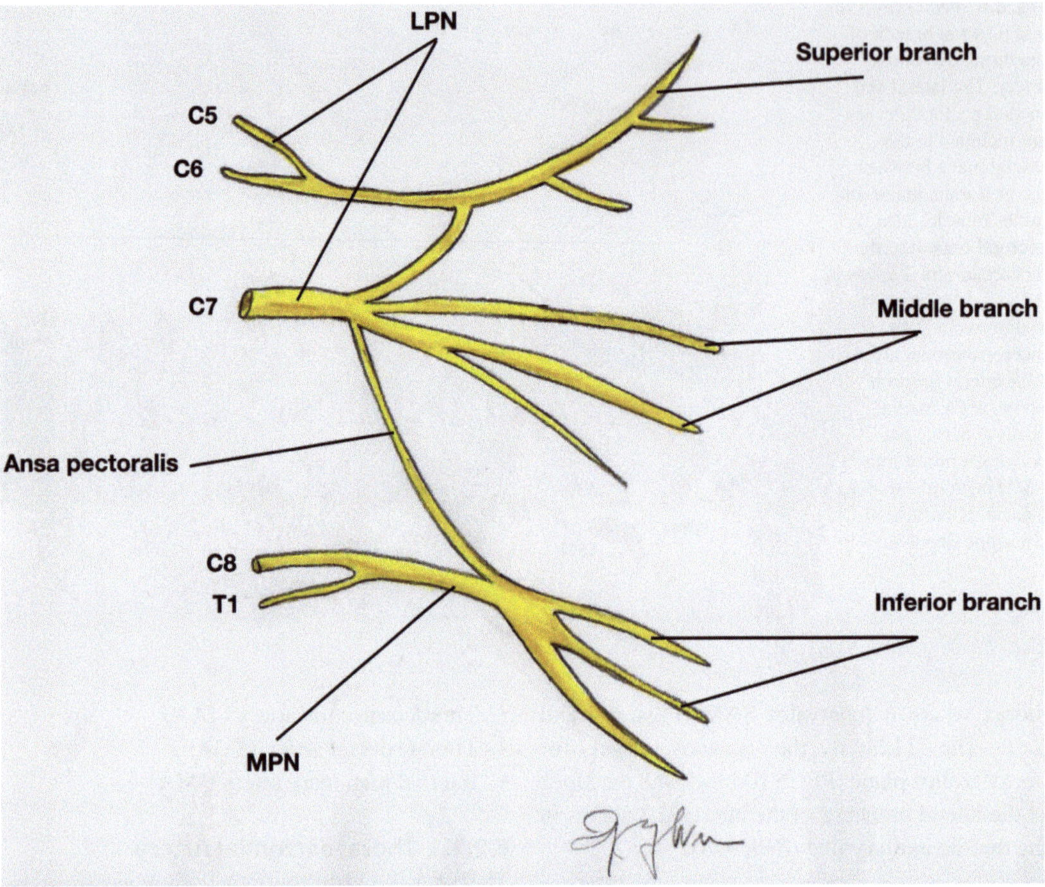

Fig. 6.7 The subpectoral plexus is formed by the lateral and medial pectoral nerves and by the three terminal branches (superior, middle, and inferior). The middle and superior branches derive from the lateral pectoral nerve, while the inferior branch derives from the pectoral loop (spinal root of C7) and the medial pectoral nerve. *MPN* medial pectoral nerve, *LPN* lateral pectoral nerve, *ansa pectoralis* ansa pectoralis. (Courtesy of Dr. Giuseppe Sepolvere)

superficial serratus anterior plane block due to its course in the fascial plane between the SAM and LDM.

6.2.3.3 Internal Mammary Artery

The internal mammary artery or IMA arises from the subclavian artery, above and behind the sternal end of the clavicle. Passing behind the first costal cartilage, close to the phrenic nerve, it goes down into the thorax. The artery descends vertically about 1 cm lateral to the sternal border, behind the first six costal cartilages. IMA is separated from the pleura at the second or third costal cartilage by a string layer of endothoracic fascia and inferiorly by the transversus thoracis muscle (TTM). It is accompanied by two mammary veins, which ascend medially and laterally, respectively. IMA runs between internal intercostal muscle (IIM) and TTM, which is a thin and hypoechogenic muscular layer close to the pleura on the inner surface of the anterior thoracic wall and always destroyed during IMA harvesting [11–13] (Fig. 6.11). This anatomical region is innervated by the anterior cutaneous branches from T2 to T6 INs, which are obliterated during cardiac surgery artery harvesting.

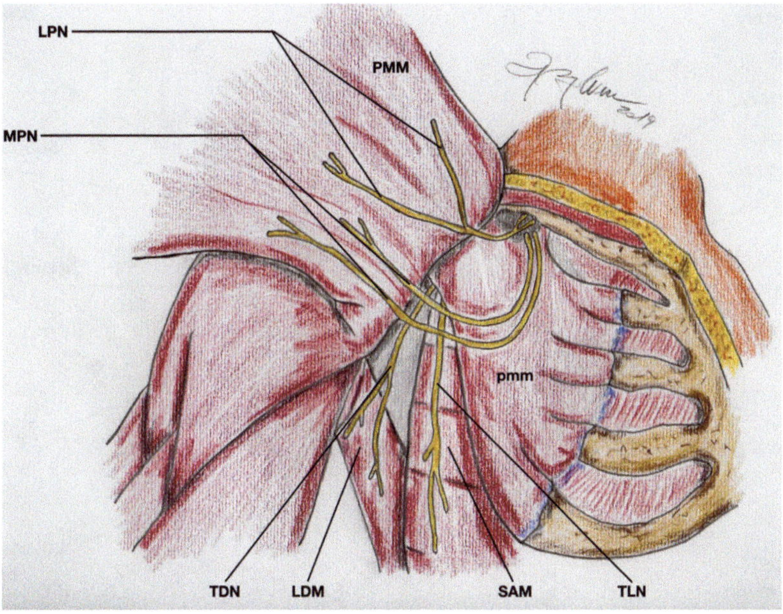

Fig. 6.8 Pectoral, thoracic long, and thoracodorsal nerves. The lateral and medial pectoral nerves run in the fascial plane between the pectoralis major and minor muscles. The thoracic long and thoracodorsal nerves innervate the serratus anterior and latissimus dorsi muscles. *LPN* lateral pectoral nerve, *MPN* medial pectoral nerve, *PMM* pectoralis major muscle, *pmm* pectoralis minor muscle, *TDN* thoracodorsal nerve, *LDM* latissimus dorsi muscle, *TLN* thoracic long nerve, *SAM* serratus anterior muscle. (Courtesy of Dr. Giuseppe Sepolvere)

Fig. 6.9 Origin and course of the thoracoacromial and thoracodorsal arteries. The thoracoacromial artery arises from the axillary artery and divides into the clavicular, acromial, deltoid, and pectoralis branches. The thoracodorsal artery is a branch of the subscapularis artery. It runs inferiorly along the lateral chest wall deep to the latissimus dorsi muscle and then moves to the outer surface of the serratus anterior muscle. (Courtesy of Dr. Giuseppe Sepolvere)

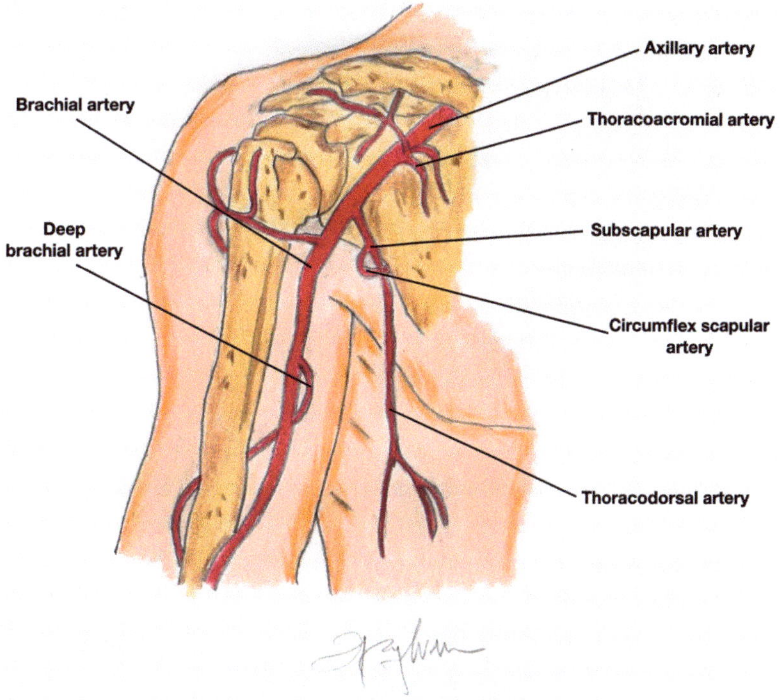

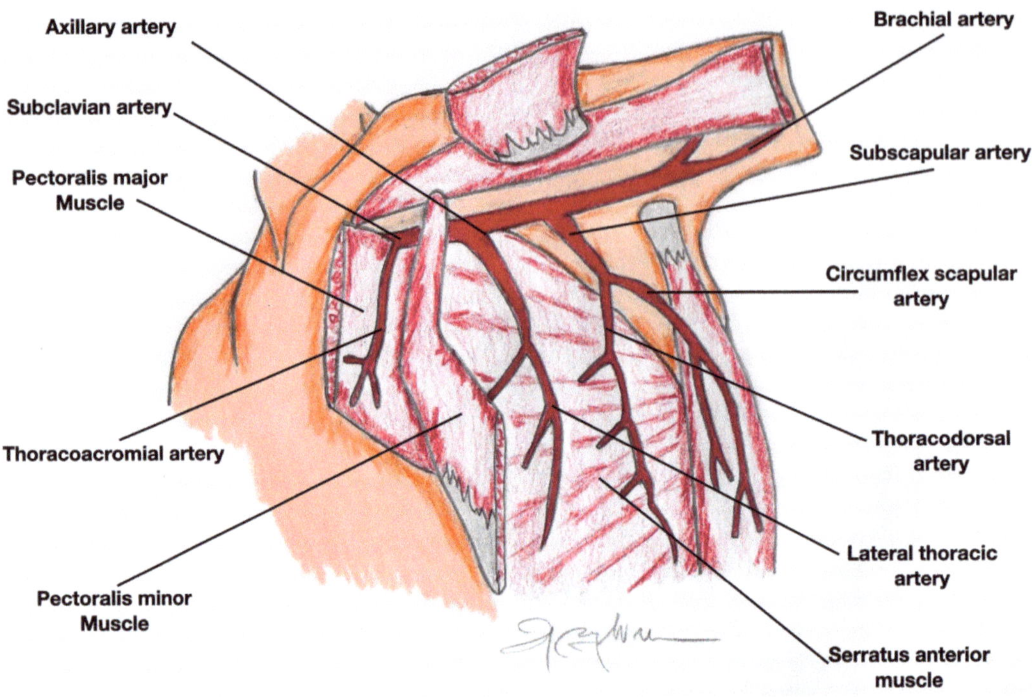

Fig. 6.10 Main arteries and their anatomical relationships with the chest wall muscles. (Courtesy of Dr. Giuseppe Sepolvere)

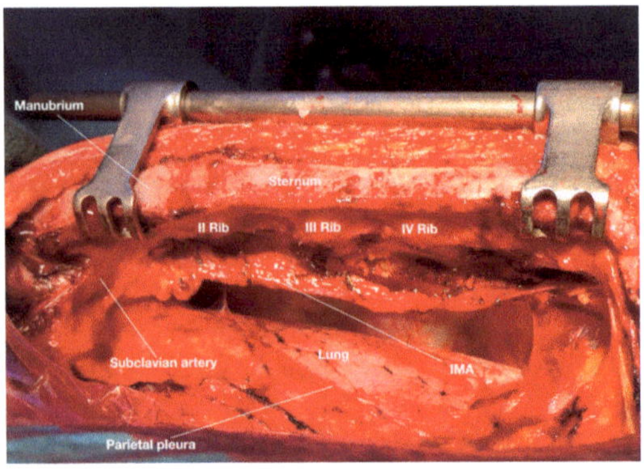

Fig. 6.11 The internal mammary artery arises from the subclavian artery. Passing behind the first costal cartilage, it goes down into the thorax. The artery descends vertically about 1 cm lateral to the sternal border, behind the first six costal cartilages. The transversus thoracis muscle is always destroyed during internal mammary artery harvesting. *IMA* internal mammary artery, *Sternum* sternum, *Rib* rib, *Manubrium* sternal manubrium, *Lung* lung, *Parietal pleura* parietal pleura, *Subclavian artery* subclavian artery. (Courtesy of Dr. Giuseppe Sepolvere)

6.3 Posterior Chest Wall Anatomy

The posterior chest wall is an anatomical region starting from the posterior axillary line up to the spinous processes including multiple different muscles lying on the thoracic cage so that many different muscular structures may be visualized depending on where the probe is placed. The most superficial and lateral muscle in the inferior region of the thorax is the LDM, while the most superficial one in the superior portion of the thorax is the trapezius muscle which covers rhomboid major and minor muscles as well as the scapula and its muscles. The latter overlie the erector spinae muscle which is composed of collective muscles represented by the spinalis, longissimus thoracis, and iliocostalis muscles, which stabilize the torso. A very important group of muscular and ligamentous structures adjacent to the bony vertebrae is represented by the multifidus, rotatores, and intertransverse muscles and the superior costotransverse ligament (SCTL), which span the gap adjacent to vertebral transverse processes. This muscular complex is also a posterior and permeable limit for the paravertebral space through which the local anesthetic may spread as observed with the retrolaminar, erector spinae, and midpoint transverse process to pleura blocks. The posterior thoracic wall is innervated by the medial, intermediate, and lateral branches arising from the dorsal rami of thoracic spinal nerves ascending through the muscles up to the superficial tissues. The posterolateral chest wall is innervated by the posterior divisions of the lateral intercostal nerves. The anatomical structures involved in the posterior chest wall blocks are represented by:

- Erector spinae muscle (ESM)
- Paravertebral space (PVS)

6.3.1 Erector Spinae Muscle

ESM is a wide and superficial muscle covered by the thoracolumbar fascia in the thoracic and lumbar area. It is not a single muscular structure but a set of muscles and tendons running along the spine from the sacrum and hips up to the base of the skull. This group of muscles rotate and straighten the back maintaining a stable posture in standing or sitting position. ESM varies in size at different vertebral regions dividing into three columns: lateral (iliocostalis), intermediate (longissimus), and medial (spinalis) decreasing in size as they ascend to be inserted on the vertebrae and ribs [14] (Fig. 6.12).

6.3.2 Paravertebral Space

PVS is a virtual wedge-shaped slot running bilaterally and continuously from T1 to L1 containing fatty tissue, dorsal, and ventral rami of the spinal nerves, arteries, and veins, the sympa-

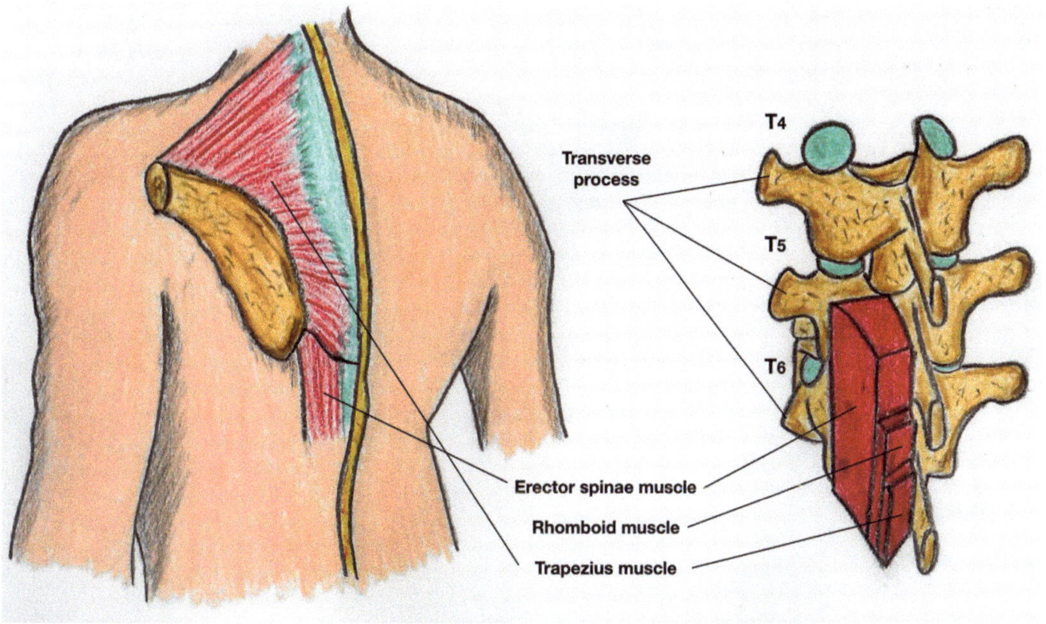

Fig. 6.12 Schematic illustration of the anatomical relationships between the transverse processes, the erector spinae, rhomboid, and trapezius muscles. (Courtesy of Dr. Giuseppe Sepolvere)

thetic trunk. It is medially formed by the lateral border of the vertebral body and transverse process and posteriorly is delimited by SCTL which runs between the rib below and the transverse process above. SCTL consists of a set of permeable and porous fibers and fenestrations responsible for the spread of the local anesthetic into the PVS. The apex of the PVS lies laterally communicating with the intercostal space. An anterolateral border is formed close to parietal pleura underneath which sits the lung [15, 16] (Figs. 6.13 and 6.14).

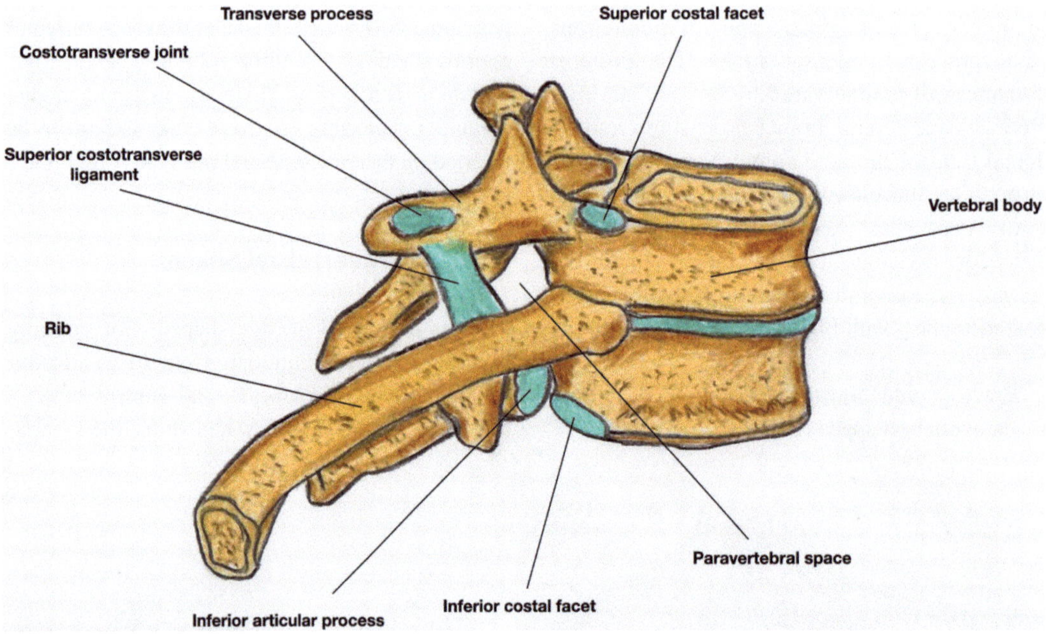

Fig. 6.13 Schematic illustration of paravertebral space and the anatomical relationships between rib, superior costotransverse ligament, and transverse process. (Courtesy of Dr. Giuseppe Sepolvere)

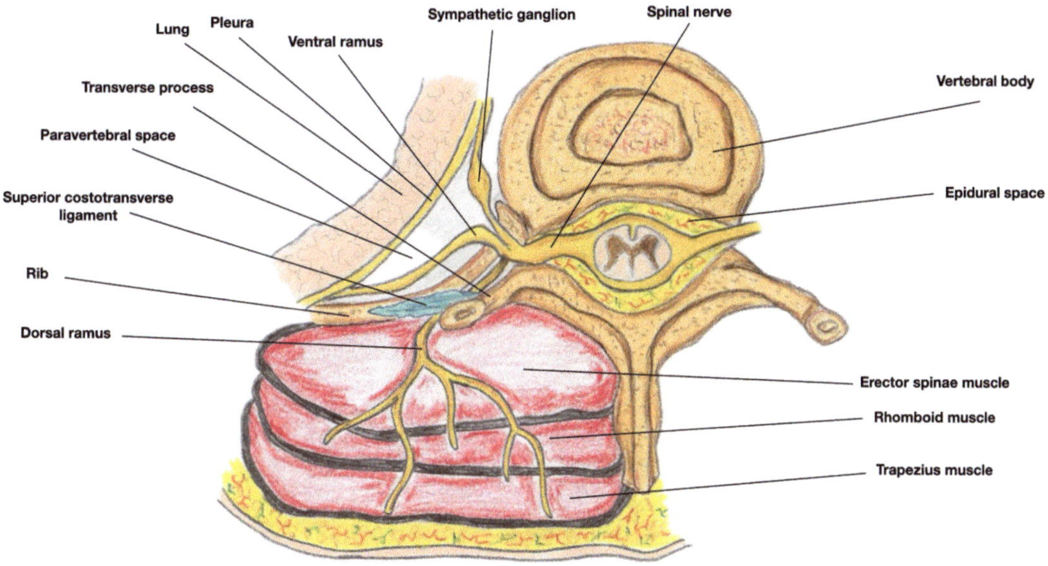

Fig. 6.14 Paravertebral space. Paravertebral space is a virtual wedge-shaped slot running bilaterally and continuously from T1 to L1 containing fatty tissue, dorsal and ventral rami of the spinal nerves, arteries, and veins, the sympathetic trunk. It is medially formed by the lateral border of the vertebral body and transverse process and posteriorly is delimited by superior costotransverse ligament which runs between the rib below and the transverse process above. The superior costotransverse ligament consists of a set of permeable and porous fibers and fenestrations responsible for the spread of the local anesthetic into the paravertebral space. The apex of the paravertebral space lies laterally communicating with the intercostal space. An anterolateral border is formed close to parietal pleura, underneath which sits the lung. (Courtesy of Dr. Giuseppe Sepolvere)

References

1. Elsharkawy H, Pawa A, Mariano ER. Interfascial plane blocks: back to basics. Reg Anesth Pain Med. 2018;43(4):341–6. https://doi.org/10.1097/AAP.0000000000000750.
2. Chin KJ, Versyck B, Pawa A. Ultrasound-guided fascial plane blocks of the chest wall: a state-of-the-art review. Anaesthesia. 2021;76(Suppl 1):110–26. https://doi.org/10.1111/anae.15276.
3. Brosnan KD, Coppens S, Ni EA. Ultrasound-guided fascial plane blocks of the chest wall: a state-of-the-art review. Anaesthesia. 2023;78(2):260–1. https://doi.org/10.1111/anae.15885. Epub 2022 Oct 7.
4. Chin KJ, Pawa A, Forero M, Adhikary S. Ultrasound-guided fascial plane blocks of the thorax: pectoral I and II, serratus anterior plane, and erector spinae plane blocks. Adv Anesth. 2019;37:187–205. https://doi.org/10.1016/j.aan.2019.08.007. Epub 2019 Sep 13.
5. Sharma R, Damiano J, Al-Saidi I, Dizdarevic A. Chest wall and abdominal blocks for thoracic and abdominal surgeries: a review. Curr Pain Headache Rep. 2023;27(10):587–600. https://doi.org/10.1007/s11916-023-01158-7. Epub 2023 Aug 25.
6. Scimia P, Gentili L, Sepolvere G. Ultrasound-guided cervical plexus block: understanding the cervical fasciae to clarify the nomenclature of this technique. Minerva Anestesiol. 2022;88(6):526–8. https://doi.org/10.23736/S0375-9393.21.16227-3. Epub 2022 Jan 24.
7. Sakamoto H, Akita K, Sato T. An anatomical analysis of the relationships between the intercostal nerves and the thoracic and abdominal muscles in man. I. Ramification of the intercostal nerves. Acta Anat (Basel). 1996;156(2):132–42. https://doi.org/10.1159/000147838.
8. Chin KJ. An anatomical basis for naming plane blocks of the anteromedial chest wall. Reg Anesth Pain Med. 2017;42(3):414–5. https://doi.org/10.1097/AAP.0000000000000575.
9. Bijkerk E, Cornelissen AJM, Sommer M, Van Der Hulst RRWJ, Lataster A, Tuinder SMH. Intercostal nerve block of the anterior cutaneous branches and the sensibility of the female breast. Clin Anat. 2020;33(7):1025–32. https://doi.org/10.1002/ca.23532. Epub 2019 Dec 23. PMID: 31837172; PMCID: PMC7540051.

10. O'Rourke MG, Tang TS, Allison SI, Wood W. The anatomy of the extrathoracic intercostobrachial nerve. Aust N Z J Surg. 1999;69(12):860–4. https://doi.org/10.1046/j.1440-1622.1999.01718.x.
11. Takahashi H, Suzuki T. Anterior thoracic medial block for administering postoperative analgesia in the internal mammary area. Reg Anesth Pain Med. 2016;41(5):660–1. https://doi.org/10.1097/AAP.0000000000000462.
12. Fujii S, Roche M, Jones PM, Vissa D, Bainbridge D, Zhou JR. Transversus thoracis muscle plane block in cardiac surgery: a pilot feasibility study. Reg Anesth Pain Med. 2019;44(5):556–60. https://doi.org/10.1136/rapm-2018-100178. Epub 2019 Mar 21.
13. Sepolvere G, Tognù A, Tedesco M, Coppolino F, Cristiano L. Avoiding the internal mammary artery during parasternal blocks: ultrasound identification and technique considerations. J Cardiothorac Vasc Anesth. 2021;35(6):1594–602. https://doi.org/10.1053/j.jvca.2020.11.007. Epub 2020 Nov 16.
14. Macaire P, Ho N, Nguyen T, Nguyen B, Vu V, Quach C, Roques V, Capdevila X. Ultrasound-guided continuous thoracic erector spinae plane block within an enhanced recovery program is associated with decreased opioid consumption and improved patient postoperative rehabilitation after open cardiac surgery-a patient-matched, controlled before-and-after study. J Cardiothorac Vasc Anesth. 2019;33(6):1659–67. https://doi.org/10.1053/j.jvca.2018.11.021. Epub 2018 Nov 19.
15. Costache I, de Neumann L, Ramnanan CJ, Goodwin SL, Pawa A, Abdallah FW, McCartney CJL. The mid-point transverse process to pleura (MTP) block: a new end-point for thoracic paravertebral block. Anaesthesia. 2017;72(10):1230–6. https://doi.org/10.1111/anae.14004. Epub 2017 Aug 1.
16. Ohgoshi Y, Ando A, Kubo EN. Paravertebral spread after different nerve blocks in the peri-paravertebral area. J Clin Anesth. 2020;62:109747. https://doi.org/10.1016/j.jclinane.2020.109747. Epub 2020 Feb 20.

Anterior and Posterior Abdominal Wall Anatomy

7

Paolo Capuano, Mario Tedesco, Andrea Tognù, and Giuseppe Sepolvere

7.1 Introduction

Abdominal wall blocks provide analgesia and anesthesia in several wide surgical fields, and they could be considered a valid and effective alternative to the use of thoracic epidural analgesia (TEA). It is known that the latter has traditionally been used in intra-abdominal surgery, but some concerns about the technique include the hypotension and the risk of bleeding and epidural hematoma with subsequent neurological damage in the presence of anticoagulated or anti-aggregate patients. On this basis, the abdominal wall blocks avoid the risk of neuraxial blockade providing an effective pain relief for abdominal surgery. Understanding the anatomy and function of the abdominal fascial plane is essential for the proper execution of the techniques and for better grasping the complexities of abdominal anatomy and providing optimal care to patients undergoing abdominal surgery. For the educational purpose, only the muscular structures involved in the abdominal fascial blocks are described.

7.2 Anatomy of the Anterior and Posterior Abdominal Wall

The anterior abdominal wall is limited superiorly by the costal arch and xiphoid process, inferiorly by the inguinal ligaments and pubic symphysis, and laterally by the posterior axillary line. The lateral anatomical region of the abdominal wall is composed of three muscles each with an associated fascial sheath. Deep to the muscles lie the transversalis fascia, extraperitoneal fat, and parietal peritoneum [1].

The anterolateral and posterior anatomy of the abdominal wall is described in Fig. 7.1.

7.2.1 Anterolateral Abdominal Wall

The anterior abdominal wall refers to the front portion of the abdomen, which is composed of layers of muscles, fascia, and other connective tissues. It serves several important functions,

P. Capuano (✉)
Department of Anesthesia and Intensive Care, Istituto Mediterraneo per i Trapianti e Terapie ad alta Specializzazione (IRCCS-ISMETT), UPMCI (University of Pittsburgh Medical Center Italy), Palermo, Italy

M. Tedesco
Department of Anesthesia and Intensive Care Unit and Pain Therapy, Mater Dei Hospital, Bari, Italy

A. Tognù
Department of Anesthesia, Intensive Care and Pain Therapy, Orthopedic University Hospital Rizzoli, Bologna, Italy
e-mail: andrea.tognu@ior.it

G. Sepolvere
Department of Anesthesia and Cardiac Surgery, Intensive Care Unit, San Michele Hospital, Maddaloni, Caserta, Italy

G. Sepolvere, S. Silvetti (eds.), *Fast-Track in Cardiac Anesthesia*,
https://doi.org/10.1007/978-3-031-70899-2_7

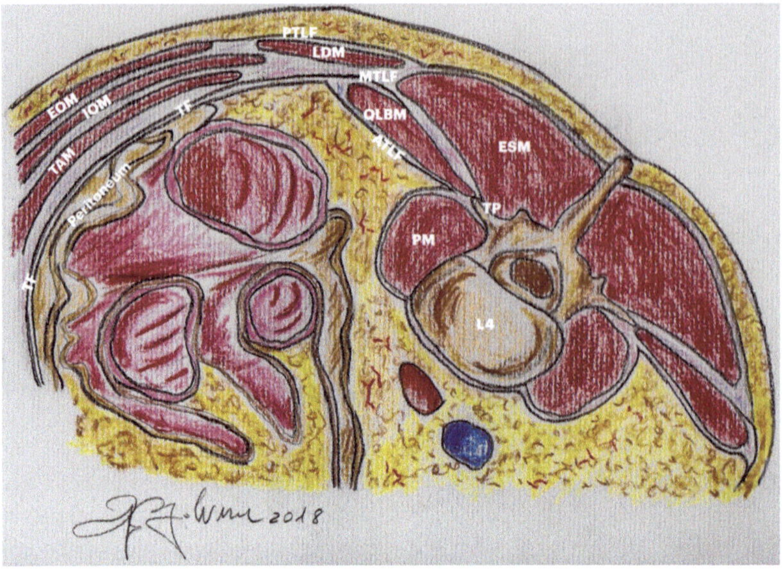

Fig. 7.1 Anterolateral and posterior anatomy of the abdominal wall. *EOM* external oblique muscle, *IOM* internal oblique muscle, *TAM* transversus abdominis muscle, *TF* transversalis fascia, *LDM* latissimus dorsi muscle, *PTLF* posterior thoracolumbar fascia, *MTLF* middle thoracolumbar fascia, *ATLF* anterior thoracolumbar fascia, *QLM* quadratus lumborum muscle, *ESM* erector spinae muscle, *PM* psoas muscle, *TP* transverse process, *L4* L4 vertebral body. (Courtesy of Dr. Giuseppe Sepolvere)

such as protecting the abdominal organs, assisting in movements such as breathing and trunk flexion, and providing structural support to the body [2].

The muscles of the anterior abdominal wall play vital roles in movement, stability, and protection, highlighting their significance in overall body function and health. Despite their broad area, these muscles serve various purposes in coordination with other body systems. They assist in defecation and urination, as well as in respiration and coughing by altering intra-abdominal and intrathoracic pressures [2]. Working in concert with back muscles, the abdominal wall muscles facilitate flexion, extension, and rotation of the torso from the hips. This allows for a wide range of movements and postures. The tension generated in the thoracolumbar fascia, along with the muscles of the back, provides stabilization for the lumbosacral spine and pelvis. This stabilization is critical for maintaining posture and preventing injury during movement. When contracted, the robust overlap of the muscular girdle provides physical protection for the underlying visceral organs. This contraction can help shield the internal organs from external trauma or pressure.

The anterolateral muscles are the following:

- **External oblique muscle (EOM)**: This is the outermost muscle layer of the anterolateral abdominal wall. It runs diagonally downward and forward, originating from the external surface of the 5th–12th ribs and the lower borders of these ribs and inserting into the linea alba, iliac crest, and pubic tubercle. The external oblique muscle aids in trunk flexion, rotation, and lateral flexion [3, 4].

- The EOM is innervated by the ventral rami (anterior divisions) of the spinal nerves T7–T12 and L1. These spinal nerves are part of the thoracoabdominal nerves and the iliohypogastric and ilioinguinal nerves, which innervate the muscles of the anterolateral abdominal wall [5, 6] (Figs. 7.2 and 7.3).
- **Internal oblique muscles (IOMs)**: The internal oblique muscle is positioned between the

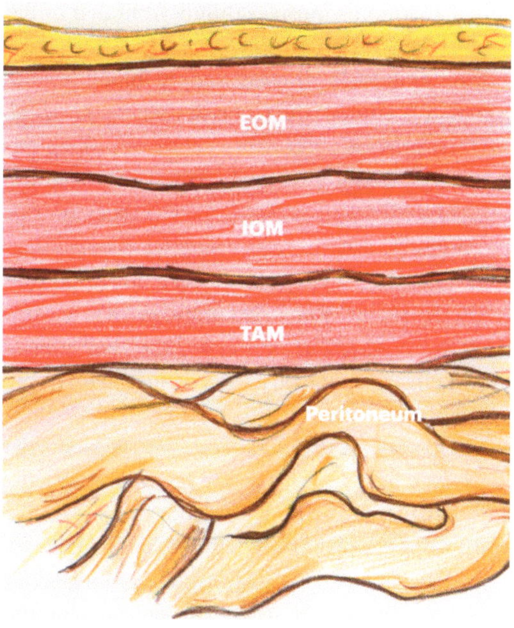

Fig. 7.2 Anatomical relationship between the lateral abdominal wall muscles. *EOM* external oblique muscle, *IOM* internal oblique muscle, *TAM* transversus abdominis muscle, *Peritoneum* peritoneum. (Courtesy of Dr. Giuseppe Sepolvere)

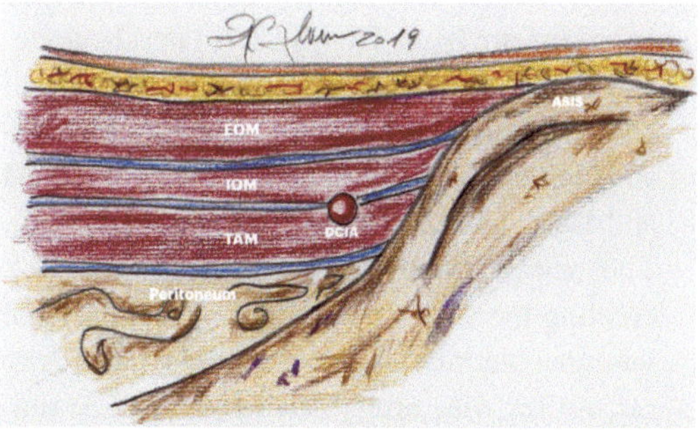

Fig. 7.3 Anatomical relationship of the lateral abdominal wall at the level of the anterior superior iliac spine. A branch of the iliohypogastric nerve pierces the internal oblique muscle. The anterior cutaneous branch of the iliohypogastric nerve, which travels within the thoracoabdominal plane, transitions to a location between the internal and external oblique muscles in proximity to the deep circumflex iliac artery around the level of the anterior superior iliac spine. *EOM* external oblique muscle, *IOM* internal oblique muscle, *TAM* transversus abdominis muscle, *DCIA* deep circumflex iliac artery, *ASIS* anterior superior iliac spine, *Peritoneum* peritoneum. (Courtesy of Dr. Giuseppe Sepolvere)

transversus abdominis muscle and the EOM. It lies ventral to the transversus abdominis muscle and dorsal to the EOM. Positioned beneath the external oblique, the internal oblique muscle runs in the opposite direction (diagonally downward and backward). It originates from the inguinal ligament, iliac crest, and thoracolumbar fascia and inserts into the linea alba and lower ribs [7]. The internal oblique muscle assists in trunk flexion, rotation, and lateral flexion, working in conjunction with the external oblique. Innervation of the IOM is provided by the ilioinguinal nerve, which typically perforates medially to accompany the spermatic cord through the inguinal canal in males or the round ligament of the uterus in females. Moreover, a branch of the iliohypogastric nerve also pierces the IOM. The anterior cutaneous branch of the iliohypogastric nerve, which travels within the thoracoabdominal plane (TAP), transitions to a location between the internal and external oblique muscles in proximity to the deep circumflex iliac artery (DCIA) around the level of the anterior superior iliac spine (ASIS) as it continues toward the rectus abdominis muscle. Moreover, the IOM and TAM work together to create tension in the thoracolumbar fascia. By contracting simultaneously, the IOM and TAM pull on the thoracolumbar fascia, generating tension that stabilizes the lumbosacral region [8] (Figs. 7.2 and 7.3). The fascial plane between the IOM and TAM is the anatomical target for the transversus abdominis plane block.

- **Transversus abdominis muscle (TAM)**: The deepest muscle layer of the anterolateral abdominal wall, the transversus abdominis runs horizontally across the abdomen. The TAM lies directly dorsal to the IOM and ventral to the transversalis fascia. It originates from the lower ribs, thoracolumbar fascia, and iliac crest and inserts into the linea alba and pubic crest. The transversus abdominis muscle primarily functions in compressing the abdominal contents and providing stability to the trunk. Nerves supplying the TAM arise from the ventral rami (anterior divisions) of the spinal nerves T6/7–L1. These spinal nerves originate from the thoracic and upper lumbar regions of the spinal cord. The nerves travel parallel to the vascular supply within the TAP, which is situated between the transversus abdominis muscle and the internal oblique muscle [9]. The TAM plays a significant functional role in the abdominal wall, particularly in conjunction with the IOM, contributing to the overall stability and support of the abdominal cavity. The TAM, along with the IOM, acts as a "corset" around the visceral sac, providing circumferential "hoop tension." This action helps maintain the integrity of the abdominal wall by compressing the abdominal contents and providing support to the organs within [10] (Fig. 7.2). The fascial plane between the IOM and TAM is the anatomical target for the transversus abdominis plane block. The fascial plane between the IOM and TAM including the DCIA at the level of ASIS represents the anatomical target of the ilioinguinal and iliohypogastric nerve block (Fig. 7.3).

- **Rectus abdominis muscle (RAM)**: This is a paired muscle that runs vertically along the midline of the abdomen. It is commonly known as the "six-pack" muscle due to its segmented appearance. The rectus abdominis muscle is responsible for flexing the lumbar spine and compressing the abdominal contents [11]. They flank the linea alba, a fibrous structure that runs down the midline of the abdomen, separating the right and left sides of the rectus abdominis muscles. The rectus abdominis muscles originate from the pubic crest, which is a bony ridge on the front of the pubic bone, and the pubic symphysis, which is a cartilaginous joint between the left and right pubic bones in the pelvis. The muscle fibers of the rectus abdominis course superiorly (upwards) and insert into the xiphoid process, which is a small cartilaginous extension at the lower end of the sternum (breastbone), as well as the anterior surface of the fifth to seventh costal cartilages [12]. The vascular supply to the rectus abdominis muscles differs from that of the anterolateral muscle group. In fact, the superior epigastric arteries supply blood to the upper portion of the rectus abdominis muscles. The superior epigastric arteries run along the anterior abdominal wall, originating from the internal thoracic artery [13]. The deep inferior epigastric arteries arise from the external iliac arteries and supply blood to the lower portion of the rectus abdominis muscles. An anastomotic connection between these two arterial systems is typically found just above the umbilical area. Each rectus abdominis is enclosed in a dense sheet of fascia called the rectus sheath. The anterior layer of the rectus sheath is formed by the aponeurosis of the EOM and the anterior half of the aponeurosis of the IOM. The posterior layer is formed by the posterior half of the aponeurosis of the IOM and the whole of the aponeurosis of the transversus abdominis. The anterior and posterior layers of the rectus sheath on both sides meet in the midline in the linea alba [14].

- The thoracoabdominal nerves derive from the anterior rami from T6 to T12. A lateral cutaneous branch covers the lateral abdominal wall and anteriorly the nerves run in the transversus abdominis plane (TAP) between the IOM and TAM with the L1 anterior ramus (Fig. 7.4). The nerves freely communicate in the TAP creating the "intercostal plexus." A significant vascular landmark is represented by the deep circumflex iliac artery (DCIA) (Fig. 7.3) running into the fascial plane between the IOM and TAM where T9 to T1 form a TAP plexus and the rectus sheath plexus alongside the deep inferior epigastric artery [15, 16] (Fig. 7.9).

Additionally, it blends with the iliac fascia as it contributes to forming the anterior layer of the femoral sheath [17].

The plane between the body of the rectus abdominis muscle and its posterior sheath is the anatomical target of the rectus abdominis sheath block. The anatomical relationship between the EOM, IOM, TAM, and RAM is described also in Figs. 7.5 and 7.6.

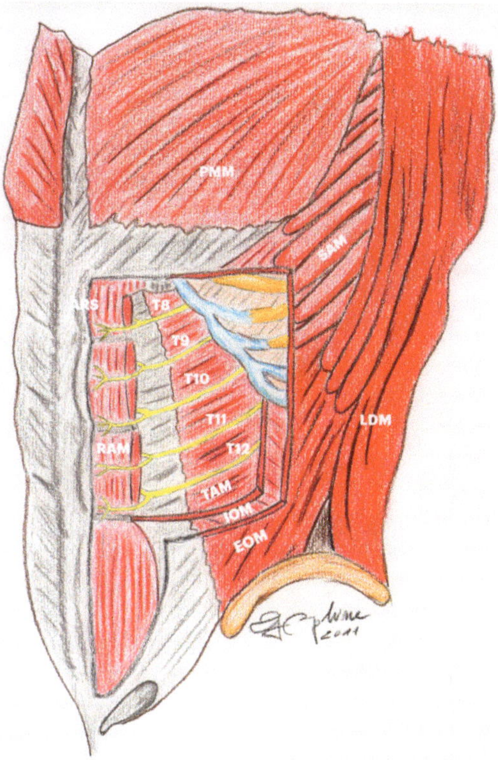

Fig. 7.4 Anterolateral abdominal relationship between the external oblique, internal oblique, and transversus abdominis muscles. Anteriorly, the nerves lie in the transversus abdominal plane between internal oblique and transversus abdominis muscles. The nerves freely communicate in the transversus abdominal plane constituting the "intercostal plexus." *EOM* external oblique muscle, *IOM* internal oblique muscle, *TAM* transversus abdominis muscle, *RAM* rectus abdominis muscle, *LDM* latissimus dorsi muscle, *SAM* serratus anterior muscle, *PMM* pectoralis major muscle, *ARS* anterior rectus abdominis sheath. (Courtesy of Dr. Giuseppe Sepolvere)

7.2.2 Posterior Abdominal Wall Muscles

The muscles of the posterior abdominal wall, such as the psoas major, quadratus lumborum, and iliacus, have functional connections with the lower limb and vertebral column. These muscles play crucial roles in both locomotion and providing support and protection for the retroperitoneal structures. Their anatomical arrangement and functional relationships with adjacent structures highlight their importance in maintaining the stability and functionality of the lower limb, vertebral column, and retroperitoneal space [18].

The posterior abdominal wall muscles are as follows:

- **Quadratus lumborum muscle (QLM)**: The quadratus lumborum muscle is a key structure in the posterior abdominal wall, with various attachments, relations, vascular supply, innervation, and actions. Inferiorly, it attaches to the iliolumbar ligament and the adjacent portion of the iliac crest. Superiorly, it attaches to the medial half of the lower border of the 12th rib and, by small tendons, to the apices of the transverse processes of the upper four lumbar vertebrae. Occasionally, a second layer of the muscle may be found in front of the first, with attachments to the upper borders of the transverse processes of the lower three or four lumbar vertebrae and the lower margin and lower part of the anterior surface of the 12th rib.

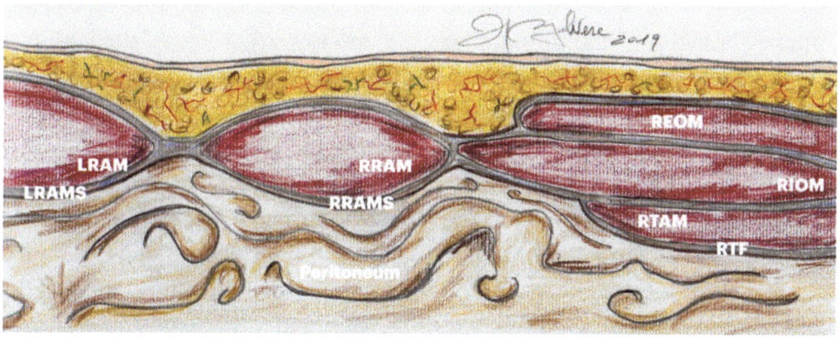

Fig. 7.5 Anatomical relationship between rectus abdominis, external oblique, internal oblique, transversus abdominis muscles, fascia transversalis, and peritoneum. *RRAM* right rectus abdominis muscle, *RRAMS* right rectus abdominis muscle sheath, *REOM* right external oblique muscle, *RIOM* right internal oblique muscle, *RTAM* right transversus abdominis muscle, *RTF* right transversalis fascia, *LRAM* left rectus abdominis muscle, *LRAMS* left rectus abdominis muscle sheath, *Peritoneum* peritoneum. (Courtesy of Dr. Giuseppe Sepolvere)

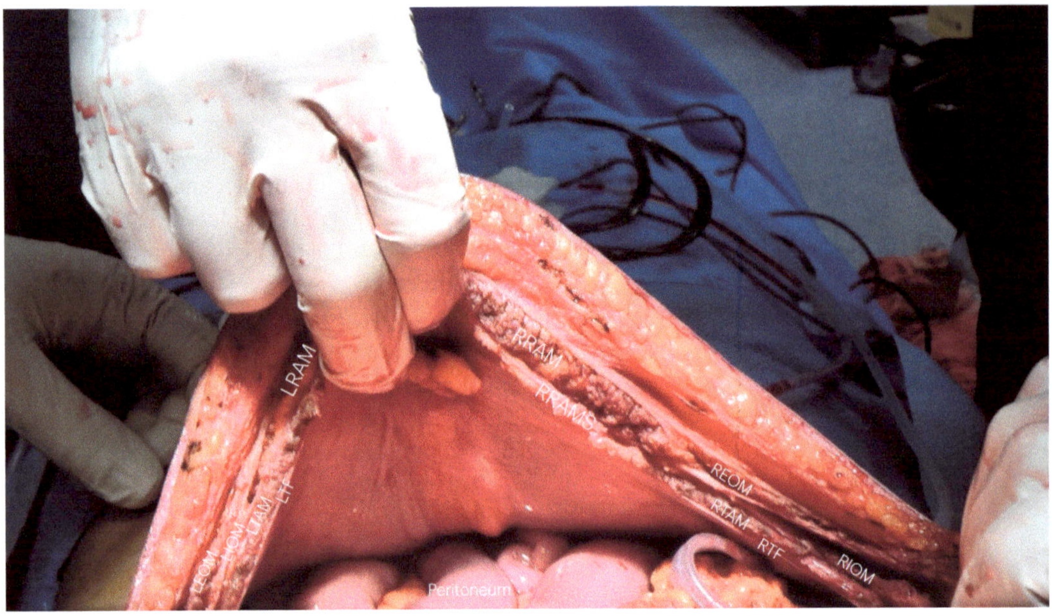

Fig. 7.6 Anatomical relationship between rectus abdominis, external oblique, internal oblique, transversus abdominis muscles, fascia transversalis, and peritoneum. It is shown the hydrodissection between the left internal oblique and left transversus abdominis muscles after the transversus abdominis plane block. *RRAM* right rectus abdominis muscle, *RRAMS* right rectus abdominis muscle sheath, *REOM* right external oblique muscle, *RIOM* right internal oblique muscle, *RTAM* right transversus abdominis muscle, *RTF* right transversalis fascia, *LRAM* left rectus abdominis muscle, *LRAMS* left rectus abdominis muscle sheath, *LEOM* left external oblique muscle, *LIOM* left internal oblique muscle, *LTAM* left transversus abdominis muscle, *LTF* left transversalis fascia, *Peritoneum* peritoneum. (Courtesy of Dr. Giuseppe Sepolvere)

Anteriorly, it is related to structures such as the colon, kidneys, psoas major and minor, and diaphragm. Nerves like the subcostal, iliohypogastric, and ilioinguinal nerves lie on the fascia anterior to the muscle, bound down to it by the medial continuation of the transversalis fascia [19]. The QLM is supplied by branches of the lumbar arteries, including the arteria lumbalis, lumbar branch of the iliolumbar artery, and branches of the subcostal artery. Innervation is provided by the ventral rami of the 12th thoracic and upper three or four lumbar spinal nerves. The QLM helps fix the last rib and stabilize the lower attachments of the diaphragm, contributing to inspiration. It may provide a fixed base for controlled relaxation of the diaphragm, aiding in precise adjustment of expiration needed for speech and singing. With the pelvis fixed, it acts upon the vertebral column, flexing it to the same side. When both muscles contract, they likely help to extend the lumbar part of the vertebral column (Fig. 7.1). The anterior and posterior surface of QLM is the anatomical target of the QLB I and QLB II blocks, respectively. The fascial plane between the QLM and the psoas muscle represents the anatomical target of QLB III.

- **Psoas major (PM)**: The psoas major muscle is attached to the transverse processes, upper and lower borders of the bodies of the lumbar vertebrae, and adjacent intervertebral discs. Its attachments form a series of fibrous arches related to the middle of the vertebral bodies. The muscle passes downward to the pelvic brim, then sweeps around its outer edge, and enters the thigh behind the inguinal ligament. Its tendon lies in front of the capsule of the hip joint and is separated from it by a bursa. The tendon is attached to the lesser trochanter of the femur [20]. The psoas major muscle has important relationships with surrounding structures, including the kidneys with their blood vessels and ureter anteriorly. It also interacts with branches of the lumbar plexus, some of which are lateral and some medial. Additionally, the inferior vena cava (on the right) and abdominal aorta (on the left) are located medially relative to the muscle. The nerve supply to the psoas major muscle comes from the ventral rami of the first three lumbar nerves. The primary action of the psoas major muscle, in conjunction with the iliacus, is to flex the thigh at the hip joint or to flex the trunk on the thigh, particularly evident in the supine position [21] (Fig. 7.1). The fascial plane between the PM and QLM represents the anatomical target of QLB III.

- **Erector spinae muscle (ESM)**: The erector spinae (ES) muscle is a key component of the back's muscular structure, playing a crucial role in maintaining posture and enabling various movements of the spine. The ES originates from the erector spinae aponeurosis (ESA), which blends with the thoracolumbar fascia. The proximal attachment is on the sacrum and the spinous processes of the lumbar vertebrae. The muscle fibers of the ES run vertically along the spine and insert onto various points along the ribs, vertebrae, and base of the skull [22].

- The ES is composed of three main muscles, each contributing to its overall function: the iliocostalis muscle (most lateral, which is involved in extending and laterally flexing the spine); the longissimus muscle (intermediate column, involved in extending the spine and in its lateral flexion); and the spinalis (most medial, involved in extending the vertebral column).

- The ES is covered by the thoracolumbar fascia, rhomboids, and trapezius muscle (Fig. 7.7).

- The fascial plane between the ES and the transverse process represents the anatomical target of ES plane block [23]: the LA injected into this fascial plane can spread through channels in the intertransverse connective tissues, reaching the ventral and dorsal ramus of the thoracic spinal nerve along with the sympathetic ramus communicans at the intervertebral foramen level [24] (Fig. 7.8).

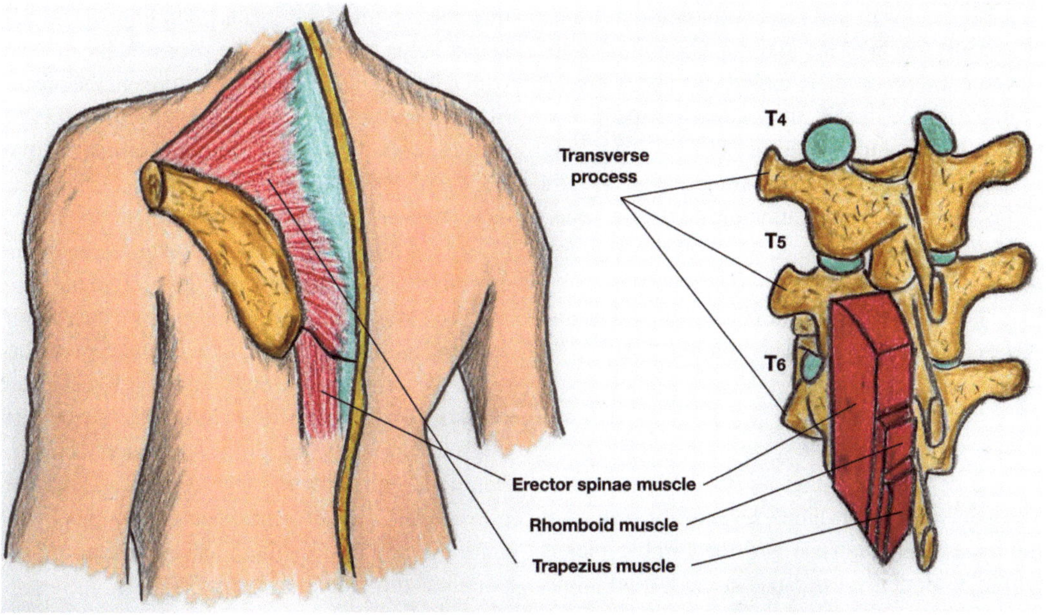

Fig. 7.7 Schematic illustration of the anatomical relationships between the transverse processes, erector spinae, rhomboid, and trapezius muscles. (Courtesy of Dr. Giuseppe Sepolvere)

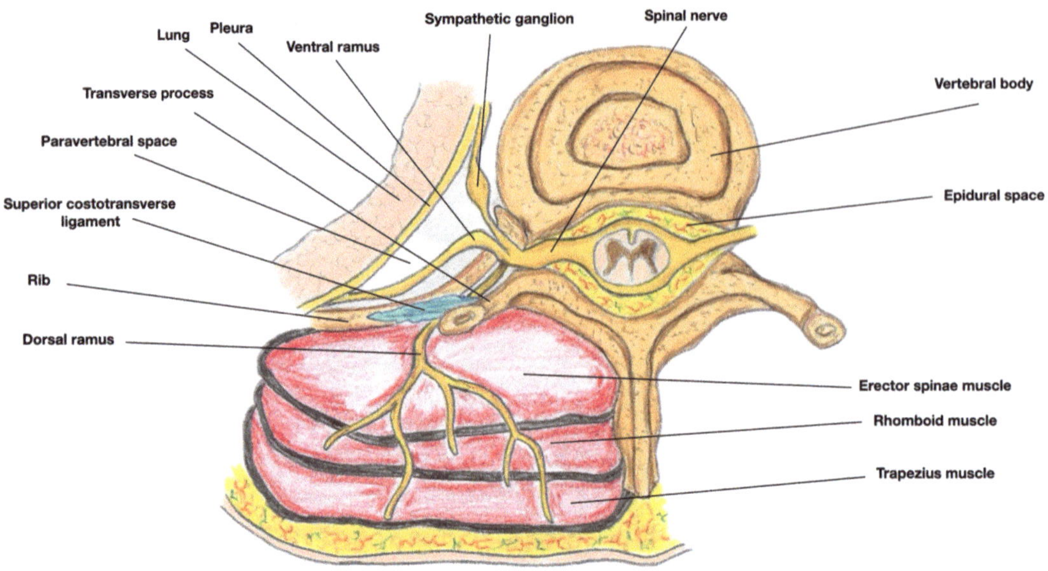

Fig. 7.8 Anatomical relationship between the erector spinae muscle, the transverse process, the superior costotransverse ligament, and the paravertebral space. (Courtesy of Dr. Giuseppe Sepolvere)

7.3 Fascial Layers

There are two fascial layers in the posterior abdominal wall and one endoabdominal [1]:

- A layer of fascia lies between the parietal peritoneum and the muscles of the posterior abdominal wall and is a continuation of transversalis fascia of the anterior abdominal wall. Over the psoas, it is called the psoas fascia, and over the iliacus, the fascia iliaca.
- The thoracolumbar fascia (TLF) is a girdling structure consisting of several aponeurotic and fascial layers that separate the paraspinal muscles from the muscles of the posterior abdominal wall.
- The transversalis fascia is an endoabdominal fascia lining the entire abdominal cavity.

7.3.1 Psoas Fascia

The psoas fascia surrounds the anterior surface of the psoas major muscle and the lumbar plexus within it. Medially, the psoas fascia is continuous with the attachments of the psoas major muscle to the transverse processes and bodies of the lumbar vertebrae. This continuity helps maintain the structural integrity of the muscle and provides attachment points for its fibers. Laterally, the psoas fascia blends with the fascia that covers the quadratus lumborum muscle superiorly and the iliac fascia inferiorly. This blending of fascial layers helps to integrate the psoas major muscle with adjacent muscles and structures in the posterior abdominal wall. Superiorly, the psoas fascia merges with the medial arcuate ligament of the respiratory diaphragm, further anchoring the psoas major muscle and contributing to the integrity of the diaphragm. Inferiorly, the psoas fascia extends into the thigh as a sheath around the iliopsoas tendon, which is formed by the psoas major and iliacus muscles. This extension helps maintain the structural continuity between the posterior abdominal wall and the structures of the thigh. Importantly, the psoas fascia acts as a barrier, dividing the psoas major muscle and lumbar plexus from the retroperitoneal organs. This separation helps protect these structures and maintain their functional integrity [25].

7.3.2 Iliac Fascia

The iliac fascia covers the anterior surface of the iliacus muscle. Superiorly and laterally, the iliac fascia attaches to the inner margin of the iliac crest. This attachment provides stability and support to the fascia [25]. Medially, it blends with the anterior layer of the thoracolumbar fascia over the quadratus lumborum muscle and contributes to the structural integrity of the abdominal wall. Additionally, the iliac fascia blends with the psoas fascia, further integrating the fascial layers of the posterior abdominal wall. At its medial border, the iliac fascia attaches to the periosteum of the ilium and the iliopubic eminence near the linea terminalis. These attachments help anchor the fascia in place and provide structural support. Inferiorly and laterally, the iliac fascia extends into the thigh. Here, it fuses with the femoral sheath, which surrounds structures passing through the femoral triangle. This extension helps maintain continuity between the fascial structures of the pelvis and thigh. Both the femoral nerve and the lateral femoral cutaneous nerve pass beneath the iliac fascia in the pelvis.

7.3.3 The Thoracolumbar Fascia

The thoracolumbar fascia (TLF) is a complex structure and plays a crucial role in providing support and stability to the lumbar spine and surrounding musculature. The TLF is a complex of several layers that separates the paraspinal muscles from the muscles of the posterior abdominal wall, quadratus lumborum (QLM), and psoas major (PM). Several anatomists have described the TLF in various ways, leading to two main models: the two-layered model and the three-layered model [26–28] (Fig. 7.1).

In the two-layered model, the TLF is described as having two layers:

- Superficial layer: This layer is located closer to the skin surface and is continuous with the fascia of the latissimus dorsi and the external oblique muscles.
- Deep layer: This layer lies deeper and is in direct contact with the paraspinal muscles, including the erector spinae group.

In contrast, the three-layered model divides the TLF into three distinct layers:

- Superficial layer: Similar to the two-layered model, this layer is continuous with the fascia of the latissimus dorsi and external oblique muscles.
- Middle layer: This layer is situated between the superficial and deep layers. It may vary in thickness and composition among individuals.
- Deep layer: Also akin to the two-layered model, this layer is in direct contact with the paraspinal muscles.

The anterior part of the TLF (or the middle part in a three-layered model) is attached to the transverse processes of the lumbar vertebrae, forming an intramuscular septum that separates paraspinal/epaxial muscles and hypaxial muscles in the posterior aspect of the abdominal wall, particularly the QL and PM muscles [29, 30].

7.3.4 The Transversalis Fascia

The transversalis fascia is a segment of the endoabdominal fascia lining the entire abdominal cavity. It contributes to forming the posterior wall of the rectus sheath and contains the deep inguinal ring, which is located midway between the anterior superior iliac spine and the symphysis pubis [31] (Figs. 7.1 and 7.9).

Positioned between the transverse abdominis muscle and the extraperitoneal fat, the transversalis fascia extends inferiorly to merge with the iliac and pelvic fascia and superiorly to blend with the fascia on the inferior surface of the diaphragm. While it is typically a thin layer on the

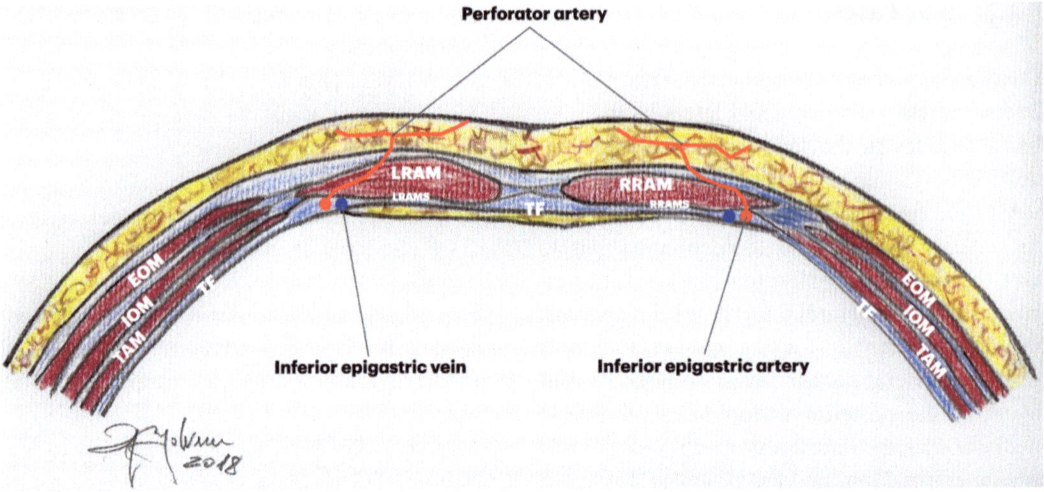

Fig. 7.9 The transversalis fascia and its anatomical relationship with the inferior epigastric artery, the perforator artery, the rectus abdominis, and the transversus abdominis muscles. The transversalis fascia is a segment of the endoabdominal fascia lining the entire abdominal cavity. It contributes to forming the posterior wall of the rectus sheath. *EOM* external oblique muscle, *IOM* internal oblique muscle, *TAM* transversus abdominis muscle, *TF* transversalis fascia, *RRAM* right rectus abdominis muscle, *RRAMS* right rectus abdominis muscle sheath, *LRAM* left rectus abdominis muscle, *LRAMS* left rectus abdominis muscle sheath. (Courtesy of Dr. Giuseppe Sepolvere)

inferior surface of the diaphragm, it thickens somewhat in the inguinal region. In the posterior abdominal wall, the transversalis fascia joins the anterior layer of the thoracolumbar fascia. It attaches to the iliac crest and the posterior margin of the inguinal ligament, as well as to the conjoint tendon and the pecten pubis. Extending around the spermatic cord in males, the transversalis fascia forms the internal spermatic fascia, which eventually merges with the parietal layer of the tunica vaginalis [17].

References

1. Chin KJ, McDonnell JG, Carvalho B, Sharkey A, Pawa A, Gadsden J. Essentials of our current understanding: abdominal wall blocks. Reg Anesth Pain Med. 2017;42(2):133–83. https://doi.org/10.1097/AAP.0000000000000545. PMID: 28085788.
2. Seeras K, Qasawa RN, Ju R, Prakash S. Anatomy, abdomen and pelvis: anterolateral abdominal wall. In: StatPearls [Internet]. Treasure Island (FL): StatPearls Publishing; 2023.
3. Schlenz I, Burggasser G, Kuzbari R, Eichberger H, Gruber H, Holle J. External oblique abdominal muscle; a new look on its blood supply and innervation. Anat Rec. 1999;255:388–95.
4. Kuzbari R, Worseg A, Burggasser G, Schlenz I, Kuderna C, Vinzenz K, Gruber H, Holle J. The external oblique muscle free flap. Plast Reconstr Surg. 1997;99:1338–45.
5. Nahas FX. Advancement of the external oblique muscle flap to improve the waistline: a study in cadavers. Plast Reconstr Surg. 2001;108(2):550–5. https://doi.org/10.1097/00006534-200108000-00043. PMID: 11496205.
6. Fan C, Fede C, Gaudreault N, Porzionato A, Macchi V, De Caro R, Stecco C. Anatomical and functional relationships between external abdominal oblique muscle and posterior layer of thoracolumbar fascia. Clin Anat. 2018;31(7):1092–8. https://doi.org/10.1002/ca.23248. Epub 2018 Oct 26. PMID: 30113090.
7. Adams L, Pace N, Heo A, Hunter I, Johnson AW, Mitchell UH. Internal and external oblique muscle asymmetry in sprint hurdlers and sprinters: a cross-sectional study. J Sports Sci Med. 2022;21(1):120–6. https://doi.org/10.52082/jssm.2022.120. PMID: 35250341; PMCID: PMC8851117.
8. Madaen K, Niknafs B. A new anatomical and surgical landmark in internal abdominal oblique muscle: fat triangle. Urol J. 2012;9(1):420–2.
9. Morris SL, Lay B, Allison GT. Transversus abdominis is part of a global not local muscle synergy during arm movement. Hum Mov Sci. 2013;32(5):1176–85. https://doi.org/10.1016/j.humov.2012.12.011. Epub 2013 Mar 5.
10. De Troyer A, Estenne M, Ninane V, Van Gansbeke D, Gorini M. Transversus abdominis muscle function in humans. J Appl Physiol (1985). 1990;68(3):1010–6.

https://doi.org/10.1152/jappl.1990.68.3.1010. PMID: 2140344.
11. Tran D, Mitton D, Voirin D, Turquier F, Beillas P. Contribution of the skin, rectus abdominis and their sheaths to the structural response of the abdominal wall ex vivo. J Biomech. 2014;47(12):3056–63.
12. Johnson TG, Von SJ, Hope WW. Clinical anatomy of the abdominal wall: hernia surgery. OA Anat. 2014;2(1):3.
13. Rizk NN. The arcuate line of the rectus sheath—does it exist? J Anat. 1991;175:1–6.
14. Miyauchi T, Ishikawa M, Miki H. Rectus sheath hematoma in an elderly woman under anti-coagulant therapy. J Med Investig. 2001;48:216–20.
15. Stecco C, Azzena GP, Macchi V, Porzionato A, Behr A, Rambaldo A, Tiengo C, De Caro R. Rectus abdominis muscle innervation: an anatomical study with surgical implications in diep flap harvesting. Surg Radiol Anat. 2018;40(8):865–72. https://doi.org/10.1007/s00276-017-1944-6. Epub 2017 Nov 10.
16. Rozen WM, Tran TM, Ashton MW, Barrington MJ, Ivanusic JJ, Taylor GI. Refining the course of the thoracolumbar nerves: a new understanding of the innervation of the anterior abdominal wall. Clin Anat. 2008;21(4):325–33. https://doi.org/10.1002/ca.20621.
17. Memon MA, Quinn TH, Cahill DR. Transversalis fascia: historical aspects and its place in contemporary inguinal herniorrhaphy. J Laparoendosc Adv Surg Tech A. 1999;9:267–72.
18. Sevensma KE, Leavitt L, Pihl KD. Anatomy, abdomen and pelvis, rectus sheath. In: StatPearls [Internet]. Treasure Island (FL): StatPearls Publishing; 2023.
19. Phillips S, Mercer S, Bogduk N. Anatomy and biomechanics of quadratus lumborum. Proc Inst Mech Eng Part H J Eng Med. 2008;222(2):151–9. https://doi.org/10.1243/09544119JEIM266.
20. Siccardi MA, Tariq MA, Valle C. Anatomy, bony pelvis and lower limb: psoas major. In: StatPearls [Internet]. Treasure Island (FL): StatPearls Publishing; 2024.
21. Sajko S, Stuber K. Psoas major: a case report and review of its anatomy, biomechanics, and clinical implications. J Can Chiropr Assoc. 2009;53(4):311–8.
22. Bonvicini D, Boscolo-Berto R, De Cassai A, Negrello M, Macchi V, Tiberio I, Boscolo A, De Caro R, Porzionato A. Anatomical basis of erector spinae plane block: a dissection and histotopographic pilot study. J Anesth. 2021;35(1):102–11. https://doi.org/10.1007/s00540-020-02881-w. Epub 2020 Dec 19. PMID: 33340344; PMCID: PMC7840626.
23. Chin KJ, El-Boghdadly K. Mechanisms of action of the erector spinae plane (ESP) block: a narrative review. Can J Anesth J Can Anesth. 2021;68:387–408. https://doi.org/10.1007/s12630-020-01875-2.
24. Capuano P, Hileman BA, Martucci G, Raffa GM, Toscano A, Burgio G, Arcadipane A, Kowalewski M. Erector spinae plane block versus paravertebral block for postoperative pain management in thoracic surgery: a systematic review and meta-analysis. Minerva Anestesiol. 2023;89(11):1042–50. https://doi.org/10.23736/S0375-9393.23.17510-9. Epub 2023 Sep 5.
25. Standring S. Gray's anatomy. Amsterdam: Elsevier; 2016.
26. Willard FH, Vleeming A, Schuenke MD, Danneels L, Schleip R. The thoracolumbar fascia: anatomy, function and clinical considerations. J Anat. 2012;221(6):507–36. https://doi.org/10.1111/j.1469--7580.2012.01511.x. Epub 2012 May 27. PMID: 22630613; PMCID: PMC3512278.
27. Macintosh JE, Bogduk N. The morphology of the lumbar erector spinae. Spine. 1987;12:658–68.
28. Macintosh JE, Bogduk N, Gracovetsky S. The biomechanics of the thoracolumbar fascia. Clin Biomech. 1987;2:78–83.
29. Gallaudet BB. A description of the planes of fascia of the human body: with special reference of the fascia of the abdomen, pelvis and perineum. New York: Columbia University Press; 1931. p. 1–32.
30. Børglum J, Hansen CK, Tanggaard KB. Quadratus lumborum block. In: Jankovic D, Peng P, editors. Regional nerve blocks in anesthesia and pain therapy. Cham: Springer; 2022. https://doi.org/10.1007/978-3-030-88727-8_33.
31. Bendavid R, Howarth D. Transversalis fascia rediscovered. Surg Clin N Am. 2000;80:25–33.

Anterior and Posterior Chest Wall Blocks

8

Giuseppe Sepolvere and Rafael Blanco

8.1 Introduction

Fascial plane blocks indeed represent a significant advancement in regional anesthesia techniques. Blanco et al.'s pioneering work, particularly in breast surgery analgesia, laid the foundation for the broader application of these blocks across various surgical fields. The concept of targeting specific fascial planes to deliver local anesthetics has shown great promise due to its effectiveness and safety [1–3]. The versatility of fascial plane blocks has led to their adoption in diverse surgical procedures beyond breast surgery. In cardiac, thoracic, and chest wall surgeries, where effective pain management is crucial for patient recovery, these techniques offer notable advantages [4–6]. By targeting the nerves within the relevant fascial planes, clinicians can provide targeted analgesia, potentially reducing the need for systemic opioids and their associated side effects. Furthermore, the relatively straightforward execution of fascial plane blocks adds to their appeal, especially in settings where rapid and effective pain relief is paramount. Their safety profile, when performed by trained practitioners using appropriate techniques and under ultrasound guidance, further enhances their attractiveness as a component of multimodal analgesia strategies. As with any medical advancement, ongoing research and refinement of techniques will likely continue to enhance the efficacy and scope of fascial plane blocks, potentially leading to even broader applications and improved patient outcomes across various surgical disciplines. These procedures involve the administration of local anesthetic into the anatomical space between two fascial layers through which nervous structures travel, achieving a conduction blockade of both sensory afferents and peripheral nociceptors in the surrounding tissue. Fascia, a connective tissue sheet that encloses and separates muscles while also housing nerves and vessels, plays a crucial role in these interventions. The planes between various muscle layers in the thorax, abdomen, and paraspinal regions, particularly near the thoracic paravertebral space and vertebral canal, are commonly targeted for ultrasound-guided local anesthetic injections [7, 8]. Stecco et al. demonstrated the presence of free nerve endings, corpuscles, and autonomic nerve fibers within the deep fascia, suggesting a comprehensive "fascial system" that plays a vital role in regulating force transmission, sensory functions, wound healing, dynamic proprioception, and pain control. This underscores the potential for the deep fascia to serve as a novel target for fascial block interventions. Current evidence regarding the clinical applications, effectiveness,

G. Sepolvere (✉)
Department of Anesthesia and Cardiac Surgery
Intensive Care Unit, San Michele Hospital,
Maddaloni, Caserta, Italy

R. Blanco
Corniche Hospital, Abu Dhabi, UAE

G. Sepolvere, S. Silvetti (eds.), *Fast-Track in Cardiac Anesthesia*,
https://doi.org/10.1007/978-3-031-70899-2_8

and safety of chest wall blocks indicates significant benefits akin to thoracic paravertebral blocks, not only in breast surgery but also in thoracic procedures. This expanding role extends to trauma, emergency, and routine cardiac surgeries, promising substantial advancements. Traditionally, cardiac surgery has relied heavily on high doses of opioids, leading to various adverse effects such as nausea, vomiting, ileus, sedation, respiratory depression, delayed extubation, pulmonary complications, and prolonged intensive care unit (ICU) stays. However, evolving practices, driven by concepts like Enhanced Recovery After Surgery (ERAS) and fast-tracking, seek to achieve rapid, high-quality recovery by leveraging regional anesthesia techniques and multimodal opioid-sparing or opioid-free protocols. In alignment with ERAS principles, Enhanced Recovery After Cardiac Surgery (ERACS) has emerged as a multidisciplinary treatment approach, aiming to optimize outcomes in cardiac surgery [9, 10]. While cardiac surgery pain typically diminishes within 24 h postoperatively, it remains classified as severe acute postoperative pain. Failure to adequately address it can lead to serious complications. Minimally invasive cardiac surgery techniques, such as minithoracotomy for procedures like coronary artery bypass grafting (CABG) or valve surgery, have been developed to mitigate pain and reduce physiological deterioration and complications associated with extensive surgical wounds. Consequently, immediate or early extubation serves as a key anesthetic goal in fast-track cardiac surgery approaches and ERAS/ERACS protocols [11–14]. The anterior and posterior chest wall blocks have emerged as safe and effective alternatives to conventional regional techniques like paravertebral, epidural, and spinal blocks. By injecting local anesthetic into a fascial plane between two muscles, through which the nerves travel, the needle tip remains distant from neuraxial structures, thus minimizing hemodynamic impact, risk of direct neural injuries, and complications such as neuraxial hematoma and bleeding, particularly in patients receiving high doses of heparin for cardiopulmonary bypass [15–20].

Table 8.1 The new nomenclature of chest wall blocks standardized by ASRA/ESRA consensus based on the anatomical target and injection identification

Fascial block ASRA/ ESRA	Nomenclature
PECS I	Interpectoral plane block
PECS II	Pectoserratus plane block
Serratus plane block	Superficial serratus anterior plane block Deep serratus anterior plane block
Parasternal block	Superficial parasternal intercostal plane block Deep parasternal intercostal plane block
Paravertebral block	Paravertebral block
Erector spinae block	Erector spinae block—ESP block

8.2 Nomenclature

In a recent international study conducted by expert consensus from the American Society of Regional Anesthesia (ASRA) Pain Medicine and the European Society of Regional Anaesthesia and Pain Therapy (ESRA), a standardized nomenclature for abdominal, paraspinal, and chest wall anesthetic techniques was established. This nomenclature is primarily based on anatomical targets and injection identification (refer to Table 8.1). In a gesture of respect towards the author, Dr. Rafael Blanco, who initially published studies on these procedures, the original nomenclatures are provided in brackets alongside the new ones [15, 21–23].

8.3 The Double V Sign and Dynamic Fascial Blocks

In Chap. 3, as previously outlined, the significance of fascia has gained widespread acknowledgment. Myofascial planes are now understood as intricate systems and distinct compartments capable of linking anatomical elements such as muscles, vessels, and nerves while also playing a pivotal role in pain perception. Despite the utilization of ultrasound, anesthesiologists may encounter challenges in achieving successful blocks, as perifascial injections can mimic cor-

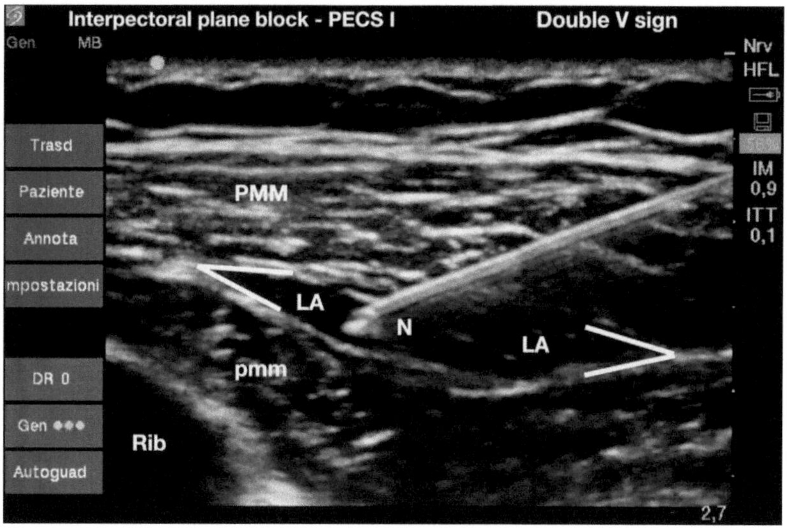

Fig. 8.1 Interpectoral plane (PECS I) block and the double V sign. If the injection is performed correctly, the local anesthetic will spread symmetrically, opening the interfascial plane and separating the two fascial compartments bilaterally, resulting in the ultrasound sign known as the double V. *PMM* pectoralis major muscle, *pmm* pectoralis minor muscle, *Rib* rib, *N* needle, *LA* local anesthetic

rect procedural execution, leading to failures. In 2019, Fusco et al. introduced the ultrasound double V sign as a means to confirm the accurate administration of a fascial block [24]. If the injection is performed correctly, the local anesthetic (LA) will spread symmetrically, opening the interfascial plane and separating the two fascial compartments bilaterally, resulting in the ultrasound sign known as the double V (see Fig. 8.1). It is important to note that the interfascial nervous target is not visible on ultrasound, necessitating higher volumes of local anesthetic for fascial blocks compared to perineural blocks, where the nervous structure is detectable. These bands serve as anatomical pathways along which the LA can "travel." When injected correctly within the fascial compartment, it can spread beyond the injection site, extending the block across multiple dermatomes. Numerous factors can impact the dispersion of LA within the fascial planes, consequently influencing the efficacy of resulting analgesia. Anatomical studies on fascia have suggested that the biomechanical properties of deep fascial planes could impede the migration of LA, halting its diffusion along the fascial compartment and nervous structures [25]. Building upon this premise, some authors have postulated that executing a dynamic block, by gradually advancing the needle within the fascial planes, may induce a stretching of the fascia. This stretching, in turn, could facilitate the active transport of LA via a pumping mechanism, supplementing its passive movement along planes of lower resistance [26, 27]. The concentration of analgesic local anesthetic varies between 0.125 and 0.25%, while the anesthetic concentration ranges from 0.375 to 0.5%. Table 8.2 summarized the parasternal intercostal plane block indications.

Table 8.2 Parasternal intercostal plane block indications

Parasternal intercostal plane block indications
• Median sternotomy
• Sternal fractures
• Subcutaneous implantable cardioverter defibrillator (S-ICD) implantation
• Internal mammary region pain after artery harvesting
• Quadrantectomies
• Tumorectomies of the medial region of the breast
• Radical mastectomies in association with PECS II and SAPB

8.4 Anterior Chest Wall Blocks

Anterior chest wall blocks encompass the anteromedial and anterolateral thoracic wall, while posterior blocks target the posterior thoracic wall, and they are widely utilized across various surgical fields including general surgery, orthopedic surgery, emergency medicine, thoracic and cardiac surgery, pain medicine, cardiology, oncology, and nephrology [28].

The anterior chest wall blocks include:

- Parasternal block or parasternal intercostal plane (PIP) block
- Interpectoral plane (IPP) block (PECS I) and interpectoral + pectoserratus plane (PSP) block (PECS II)
- Serratus anterior plane block (SAPB)

8.4.1 Parasternal Block: Parasternal Intercostal Plane (PIP) Block

The PIP block targets the anterior cutaneous branches from T2–T6 intercostal nerves, innervating the anteromedial chest wall and penetrating the intercostal (IM) and pectoralis major muscles (PMM). The procedure involves superficial and deep PIP blocks, depending on whether the injection is above or below the IM. Bilateral injection is necessary for complete sternal area coverage due to nervous overlap. PIP block provides analgesia and anesthesia for various procedures, including median sternotomy, sternal fractures, subcutaneous implantable cardioverter defibrillator (S-ICD) implantation, and internal mammary region interventions [22, 29–32]. Further indications include quadrantectomy and tumorectomy of the medial breast region, often in combination with PECS I, PECS II, and SAPB blocks.

8.4.2 Superficial Parasternal Intercostal Plane Block

This was first introduced by Torre et al. in 2014 as the "pecto-intercostal fascial plane block" and later redefined by Fusco et al. in 2017 as an analgesic technique for breast surgery's medial region [33, 34]. Combined with interfascial blocks such as PECS I, PECS II, and SAPB, it ensures analgesia of the entire anterior chest wall and mammary gland. Patient and probe positioning, as well as the approach and needle insertion, remain consistent for both superficial and deep blocks. The patient lies supine with arms extended alongside the body and head in a neutral position. A high-frequency linear probe is positioned approximately 2 cm parallel and lateral to the sternum's border, first at the second and then at the fourth intercostal space level. The needle is inserted using the in-plane (IP) approach in a cranial-to-caudal or caudal-to-cranial direction (Fig. 8.2). Ultrasound landmarks include the PMM and external intercostal muscle (EIM), visualization of ribs and their posterior shadow cones, and pleura sliding (Fig. 8.3). 5–10 mL of local anesthetic is injected into the fascial plane between the PMM and EIM at the second and fourth intercostal spaces (Fig. 8.4). Sepolvere et al. [35] suggested a modified

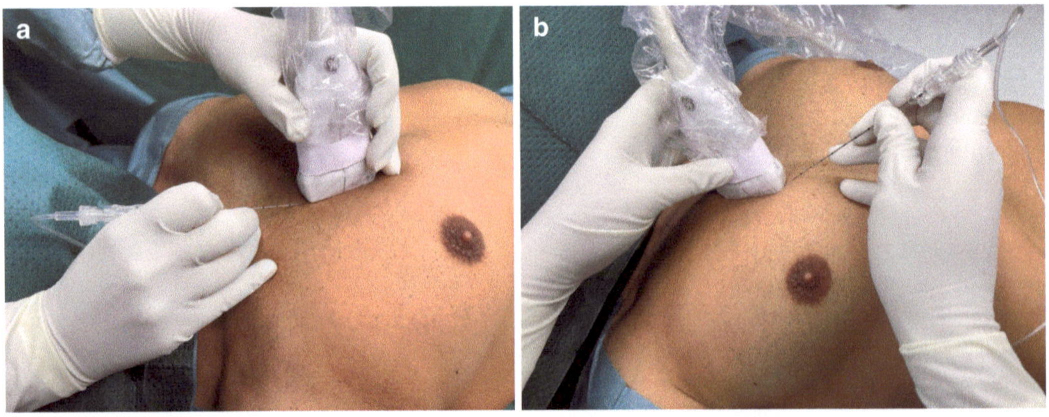

Fig. 8.2 Superficial and deep parasternal block. Patient and probe position. (**a**) The needle is inserted with the in-plane approach in a cranial-to-caudal direction. (**b**) The needle could also be inserted in a caudal-to-cranial direction

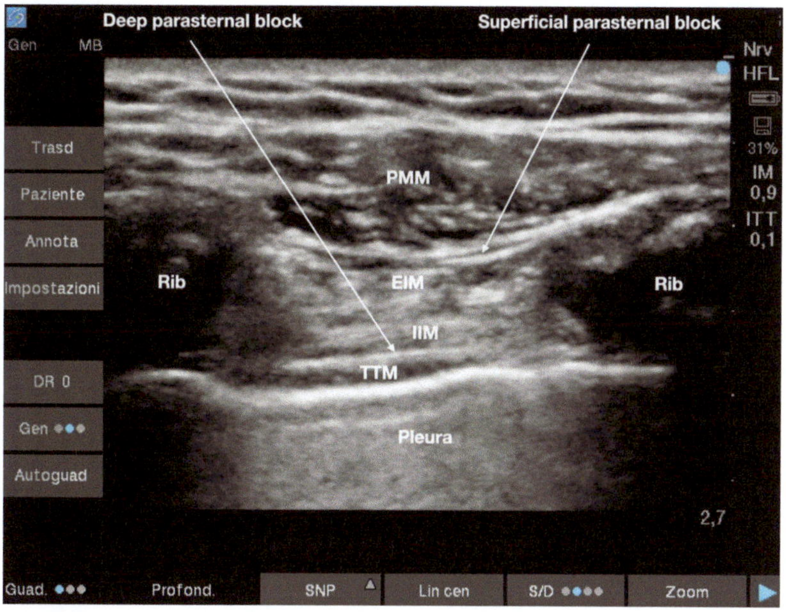

Fig. 8.3 Ultrasound landmarks and target of superficial and deep parasternal block. From top to bottom: pectoralis major muscle, external intercostal muscle, internal intercostal muscle, transversus thoracis muscle, pleura, ribs laterally. *PMM* pectoralis major muscle, *EIM* external intercostal muscle, *IIM* internal intercostal muscle, *TTM* transversus thoracis muscle, *Pleura* pleura, *Rib* rib

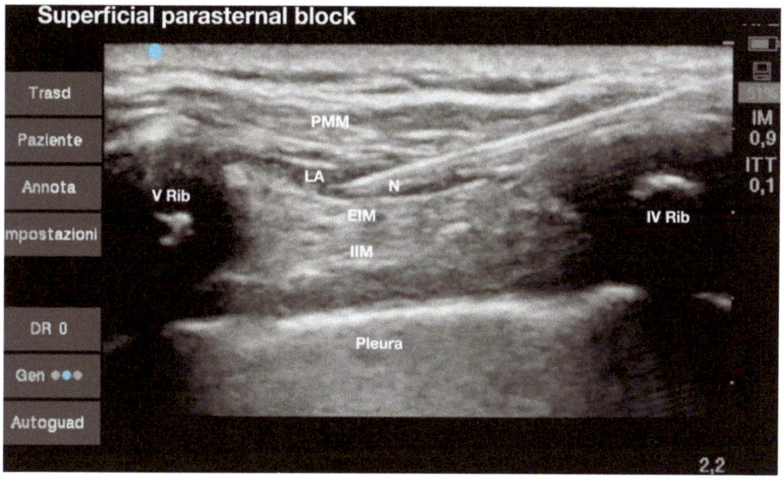

Fig. 8.4 Superficial parasternal block. At the level of second and fourth intercostal spaces, the local anesthetic is injected between the pectoralis major muscle and the external intercostal muscles. *PMM* pectoralis major muscle, *EIM* external intercostal muscle, *IIM* internal intercostal muscle, *Pleura* pleura, *Rib* rib, *N* needle, *LA* local anesthetic

approach, positioning the needle tip on the rib dome to reduce local anesthetic volume and achieve a more homogeneous and longitudinal spread into the target fascial compartment (Figs. 8.5 and 8.6). The evolution of the superficial PIP block has significantly advanced in recent years. Initially proposed for managing intra- and postoperative pain from cardiac sternotomy, it is now widely used as an anesthetic procedure for sternal surgery, particularly on spontaneously breathing patients with high comorbidities, avoiding serious pulmonary complications associated with general anesthesia and intubation [36–39].

8.4.3 Deep Parasternal Intercostal Plane (DPIP) Block or Transversus Thoracis Plane (TTP) Block

The anterior cutaneous nerves run over the deep transversus thoracis muscle (TTM) before crossing the internal and parasternal muscles near the sternal border to reach the superficial plane. This anatomical arrangement allows for a deeper injection and block, initially described in 2015 by Ueshima et al. as the transversus thoracis plane (TTP) block [40]. The patient and probe positioning, as well as the approach and needle

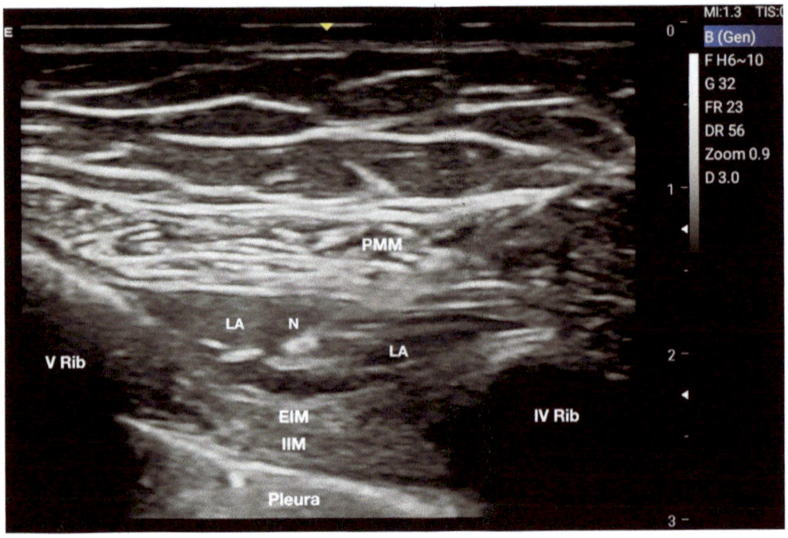

Fig. 8.5 Superficial parasternal block. The convexity of the rib may stop the longitudinal spread of local anesthetic collecting the volume of the injectate inside a single intercostal space. *PMM* pectoralis major muscle, *EIM* external intercostal muscle, *IIM* internal intercostal muscle, *Rib* rib, *N* needle, *LA* local anesthetic, *Pleura* pleura

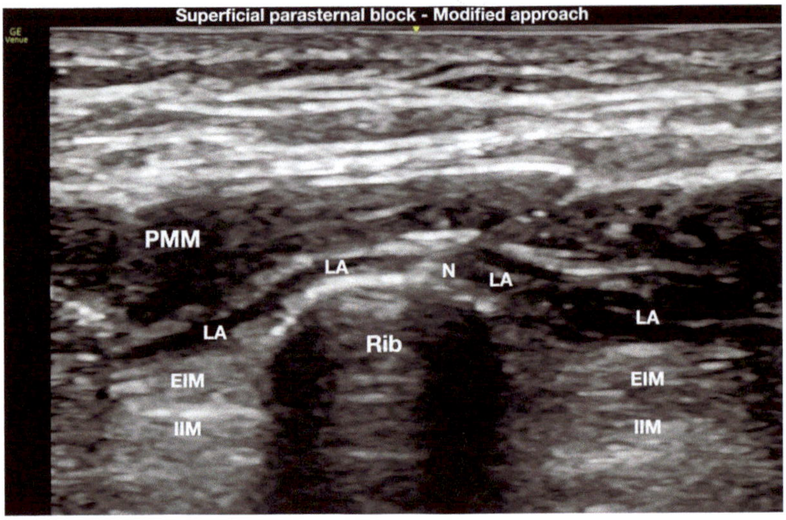

Fig. 8.6 Superficial parasternal block—modified approach. The injection on the dome of the rib allows a more homogeneous and longitudinal diffusion of local anesthetic obtaining a better dermatomal coverage. *PMM* pectoralis major muscle, *EIM* external intercostal muscle, *IIM* internal intercostal muscle, *Rib* rib, *N* needle, *LA* local anesthetic, *Pleura* pleura

insertion, remain consistent for both superficial and deep blocks (see Fig. 8.2). The ultrasound anatomy of the deep parasternal block is depicted in Fig. 8.3. Local anesthetic (LA) is injected between the internal intercostal muscle (IIM) and the TTM (see Fig. 8.7). The analgesic efficacy of deep PIP block post-cardiac surgery has been well established, contributing to patient satisfaction, opioid sparing, and reduced extubation time, as well as shorter stays in ICU and hospital [41–44]. Both superficial and deep PIP blocks exhibit similar analgesic and anesthetic efficacy, although some notable anatomical considerations arise. The TTM is often a small and variable muscle, challenging to visualize with ultrasound. At the fourth parasternal rib intercostal space level, the internal mammary artery (IMA) and internal mammary vein (IMV) can be identified between the IIM and TTM as a longitudinal pulsatile structure approximately 1.5 cm from the lateral border of the sternum. This anatomical proximity to the IMA and IMV underscores the need for caution to mitigate risks such as pneumothorax, local anesthetic systemic toxicity (LAST), and IMA injury or hematoma during deep PIP block procedures (see Fig. 8.8). Additionally, patients who have undergone IMA harvesting may experience tissue disruption in

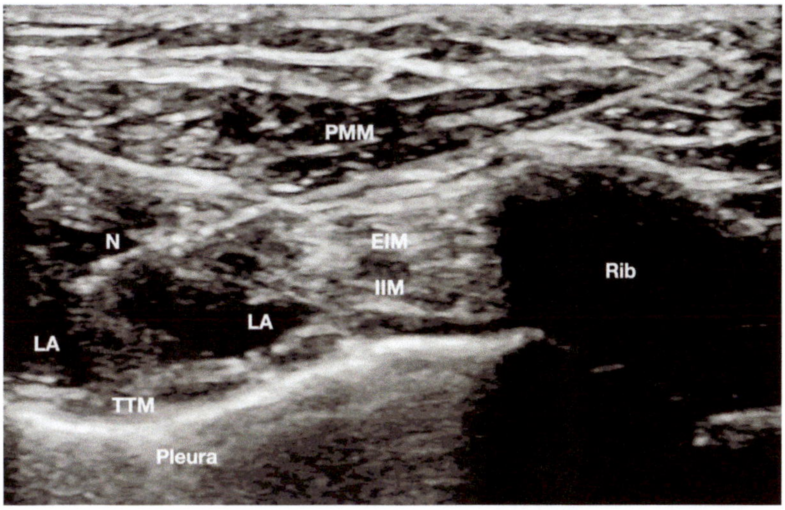

Fig. 8.7 Deep parasternal block or transversus thoracis plane block. The local anesthetic is injected between the internal intercostal and transversus thoracis muscles. *PMM* pectoralis major muscle, *EIM* external intercostal muscle, *IIM* internal intercostal muscle, *TTM* transversus thoracis muscle, *Pleura* pleura, *Rib* rib, *N* needle, *LA* local anesthetic

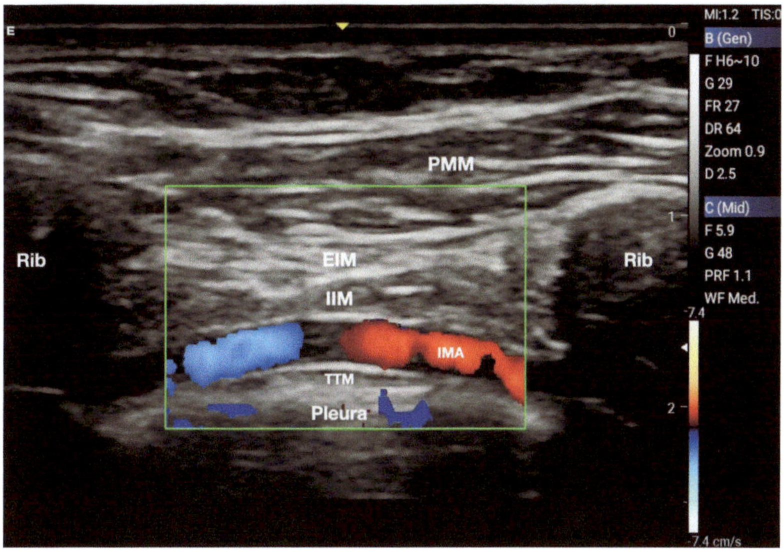

Fig. 8.8 The internal mammary artery can be identified between the internal intercostal and transversus thoracis muscles. This anatomical plane represents the target of the transversus thoracis plane block. *PMM* pectoralis major muscle, *EIM* external intercostal muscle, *IIM* internal intercostal muscle, *TTM* transversus thoracis muscle, *IMA* internal mammary artery, *Pleura* pleura, *Rib* rib

the transversus thoracis plane, complicating TTM identification and making deep PIP block challenging or impractical (see Fig. 8.9a, b). Furthermore, performing the block before cardiac surgery raises concerns about potential damage to both the right and left IMAs, rendering them unsuitable for bypass grafting. Conversely, if performed after left IMA harvesting at the end of coronary artery bypass grafting, only the right internal mammary artery might be at risk. Considering these factors, superficial PIP block may be considered a safer technique for IMA protection compared to a deep PIP block [45] as it is performed farther from vascular structures, pleura, and the heart (see Fig. 8.10). Liu et al. in a systematic review and meta-analysis of randomized controlled trials, found that while deep PIP effectively provides postoperative analgesia and shows inconclusive incidence of postoperative nausea and vomiting (PONV), no significant complications or side effects were reported [46, 47]. A current and debated topic in cardiac surgery revolves around the timing of PIP block administration, whether before or at the end of surgery. Padala et al. compared pre-incisional and post-incisional PIP

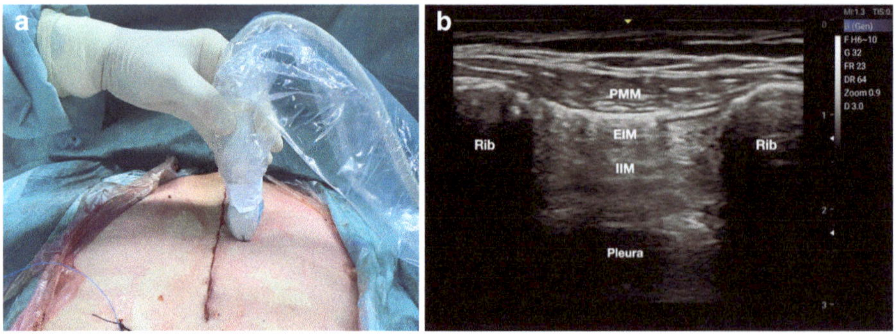

Fig. 8.9 Ultrasound anatomy after left internal mammary artery harvesting. (**a**) Probe scanning after left internal mammary artery harvesting. (**b**) Patients could have tissue disruption in the transversus thoracis plane muscle after the internal mammary artery harvest, making transversus thoracis muscle identification more difficult and the deep parasternal intercostal plane block challenging or impractical. *PMM* pectoralis major muscle, *EIM* external intercostal muscle, *IIM* internal intercostal muscle, *Pleura* pleura, *Rib* rib

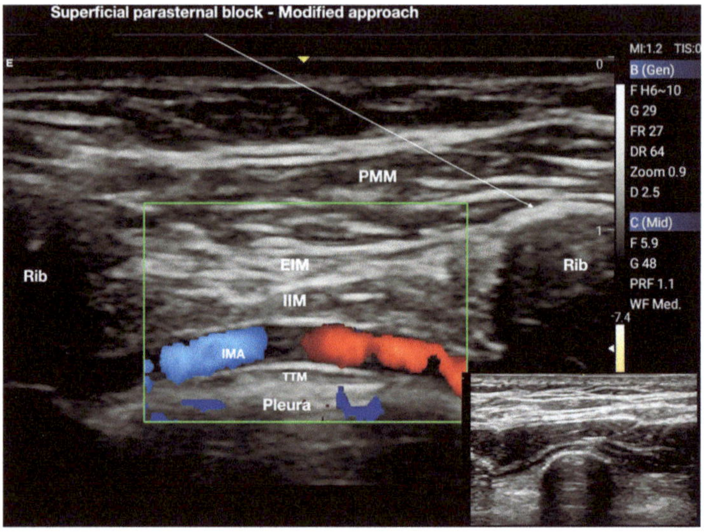

Fig. 8.10 Anatomical relationship between the superficial parasternal block and the internal mammary artery, pleura, and transversus thoracis muscle. The modified superficial parasternal block could be performed on the dome of the rib far from the vascular structures and pleura, obtaining a more homogeneous longitudinal spread of local anesthetic. *PMM* pectoralis major muscle, *EIM* external intercostal muscle, *IIM* internal intercostal muscle, *TTM* transversus thoracis muscle, *IMA* internal mammary artery, *Pleura* pleura, *Rib* rib

blocks, concluding that both options offer equivalent pain relief during the postoperative period [48]. Zou et al. in a double-blind, randomized controlled trial, observed that preemptive PIP block reduces intraoperative opioid requirements and provides effective analgesia for the initial 12 postoperative hours in patients undergoing off-pump coronary artery bypass grafting, maintaining hemodynamic stability [49]. Key tips and tricks for parasternal block are summarized in Table 8.3.

Table 8.3 Parasternal block tips and tricks

Parasternal block tips and tricks
• The injection of local anesthetic between the pectoralis major and intercostal muscles may result inadequate in terms of spread of injectate due to the anatomical convexity of the ribs, which may hinder the fascial hydrodissection • Placing the tip of the needle on the dome of the rib allows an easier and more homogeneous diffusion of local anesthetic obtaining a wider dermatomal coverage

8.4.4 Rectus Sheath Block

Although the rectus sheath block (RSB) is categorized as an abdominal block, it provides comprehensive analgesia to the anterior chest wall when combined with the parasternal block. RSB offers somatic analgesia to the anteromedial abdominal wall and periumbilical area following midline laparotomy abdominal surgery by targeting the anterior cutaneous branches from T9 to T12 intercostal nerves. Initially described as a blind technique in 1899 by Schleich, the introduction of ultrasound has transformed RSB into a safe and effective Enhanced Recovery After Surgery (ERAS) procedure, reducing opioid requirements and mitigating complications associated with neuraxial techniques and vascular injury. In addition to pain following median sternotomy, the insertion sites of drainage catheters are significant sources of discomfort after cardiac surgery. Pain from subxiphoid drainage tubes may stem from various factors, including skin incision, friction during insertion, ongoing irritation between adjacent tissues and the tube, and direct injury to the rectus abdominis muscles. Effective pain control at tube insertion sites plays a crucial role in overall pain management after cardiac surgery. The high incidence of severe postoperative pain reported in the epigastric region compromises the patient's respiratory dynamics, increasing the risk of respiratory complications, particularly in patients with severe chronic obstructive pulmonary disease, and delaying extubation [50, 51]. RSB is typically performed at the conclusion of surgery following the placement of subxiphoid drains. With the patient in the supine position, a high-frequency linear probe is positioned just below the tube emergence from the skin (Fig. 8.11a). Ultrasound landmarks include the skin, the right (RAM) and left (LAM) rectus abdominis muscles, the rectus abdominis muscle sheath (RAMS), and the peritoneum (Fig. 8.11b). Using an infraumbilical-pararectus approach and bilateral injection (from lateral to medial followed by medial to lateral), a volume of 15–20 mL of local anesthetic is deposited between the rectus muscle and its sheath (Fig. 8.12). RSB is now an integral part of an effective multimodal opioid-sparing approach, often combined with superficial or deep pectoral-intercostal plane (PIP) blocks, to manage pain stemming from median sternotomy and subxiphoid drainages, with the goal of reducing complications associated with delayed extubation in both pediatric and adult populations [52, 53]. Toscano et al. have suggested that the combined use of PIP and RSB blocks, referred to as the pectoralis-intercostal rectus sheath (PIRS) plane block, may serve as a valid and effective analgesic strategy for patients undergoing mediastinal revision via subxiphoid access due to deep sternal wound infection [54]. During the induction of general anesthesia, this

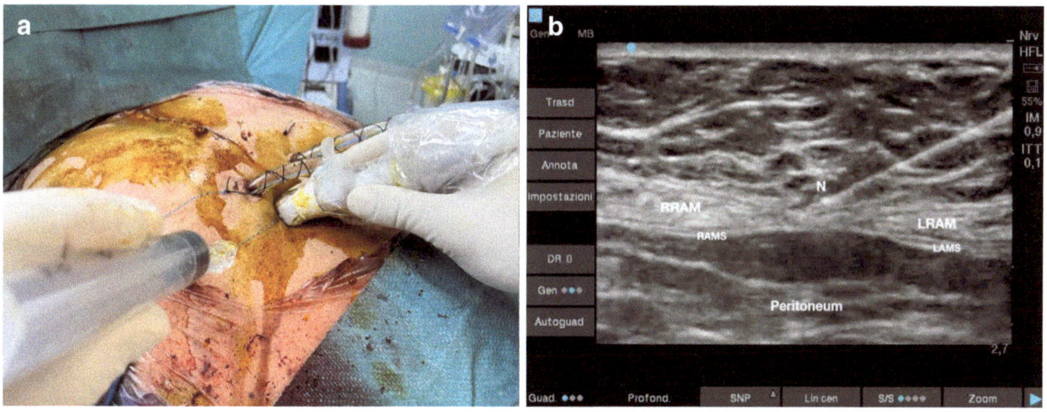

Fig. 8.11 Rectus sheath block. (**a**) Patient and probe position. The patient is in the supine position, and a high-frequency linear probe is placed just below the tube emergence from the skin. (**b**) The ultrasound landmarks are represented by the skin, the right and left rectus abdominis muscles, the rectus abdominis muscle sheath, and the peritoneum. *RRAM* right rectus abdominis muscle, *LRAM* left rectus abdominis muscle, *LRAS* left rectus abdominis muscle sheath, *RAMS* right rectus abdominis muscle sheath, *Peritoneum* peritoneum, *N* needle

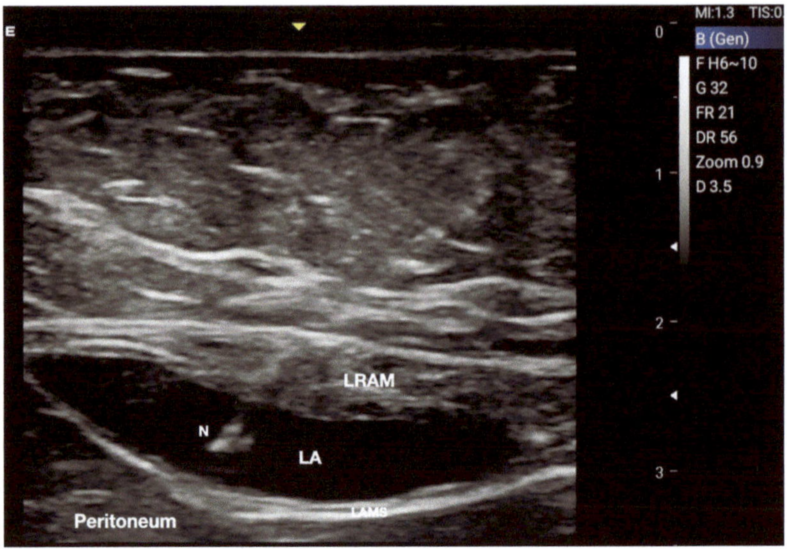

Fig. 8.12 Rectus sheath block. The local anesthetic is injected between the rectus abdominis muscle and its sheath. *LRAM* left rectus abdominis muscle, *LAMS* left abdominis muscle sheath, *N* needle, *Peritoneum* peritoneum

technique can also be executed by introducing bilateral indwelling catheters running from the epigastrium, where a single-shot RSB is initially performed bilaterally, to the sternal notch, covering from T1 to T10 dermatomes, through continuous infusion of local anesthetic in patients undergoing cardiac surgery via sternotomy and receiving subxiphoid drainages [55]. An additional significant and innovative application for pain management following left ventricular assist device (LVAD) implantation via median sternotomy involves combining bilateral deep PIP (TTP) block to provide analgesia to the sternal region and unilateral RSB to ensure pain relief to the left abdominal structures through which the LVAD driveline was inserted, facilitating prompt discharge from the intensive care unit (ICU) without the need for rescue analgesia administration [56].

8.4.5 Interpectoral Plane Block (PECS I) and Interpectoral-Pectoserratus Plane Block (PECS II)

The interpectoral plane block (PECS I) and interpectoral-pectoserratus plane block (PECS II) were initially introduced by Rafael Blanco in 2011 and 2012, respectively, as effective alternatives to thoracic epidural and paravertebral blocks for postoperative analgesia in breast surgery. PECS I targets the lateral (LPN) and medial (MPN) pectoral nerves, innervating the PMM and pmm muscles. LPN is typically proximate to the pectoral branch of the thoracoacromial artery (TAA), serving as a vascular landmark for PECS I. Blanco later introduced a modified version, known as "PECS II," which extends the focus on the lateral branches of the intercostal nerves from T2 to T6, along with other nerves crucial for axillary surgery. Although PECS II technically consists of two blocks (IPP and PSP), it is sometimes mistakenly described as separate procedures. In cardiac surgery, however, they may be employed as distinct techniques based on surgical requirements. PECS blocks, when compared to parenteral analgesia alone, offer superior postoperative pain relief in cardiac surgery patients as part of multimodal protocols. Combining PSP block (PECS II) with serratus anterior plane block (SAPB) further extends analgesic effects after thoracotomy in cardiac surgery patients [57, 58].

The indications for both PECS I and PECS II are summarized in Table 8.4.

8.4.6 Interpectoral Plane (IPP) Block (PECS I)

The patient is positioned supine with the head rotated to expose the deltoid-pectoral groove opposite the injection site. Using a linear high-

Table 8.4 Interpectoral plane block (PECS I) and pectoserratus plane block (PECS II) indications

Interpectoral plane block (PECS I) indications	Pectoserratus plane block (PECS II) indications
• Breast surgery: breast expanders, subpectoral implants, radical mastectomies, axillary lymphadenectomy	• Breast surgery: radical mastectomies, tumorectomies, axillary lymphadenectomy, upper-external quadrantectomies
• Thoracic surgery: postoperative analgesia, placement of chest drains, post-traumatic chest injuries	• Thoracic surgery: pain management after thoracotomy in cardiac surgery in association with SAPB block
• Other: pacemaker implant, ICD, port-a-caths	

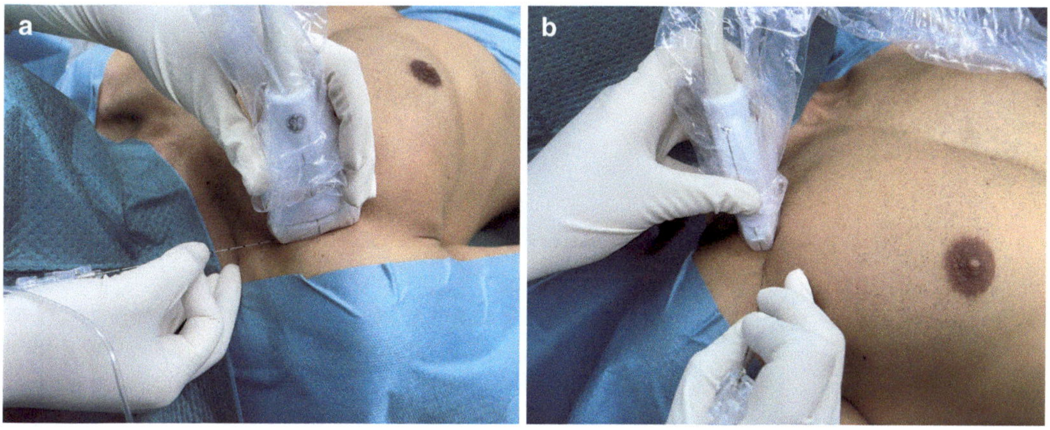

Fig. 8.13 Interpectoral plane (PECS I) block. Patient and probe position. The patient is in the supine position with the head rotated in the opposite injection site exposing the deltoid-pectoral groove. A linear high-frequency probe is positioned in the deltoid-pectoral groove. (**a**) The needle is inserted with the in-plane approach in a medial-to-lateral direction or (**b**) in a lateral-to-medial direction

frequency probe, positioned in the deltoid-pectoral groove akin to the infraclavicular block, the needle is inserted with an in-plane approach from medial to lateral direction. Alternatively, a lateral to medial approach may be chosen for patient and practitioner comfort (Fig. 8.13). Ultrasound landmarks include the PMM, pmm, TAA, and rib (Fig. 8.14). Following TAA visualization, 10 mL of LA is injected into the fascial plane between the PMM and pmm (Fig. 8.15). Tips and tricks for the interpectoral plane block (PECS I) are summarized in Table 8.5.

8.4.7 Pectoserratus Plane (PSP) Block (Second Part of the PECS II)

The patient and probe positioning remain similar to the IPP (PECS I) block. By tilting the probe medially towards the thorax, the axillary artery and vein are identified, with the second rib visualized beneath these vessels. Moving the probe distally and laterally towards the axilla, the lateral margin of the PMM is located beneath which lie the third and fourth ribs. Near the fourth rib, landmarks such as the ligament of Gerdy, indicating the axillary cavity entrance, along with the pmm and the serratus anterior muscle (SAM), are identified (Fig. 8.16). Sonoanatomy includes PMM, pmm, SAM, IM, ribs, and pleural sliding (Fig. 8.17). Following PECS I block, a PECS II involves an additional 20 mL of LA between pmm and SAM (Fig. 8.18a), and optionally below SAM and above IM, referencing the bone plane of the fourth rib (Fig. 8.18b). Both techniques facilitate LA spread to the axilla, encompassing the TLN, TDN, and IBN. For educational clarity in cardiac surgery, PECS I and PECS II are described as distinct procedures. PECS II's extension to the axilla, not a cardiac surgical target, may result in LA loss; hence, it is often com-

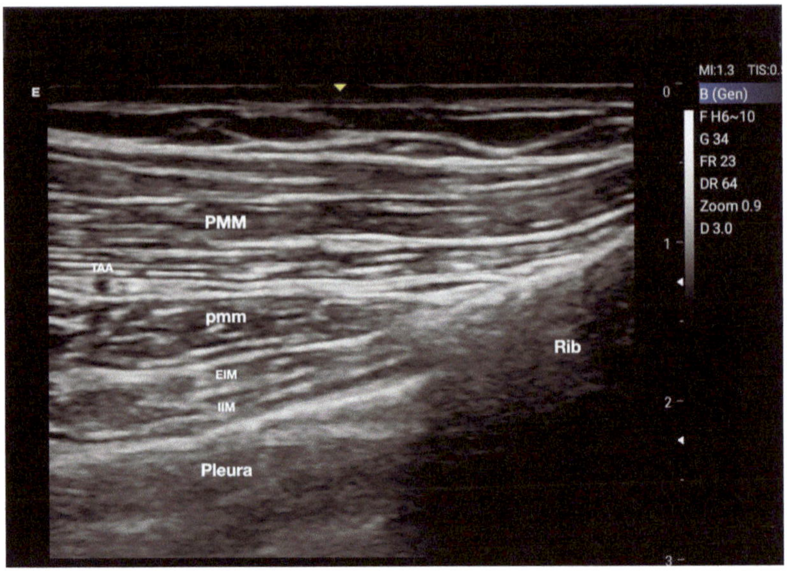

Fig. 8.14 Interpectoral plane (PECS I) ultrasound landmarks. From the top to bottom: pectoralis major muscle, pectoralis minor muscle, pectoral branch of the thoracoacromial artery, rib, external and internal intercostal muscles, pleura. *PMM* pectoralis major muscle, *pmm* pectoralis minor muscle, *TAA* pectoral branch of the thoracoacromial artery, *EIM* external intercostal muscles, *IIM* internal intercostal muscles, *Rib* rib, *Pleura* pleura

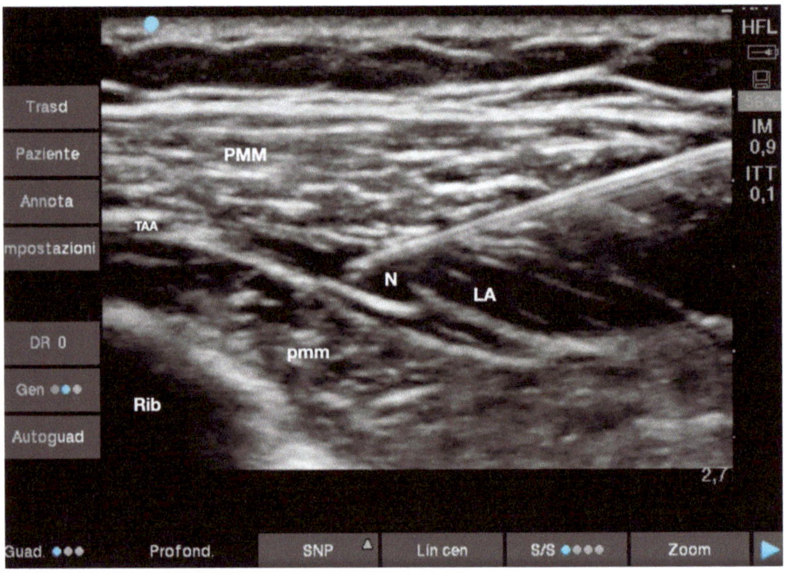

Fig. 8.15 Interpectoral plane (PECS I) block. The local anesthetic is injected between the pectoralis major and minor muscles following the pectoral branch of the thoracoacromial artery. *PMM* pectoralis major muscle, *pmm* pectoralis minor muscle, *TAA* pectoral branch of the thoracoacromial artery, *N* needle, *LA* local anesthetic, *Rib* rib

Table 8.5 Interpectoral plane block (PECS I) tips and tricks

Interpectoral plane block (PECS I) tips and tricks
• The lateral-to-medial approach to interpectoral plane (PECS I) block allows the patient and anesthesiologist to assume a more comfortable position than the medial-to-lateral approach • The pectoral branch of the thoracoacromial artery is an important vascular landmark to identify the interfascial plane • An effective block is realized when the ultrasound double V sign is visualized

bined with an overlapping technique like the serratus anterior plane block. Tips and tricks for the interpectoral-pectoserratus plane block (PECS II) are summarized in Table 8.6.

8.4.8 Serratus Anterior Plane Block

Introduced by Blanco as a modification of PECS blocks, the serratus anterior plane block (SAPB)

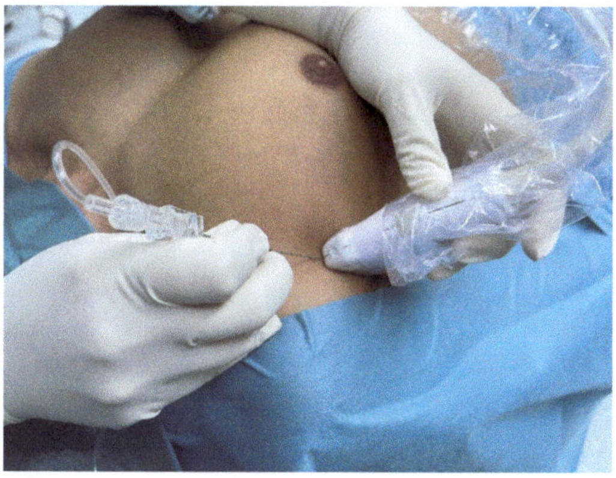

Fig. 8.16 Pectoserratus plane (PECS II) block. Patient and probe position. Starting from the deltoid-pectoral groove, the probe slides towards the Gerdy ligament and the axilla at the level of the fourth rib. The needle is inserted with the in-plane approach in a medial-to-lateral direction

targets lateral intercostal nerves from T2 to T6–T9, providing analgesia for most of the hemithorax. Indications span breast cancer and thoracic surgery to cardiac procedures like mitral valve surgery. Other indications like minithoracotomies or implantation of subcutaneous defibrillators (S-ICD) are listed in Table 8.7. SAPB can be superficial (SSAPB) or deep (DSAPB), depending on whether LA is injected above or below the serratus anterior muscle (Figs. 8.19 and 8.20). Ultrasound landmarks include latissimus dorsi (LDM), serratus anterior (SAM) muscles, ribs, and pleura. The thoracodorsal artery (TDA) visualization allows the identification of the SAM superficial plane (Fig. 8.21). SSAPB involves injecting 30 mL of LA between LDM and SAM, while DSAPB

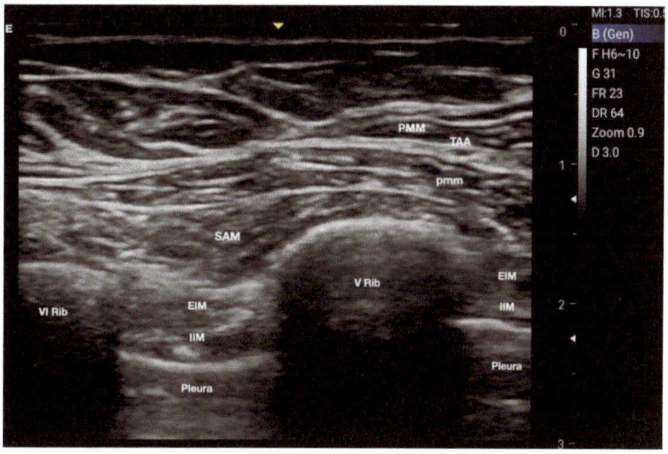

Fig. 8.17 Pectoserratus plane (PECS II) block landmarks. *PMM* pectoralis major muscle, *pmm* pectoralis minor muscle, *SAM* serratus anterior muscle, *IIM* internal intercostal muscle, *TAA* pectoral branch of the thoracoacromial artery, *EIM* external intercostal muscle, *IIM* internal intercostal muscle, *Rib* rib, *Pleura* pleura

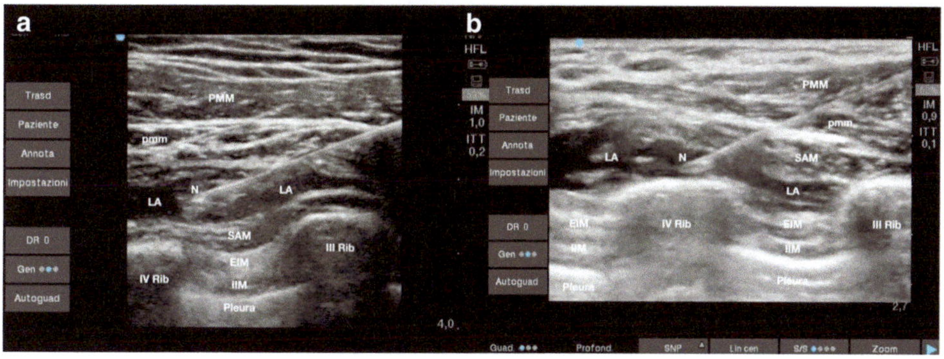

Fig. 8.18 Pectoserratus plane (PECS II) block. (**a**) Pectoserratus plane block above the serratus anterior muscle. Local anesthetic is injected between the pectoralis minor muscle and the serratus anterior muscle at the level of the fourth rib. (**b**) Pectoserratus plane block under the serratus anterior muscle. Local anesthetic is injected between the serratus anterior muscle and the intercostal muscle at the level of the fourth rib. *PMM* pectoralis major muscle, *pmm* pectoralis minor muscle, *SAM* serratus anterior muscle, *EIM* external intercostal muscle, *IIM* internal intercostal muscle, *Rib* rib, *Pleura* pleura, *N* needle

Table 8.6 Pectoserratus plane block (PECS II) tips and tricks

Pectoserratus plane block (PECS II) tips and tricks
• Placing the patient in opposite decubitus to the surgical site, the probe can be placed on the midaxillary line. At the level of the fourth rib, the local anesthetic can be injected below the plane of serratus muscle realizing a deep serratus anterior plane block or BRILMA (blocking the branches of intercostal nerves in the middle axillary line)

Table 8.7 Serratus anterior plane block indications

Serratus anterior plane block indications
• Breast surgery: radical mastectomies, external quadrants, axillary lymphadenectomies (lymph node emptying), placement of implants or expanders, additive or reduction mammoplasty
• Thoracic surgery: pain management after rib fractures or thoracic trauma, placement of chest drains, lobectomies, continuous analgesia for thoracotomies, video-assisted thoracoscopic surgery • Cardiac surgery: pain management after mitral valve surgery, minithoracotomies, implantation of subcutaneous defibrillators (S-ICD)

entails injecting the same volume between SAM and the fifth rib (Fig. 8.22). Notably, DSAPB's target area aligns with the PSP (PECS II) block below SAM, making them anatomically similar. The SAM plane is suitable for catheter place-

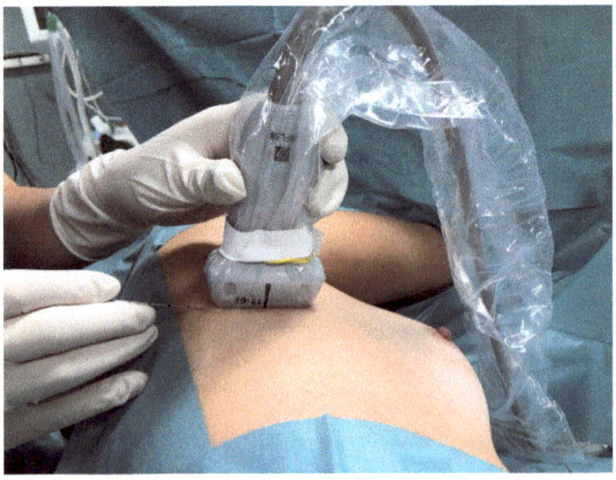

Fig. 8.20 Serratus anterior plane block and transverse approach. Probe and patient position

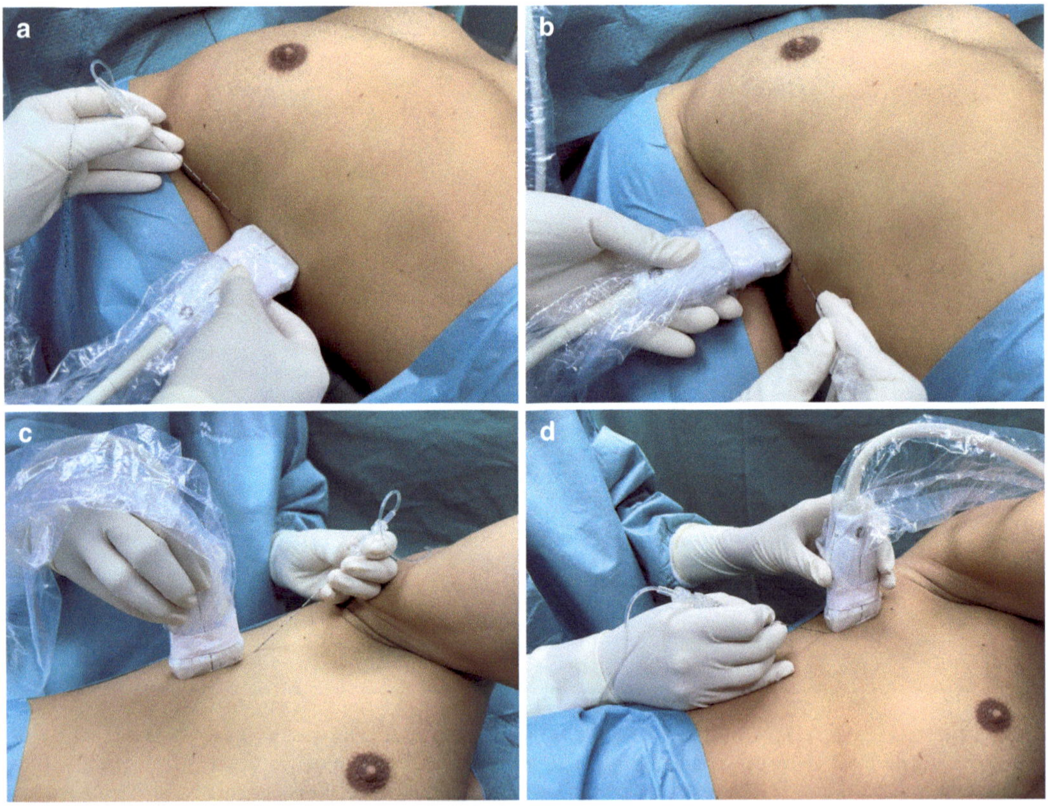

Fig. 8.19 Serratus anterior plane block. Probe and patient position. (**a, b**) Supine position and cranial-to-caudal or caudal-to-cranial approach. (**c, d**) Lateral position and cranial-to-caudal or caudal-to-cranial approach

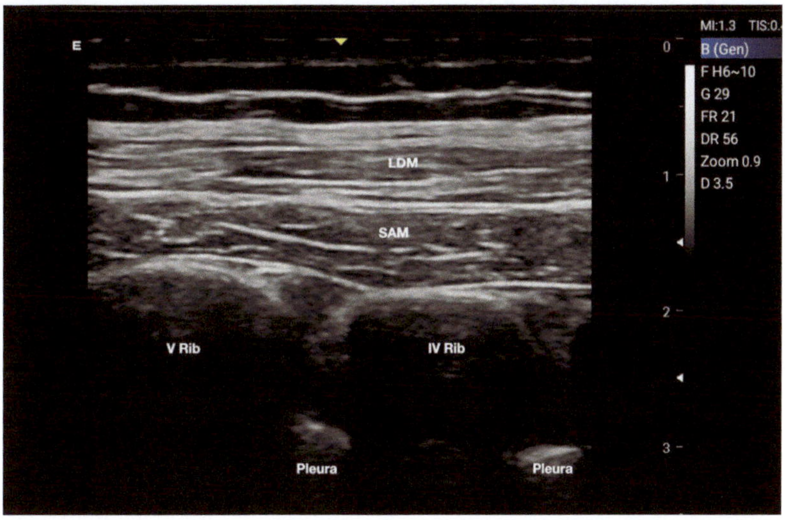

Fig. 8.21 Serratus anterior plane block landmarks. Latissimus dorsi muscle, serratus anterior muscle, ribs, and pleura. *LDM* latissimus dorsi muscle, *SAM* serratus anterior muscle, *Rib* rib, *Pl* pleura

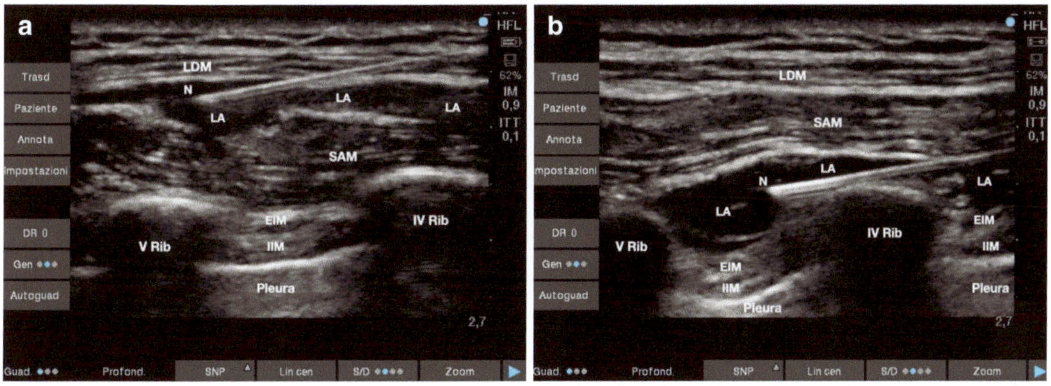

Fig. 8.22 Serratus anterior plane block. (**a**) The superficial serratus anterior plane block is performed by the injection of local anesthetic between latissimus dorsi and serratus anterior muscle (above the surface of serratus anterior muscle). (**b**) The deep serratus anterior plane block is performed by the injection of local anesthetic between serratus anterior and fifth rib (below the surface of serratus anterior muscle)

ment to manage intra- and postoperative pain via continuous LA infusion. The plane of the SAM is anatomically suitable for the placement of a catheter in order to manage the intra- and postoperative pain through the continuous infusion of LA (patient-controlled analgesia, PCA) [59]. Placing the catheter along the midaxillary line produces a wider spread of local anesthetic (Fig. 8.23a, b). Some authors suggest single-shot DSAPB with dexmedetomidine for effective postoperative pain control after minithoracotomy heart surgery [60, 61]. Tips and tricks for the serratus anterior plane block are summarized in Table 8.8.

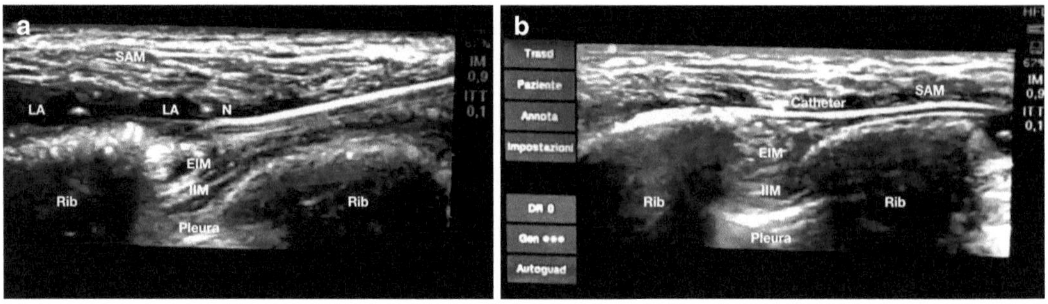

Fig. 8.23 Continuous deep serratus anterior plane block. (**a**) Local anesthetic is injected below the serratus anterior muscle. (**b**) The continuous infusion catheter is placed between the anterior muscle and the ribs. *SAM* serratus anterior muscle, *EIM* external intercostal muscle, *IIM* internal intercostal muscle, *Rib* rib, *Pleura* pleura, *LA* local anesthetic, *N* needle, *Catheter* catheter

Table 8.8 Serratus anterior plane block tips and tricks

Serratus anterior plane block tips and tricks
• The anatomical target of PSP (PECS II) block under the serratus anterior muscle is the same as that of deep SAPB making the two procedures very similar in terms of dermatomal coverage and efficacy. The only difference between them is the level of injection and the volume of local anesthetic: Fourth rib for the PSP (PECS II) block under the serratus anterior muscle and fifth rib for deep SAPB. 20 mL for PSP (PECS II) block and 30 mL for deep SAP block • If the probe is positioned along the midaxillary line and the local anesthetic is deposited below the serratus muscle plane, the technique could also be named BRILMA
• Placing the tip of the needle on the surface of the rib represents an anatomical protection to avoid pleural punctures and obtain a better and longitudinal diffusion of local anesthetic

8.5 Posterior Chest Wall Blocks

Posterior chest wall blocks, also known as paraspinal fascial blocks, aim to distribute local anesthetic as close as possible to the paravertebral space without directly inserting the needle into this space, where the dorsal and ventral branches of the spinal roots emerge, providing both somatic and visceral anesthesia and analgesia. For these reasons, they are also referred to as "paravertebral by proxy."

The posterior chest wall blocks include:

1. Erector spinae plane (ESP) block
2. Paravertebral block (PVB)
3. Retrolaminar blocks
4. Midpoint transverse process-to-pleura (MTP) block
5. Paraspinal-intercostal plane blocks
6. Rhomboid intercostal subserratus plane (RISS) block

8.5.1 Erector Spinae Plane Block

The erector spinae plane (ESP) block was first described by Forero et al. in 2016 as a novel analgesic procedure for managing neuropathic pain resulting from metastatic disease of the ribs and multiple rib fractures, providing an extensive dermatomal sensory block [62]. It is increasingly performed across various surgical fields due to its safety and simplicity compared to established thoracic paravertebral or epidural blocks, which carry risks such as pneumothorax, hematomas, and neural injury related to anticoagulation in cardiac surgery [63]. Indications include a wide range of surgical procedures, including breast surgery, cardiac and thoracic surgery, abdominal surgery, urological surgery, orthopedic surgery, and spine surgery (Table 8.9). The mechanism of the ESP block involves the spread of local anesthetic close to or into the paravertebral space, where the ventral and dorsal rami of the spinal nerves emerge and diverge. Catheter insertion into the ESP block site allows for continuous infusion of local anesthetic, providing lasting intra- and postoperative analgesia, especially for pain deriving from minithoracotomy in cardiac surgery. It is believed to relieve pain in a large area of the posterior, lateral, and anterior chest and lumbar walls, also preventing visceral pain. It can be used for acute and chronic pain of the trunk, as well as for upper and lower limbs. However, it may not be as effective for managing pain from midline sternotomy, as demonstrated in a systematic review and meta-analysis by King et al. Supporting these findings, Dost et al. demonstrated superior efficacy of a combined superficial parasternal-intercostal plane (PIP) plus ESP blocks compared to bilateral ESP block alone in acute post-sternotomy pain following cardiac surgery [64, 65].

Table 8.9 Erector spinae block indications

Erector spinae block indications
• Whiplash
• Chronic shoulder pain syndrome
• Cervicogenic headache
• Rib fracture (unilateral or bilateral ESP)
• Open thoracotomy and VATS lobectomy
• Rescue after thoracic epidural failure
• Cardiac surgery—minithoracotomy
• Breast surgery with axillary lymph node dissection
• Chronic postherpetic neuralgia
• Chronic post-thoracotomy pain syndrome
• Metastatic cancer of the rib
• Nephrectomies (unilateral ESP)
• Hysterectomies (bilateral ESP)
• Laparoscopic ventral hernia repair with mesh
• Laparotomies (bilateral ESP)
• Chronic postherpetic neuralgia
• Chronic myofascial pain syndrome
• Facet pain
• Vertebral surgery

The block is typically performed with the patient in the seated, prone, or lateral position, using ultrasound guidance to identify landmarks and administer local anesthetic. The steps are as follows:

1. A high-frequency linear probe is placed approximately 3 cm lateral to the interspinous line at the level of T3–T4 or T5–T6 transverse processes (Fig. 8.24).
2. In the paraspinal area, the correct landmarks are trapezius, rhomboid, erector spinae muscles, transverse processes, and pleura (Fig. 8.25).
3. Starting from the spinous processes, the anesthesiologist slides the probe in the medial-to-lateral direction to visualize the convex shape of the rib and the squared shape of the transverse process (Fig. 8.26).
4. The needle is inserted through an IP approach, and a volume of 20 mL of LA is injected into the plane between the edge of the transverse process (TP) and the erector spinae muscle (ESM) (Fig. 8.27).

The mechanism of the ESP block appears related to the spread of LA close or into the paravertebral space where the ventral and dorsal rami

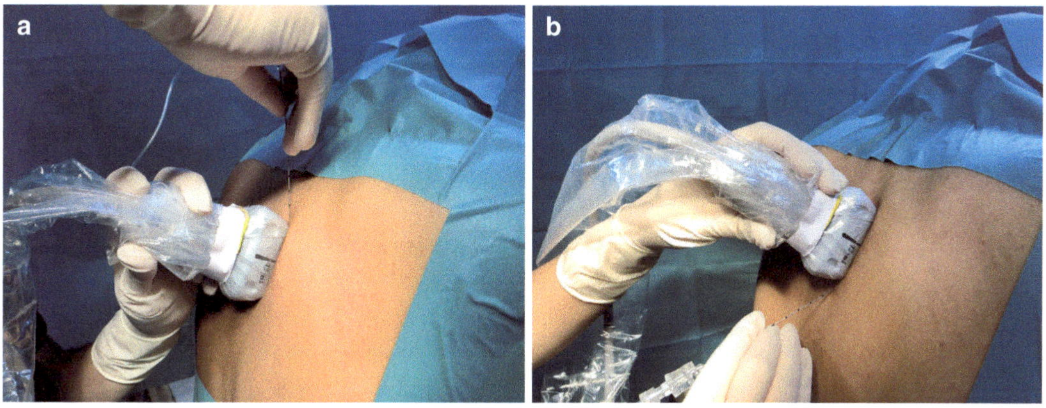

Fig. 8.24 ESP block patient and probe position. The patient may assume the seated, prone, or lateral position. A high-frequency linear probe is placed approximately 3 cm lateral to the interspinous line at the level of T3–T4 or T5–T6 transverse processes. (**a**) The needle is inserted with the in-plane approach in a cranial-to-caudal direction or (**b**) in a caudal-to-cranial direction

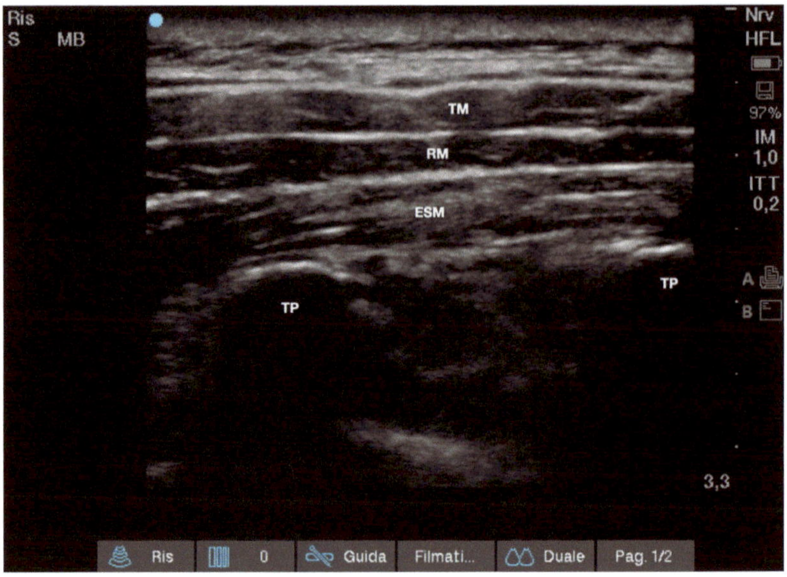

Fig. 8.25 Ultrasound erector spinae muscle landmarks. From top to bottom: trapezius, rhomboid, and erector spinae muscles. *TM* trapezius muscle, *RM* rhomboid muscle, *ESM* erector spinae muscle, *TP* transverse process

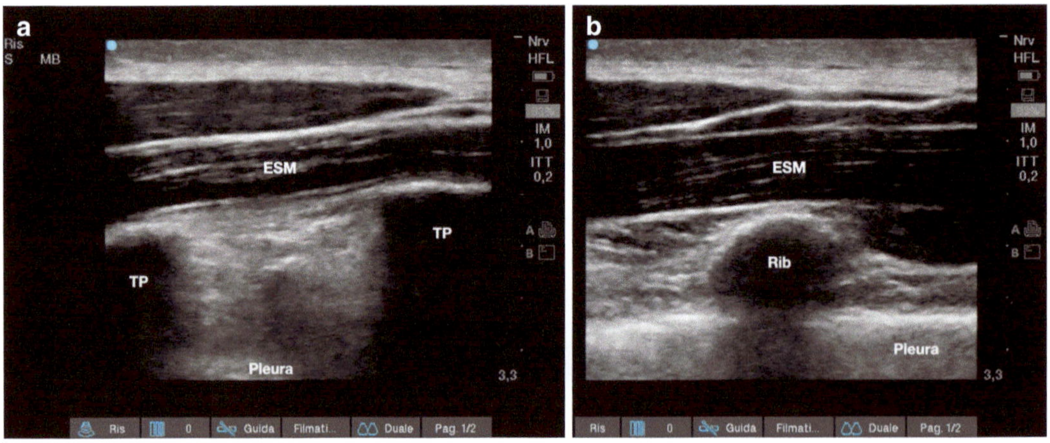

Fig. 8.26 Ultrasound differences between transverse process and rib. (**a**) Squared shape of the transverse process. (**b**) Convex shape of the rib

of the spinal nerves emerge and diverge. Most likely, the injectate spreads through the costotransverse foramen and several slits of the superior costotransverse ligament (SCTL), which represents the posterior wall of the paravertebral space [66, 67]. On this basis, several techniques deriving from the intertransverse process (ITP) blocks have been introduced under different nomenclatures with the aim to inject the LA a little closer to the slits of the SCTL than the ESP block to obtain a more effective diffusion of the volume to the paravertebral space. The plane between the ESM and the transverse processes represents an optimal anatomical site in which a catheter may be inserted to perform a continuous infusion of LA and provide a lasting intra- and postoperative analgesia in cardiac surgery especially for pain deriving from minithoracotomy (Fig. 8.28). The catheter may be inserted with the patient in seated position, but it is preferable performing the continuous ESP block before general anesthesia with the patient in lateral decubitus to minimize dangerous hemodynamic instability such as hypertension, hypotension, arrhythmia, lipothymia, and bradycardia which may occur in cardiac critically ill patients in a sit-

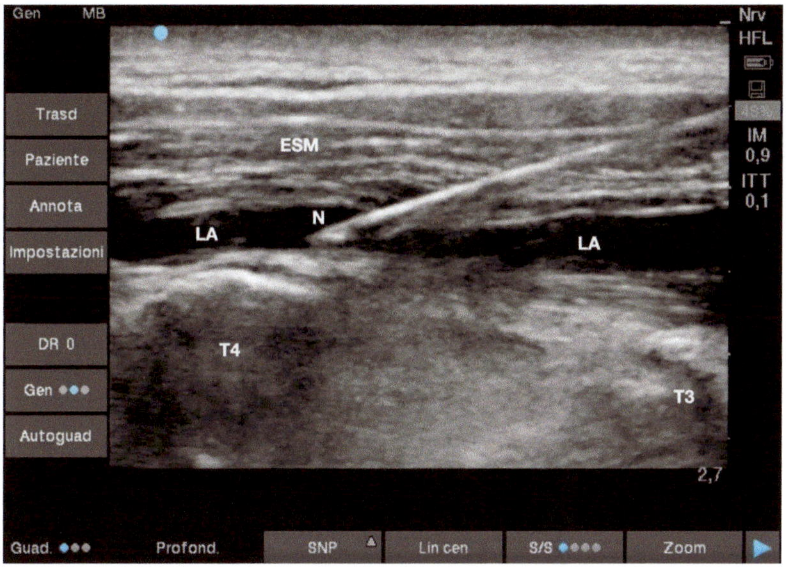

Fig. 8.27 ESP block. The local anesthetic is injected between the transverse process and the erector spinae muscle. *ESM* erector spinae muscle, *T4* T4 transverse process, *T3* T3 transverse process, *N* needle, *LA* local anesthetic

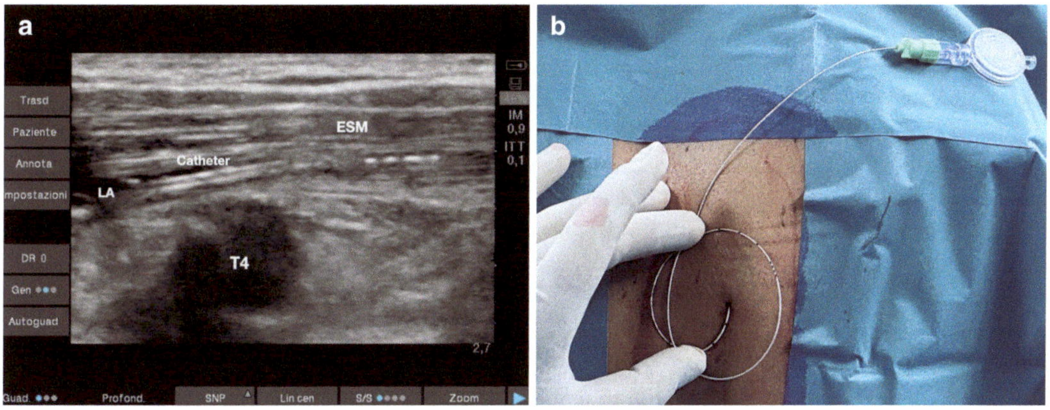

Fig. 8.28 Continuous erector spinae block. (**a**) The catheter is inserted between the erector spinae muscle and the transverse processes. (**b**) Skin catheter fixation. *ESM* erector spinae muscle, *T4* T4 transverse process, *N* needle, *LA* local anesthetic, *Catheter* catheter

ting position. The alternative is represented by the continuous DSAPB performed before the induction or at the end of surgery with the patient already in supine position [68].

The ESP block tips and tricks are summarized in Table 8.10.

8.5.2 Paravertebral Block

The thoracic paravertebral block (TPVB) was first described by Hugo Sellheim of Leipzig in 1905 and developed as the currently blind technique by Kappis in 1919. It involves injecting local anesthetic into the paravertebral space, providing anesthesia and analgesia for both somatic and visceral acute and chronic pain. The TPVB is mostly performed for thoracic and abdominal surgeries, although its use in cardiac surgery remains controversial due to patient anticoagulation [69]. Naganuma et al. demonstrated that preoperative bilateral TPVB combined with general anesthesia reduced extubation time and intraoperative and postoperative opioid con-

Table 8.10 Erector spinae block tips and tricks

Erector spinae block tips and tricks
• The rib has a convex ultrasound shape, while the transverse process has a squared ultrasound shape • During scanning, the visualization of ribs indicates the excessive laterality of the probe as compared to the interspinous line • Placing the tip of the needle on the transverse process represents a safety stop for several complications • An effective ESP block is realized when the ultrasound erector spinae muscle lift is observed during the injection of local anesthetic

sumption in adult patients undergoing aortic valve replacement and coronary artery bypass grafting (CABG) with full sternotomy [70]. El Shora et al. found that bilateral TPVB provides effective pain relief after median sternotomy, although it is not superior to thoracic epidural anesthesia [71]. Continuous TPVB has been shown to have equivalent analgesic efficacy compared to epidural analgesia but with a lower incidence of postoperative nausea and vomiting, hypotension, and urinary retention [72]. Cardiac surgery often entails significant acute and chronic pain, necessitating consideration of continuous analgesia infusion, particularly when performing a thoracic paravertebral block (TPVB). Continuous TPVB has demonstrated comparable analgesic efficacy to epidural analgesia but with a lower incidence of postoperative nausea and vomiting (PONV), hypotension, and urinary retention compared to epidural analgesia [72]. Continuous TPVB has also been employed in managing pain resulting from minithoracotomy for minimally invasive cardiac surgery (MICS) without complications or post-extubation pulmonary failure. Minor bleeding associated with continuous TPVB has been linked to preoperative prolongation of prothrombin time-international normalized ratio (PT-INR) [73]. Okitsu et al. sought to assess the risk of hematoma related to TPVB in cardiac surgery patients and found it to be close to 0%. However, they emphasized the necessity of carefully evaluating the risk-to-benefit ratio to determine TPVB's appropriateness [74]. TPVB is regarded as an advanced technique requiring experienced anesthesiologists. Unilateral TPVB is sufficient for managing pain from minithoracotomy, whereas a bilateral procedure is necessary for pain relief from median sternotomy. Additionally, a single puncture at the T4 or T5 level with 20 mL of LA may serve as an alternative to double puncture, albeit with potential unpredictable cranial spread of volume and variable coverage of dermatomes. Performing TPVB can pose challenges, both with the patient in the sitting position due to hemodynamic complications and in lateral decubitus due to the risk of losing ultrasound landmarks and needle-probe alignment. Despite some scientific publications, the level of evidence remains low. While ultrasound use reduces complication rates, limited data in the literature hinders drawing definitive conclusions. Future trials are warranted to evaluate TPVB's indications and safety in patients receiving anticoagulant or antiplatelet therapy. Consequently, concerns about hematoma and neuraxial injury have spurred interest in simpler and safer regional procedures like erector spinae plane (ESP) block and retrolaminar procedures [75]. The indications and contraindications for TPVB are outlined in Table 8.11. The patient is positioned either sitting, prone, or in lateral decubitus, with the surgical site facing upward. Key skin landmarks include the cranial boundary represented by the roof of the scapula, corresponding to the T3 spinous process, and the caudal boundary represented by its apex, aligning with the T6–T7 spinous processes (Fig. 8.29). The high-frequency linear probe can be positioned in the paravertebral region longitudinally, transversally, or with a 45° rotation from the interspinous line. Ultrasound imaging reveals the trapezius (TM), rhomboid (RM), erector spinae (ESM) muscles, transverse processes, ribs, intercostal muscles (IM), superior costotransverse ligament (SCTL), and sliding motion of the pleura. The SCTL and ribs are visualized inferiorly using the intermediate longitudinal or transverse approach (Fig. 8.30). Thoracic paravertebral block (TPVB) can be performed using both the in-plane (IP) and out-of-plane (OOP) techniques. The IP technique encompasses three distinct approaches (Fig. 8.31).

Table 8.11 Thoracic paravertebral block indications and contraindications

Thoracic	Paravertebral block
Indications	Contraindications
Pain therapy: rib fractures, neuralgia, pleuritic pain	Infection at the site of *injection*, allergy to local anesthetic drug, empyema, and a neoplastic mass occupying the paravertebral space
Breast surgery: all breast surgery (oncological-aesthetic-reconstructive) that does not include the axillary cavity (in this case, it is advisable to associate a general anesthesia)	Coagulopathy, bleeding disorders, or patients receiving *anticoagulant* drugs are relative contraindications for TPVB
Thoracic surgery: thoracotomies, thoracoscopy	One must exercise caution in patients with kyphoscoliosis or deformed spines and those who have had previous thoracic surgery
Minimally invasive cardiac surgery in minithoracotomy: mitral valve surgery, bypass single- and two-vessel coronary artery	The chest deformity in the former may predispose to inadvertent thecal or pleural puncture, and the altered paravertebral anatomy due to fibrotic obliteration of the paravertebral space or adhesions of the lung to the chest wall in the latter may predispose to pulmonary puncture
Liver surgery: thermal ablation of liver tumors, placement of percutaneous biliary drainage. Renal and gynecological surgery	
Other: cholecystectomy, inguinal hernia	

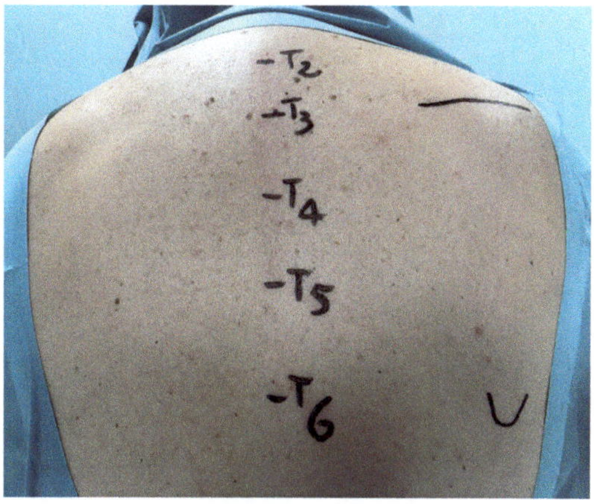

Fig. 8.29 Thoracic paravertebral block skin landmarks. Key skin landmarks include the cranial boundary represented by the roof of the scapula, corresponding to the T3 spinous process, and the caudal boundary represented by its apex, aligning with the T6–T7 spinous processes

1. Longitudinal approach: The probe is positioned approximately 1.5 cm laterally and parallel to the interspinous line, intercepting two adjacent transverse processes (T3–T4 or T5–T6). The needle is inserted in an IP approach, directed from caudal to cranial (Fig. 8.31a).
2. Intermediate longitudinal approach: Starting from the longitudinal position, the probe is rotated laterally by 45° to intercept the transverse process cranially and the rib inferiorly. This approach facilitates a more comfortable trajectory for needle insertion into the paravertebral space (PVS). The needle is inserted in an IP approach from lateral to medial (Fig. 8.31b).
3. Transverse approach: The probe is positioned transversely to the interspinous line, intercepting the transverse process, rib, and PVS. The needle is inserted in an IP approach from lateral to medial. While effective, this approach is limited due to the higher incidence of epidural spread of LA (Fig. 8.31c).
4. In the OOP technique, the probe is positioned longitudinally to the interspinous line at the level of T3–T4 or T5–T6 transverse processes. The needle is inserted with an IP approach from posterior to anterior (Fig. 8.31d).

Upon needle placement in the PVS, crossing the SCTL, the spread of LA leads to simultaneous downward displacement of the pleura, indicating successful TPVB (Fig. 8.32).

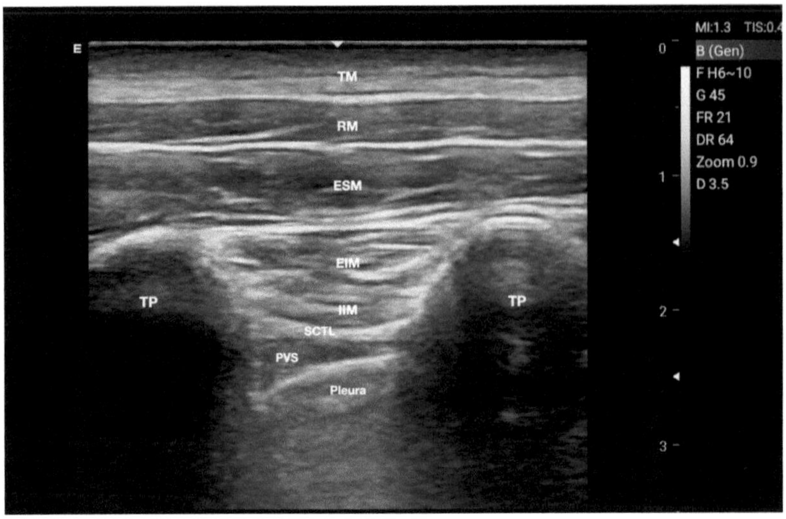

Fig. 8.30 Ultrasound paravertebral block landmarks. The ultrasound anatomy is represented by the trapezius, rhomboid, and erector spinae muscles; transverse processes; rib; intercostal muscle; superior costotransverse ligament; and pleura. *TM* trapezius muscle, *RM* rhomboid muscle, *ESM* erector spinae muscle, *TP* transverse process, *PVS* paravertebral space, *SCTL* superior costotransverse ligament, *Pleura* pleura, *IIM* internal intercostal muscle, *EIM* external intercostal muscle

Tips and tricks for thoracic paravertebral block are summarized in Table 8.12.

8.5.3 Retrolaminar Block

The retrolaminar block was first reported in 2013 by Voscopoulos et al. as a technique to manage pain after multiple rib fractures [76]. Like the ESP block, it involves using ultrasound guidance to visualize anatomical landmarks and inject local anesthetic between the lamina and erector spinae muscle (ESM) as seen in Fig. 8.33. The mechanism of action is similar to that of the ESP block, with the aim of spreading local anesthetic anteriorly into the paravertebral space. Limited evidence exists for the efficacy of retrolaminar blocks, with further research needed to establish its role in pain management (Table 8.13).

8.5.4 Midpoint Transverse Process Blocks

The midpoint transverse process block (MTPB) serves as an intermediary technique between the ESP block and the TPVB. It involves placing the needle tip and injecting the local anesthetic (LA) into the intertransverse muscular layer posterior to the SCTL [77], resulting in downward displacement of the pleura and effective diffusion of the injectate into the PVS (Fig. 8.34). Other similar techniques, such as the costotransverse block, the multiple-injection costotransverse (MIC) block, and the subtransverse process interligamentary block, have been reported in the literature with varying nomenclatures [78, 79]. Cadaveric studies suggest that these procedures may be more effective than the ESP block because the LA is injected closer to the PVS, making it more feasible for the anesthetic solution to cross the slits of the SCTL. However, currently, supporting literature consists mainly of small case series and case reports evaluated in breast and thoracic surgery and chest traumatology [80].

8.5.5 Paraspinal-Intercostal Plane Block

The term "paraspinal-intercostal plane block" refers to a group of regional procedures targeting the fascial plane lying on the ribs and intercostal

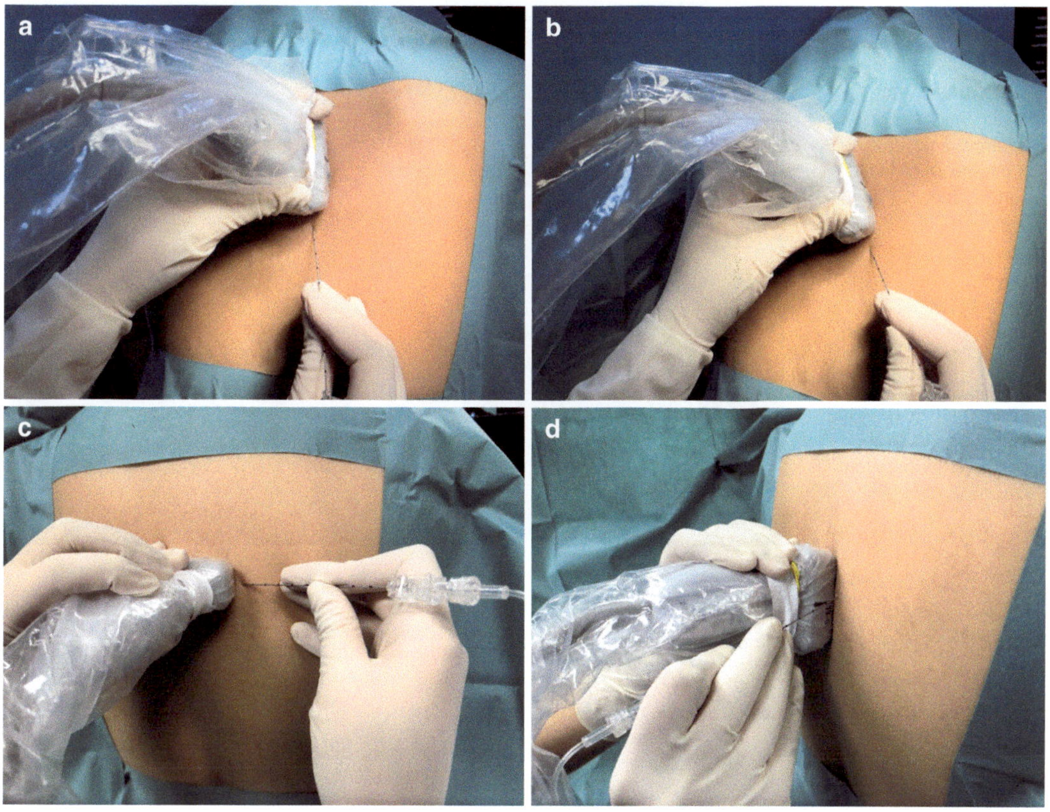

Fig. 8.31 (**a**) Thoracic paravertebral block. Longitudinal approach: the probe is positioned approximately 1.5 cm laterally and parallel to the interspinous line, intercepting two adjacent transverse processes (T3–T4 or T5–T6). The needle is inserted in an IP approach, directed from caudal to cranial. (**b**) Intermediate longitudinal approach: starting from the longitudinal position, the probe is rotated laterally by 45° to intercept the transverse process cranially and the rib inferiorly. This approach facilitates a more comfortable trajectory for needle insertion into the paravertebral space. The needle is inserted in an IP approach from lateral to medial. (**c**) Transverse approach. The probe is positioned transversely to the interspinous line, intercepting the transverse process, rib, and paravertebral space. The needle is inserted in an in-plane approach from lateral to medial. (**d**) Paravertebral block. The probe is positioned longitudinally to the interspinous line at the level of T3–T4 or T5–T6 transverse processes. The needle is inserted with an IP approach from posterior to anterior

muscles, as well as the overlying erector spinae muscle (Fig. 8.35). Depending on the lateral positioning of the injection point from the midline, the longissimus thoracis or iliocostalis muscles may be involved. This block targets the lateral cutaneous branches from T2 to T7 intercostal nerves. The first described technique involved the insertion of a multi-orifice catheter into this plane, providing continuous analgesia equivalent to thoracic epidural anesthesia for rib fractures. Similar approaches to the same target have been introduced under different names, including the rhomboid intercostal block, intercostal/paraspinal block, extrathoracic subparaspinal block, continuous intercostal nerve block, and posterior paramedian subrhomboidal block.

8.5.6 Rhomboid Intercostal Subserratus Plane Block

The rhomboid intercostal subserratus plane (RISS) block was initially described as a single-

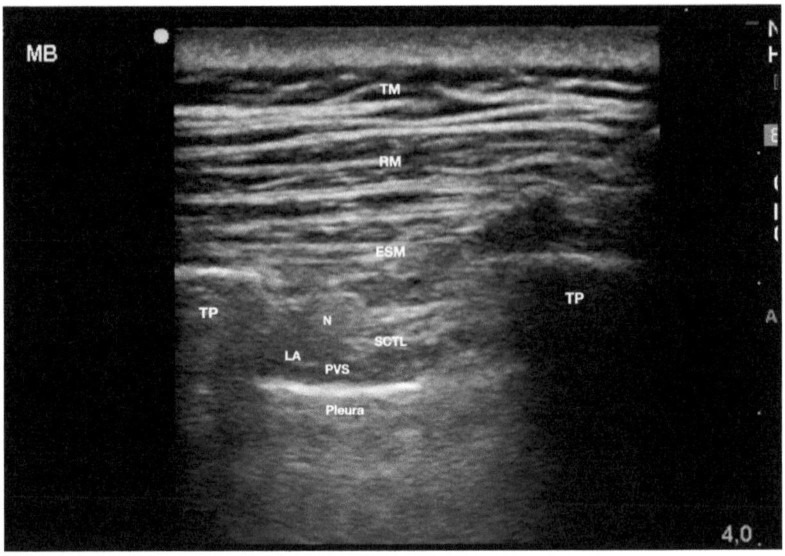

Fig. 8.32 Paravertebral block. The tip of the needle is placed in the paravertebral space crossing the superior costotransverse ligament, and the spread of local anesthetic determines the downward displacement of the pleura. *TP* transverse process, *TM* trapezius muscle, *RM* rhomboid muscle, *ESM* erector spinae muscle, *N* needle, *PVS* paravertebral space, *LA* local anesthetic, *SCTL* superior costotransverse ligament, *Pleura* pleura

Table 8.12 Thoracic paravertebral block tips and tricks

Thoracic paravertebral block tips and tricks
• The thoracic paravertebral block belongs to the advanced block, and it requires significant experience and skills
• The intermediate longitudinal approach is easier to perform as it enhances the pathway for the needle up to the paravertebral space
• The spread of local anesthetic into the paravertebral space and the subsequent downward displacement of the pleura may trigger a visceral reflex and vagal complications
• The patient is also asked to breathe deeply to allow better cranial and caudal diffusion of local anesthetic and reduce the visceral reflex of the block

injection or continuous technique for thoracic and breast surgery and for rib fractures [81, 82]. The most recent procedure involves the RISS combined with a deep SAP block to increase dermatomal coverage, involving the lateral branches from T2 to T7 up to T10 intercostal nerves. The first injection is performed at a specific site known as the anatomical "triangle of auscultation" between the ribs, plus the IM and the rhomboid major muscle, and the ESM (Fig. 8.36). The second injection (subserratus) is a deep SAP block used to cover the lower branches of the intercostal nerves.

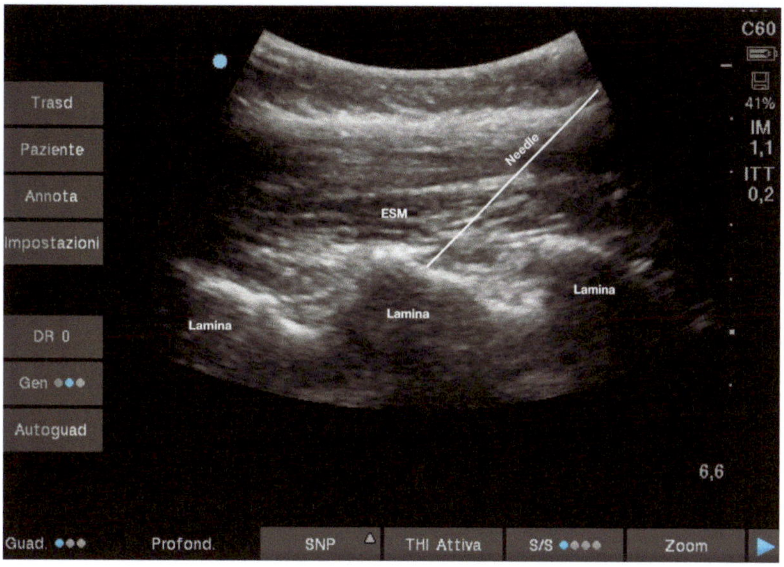

Fig. 8.33 Retrolaminar block. Through an in-plane approach, the tip of the needle is placed on the surface of the lamina, and the local anesthetic is injected between the lamina and the erector spinae muscle. *ESM* erector spinae muscle, *Lamina* lamina, *Needle* needle

Table 8.13 Summary of nervous and anatomical targets, injection site, local anesthetic volume, and concentrations of the main chest wall blocks

Technique	Nervous and anatomical targets	Injection site	Local anesthetic volume	Local anesthetic concentration
Parasternal intercostal plane (PIP) block	Anterior cutaneous branches of T2–T6 intercostal nerves. Medial chest region	Second and fourth intercostal spaces. Bilaterally for sternotomy	5–10 mL	Analgesia 0.125–0.25% Anesthesia 0.375–0.5%
Interpectoral plane block (PECS I)	Lateral and medial pectoral nerves. Pectoral muscles. Anterior chest region	Between pectoralis major and minor muscles	10 mL	Analgesia 0.125–0.25% Anesthesia 0.375–0.5%
Pectoserratus plane block (PECS II)	Lateral and medial pectoral nerves Lateral cutaneous branches of T2–T6 intercostal nerves Lateral chest region. Intercostobrachial, thoracodorsal, and thoracic longus nerves. Armpit	Fourth rib	20 mL	Analgesia 0.125–0.25% Anesthesia 0.375–0.5%
Serratus anterior plane block (SAPB)	Lateral cutaneous branches of T2–T7 intercostal nerves. Lateral chest region	Fifth rib. Superficial or deep to serratus anterior muscle	30 mL	Analgesia 0.125–0.25% Anesthesia 0.375–0.5%
Erector spinae block (ESP)	Ventral rami of the spinal nerves. Also dorsal rami when local anesthetic spread into the paravertebral space. Posterior and lateral chest wall. Intercostobrachial nerve	Cardiac surgery T4–T5 transverse processes	20–25 mL	Analgesia 0.125–0.25% Anesthesia 0.375–0.5%
Paravertebral block (PVB)	Ventral and dorsal rami of the spinal nerves. Posterior, anterior, and lateral chest wall. Intercostobrachial nerve	Two injections: T3–T4 and T6–T7	12–15 mL each injection	Analgesia 0.125–0.25% Anesthesia 0.375–0.5%
Retrolaminar block	Dorsal and ventral rami of spinal nerves. Posterior, anterior, and lateral chest wall	Injection in the plane between the vertebral lamina and the overlying muscle (transversospinalis and erector spinae muscle groups)	20–25 mL	Analgesia 0.125–0.25% Anesthesia 0.375–0.5%
Midpoint transverse process-to-pleura (MTP) block	Dorsal and ventral rami of spinal nerves. Posterior, anterior, and lateral chest wall	Injection deep and posterior to the transverse process but superficial and next to the superior costotransverse ligament	20–25 mL	Analgesia 0.125–0.25% Anesthesia 0.375–0.5%

(continued)

Table 8.13 (continued)

Technique	Nervous and anatomical targets	Injection site	Local anesthetic volume	Local anesthetic concentration
Paraspinal-intercostal plane blocks	Lateral cutaneous branches of T2–T7 intercostal nerves	Injection in the plane between the bony ribs plus intercostal muscles and the overlying erector spinae	20–25 mL	Analgesia 0.125–0.25% Anesthesia 0.375–0.5%
Rhomboid intercostal subserratus plane (RISS) block	Lateral cutaneous branches of T2–T7 intercostal nerves	First injection between the bony ribs plus intercostal muscles and the rhomboid major muscle plus erector spinae muscle. Second injection is into the same plane at a site that is more lateral and more inferior, where the overlying muscle is now serratus anterior muscle	20–25 mL	Analgesia 0.125–0.25% Anesthesia 0.375–0.5%

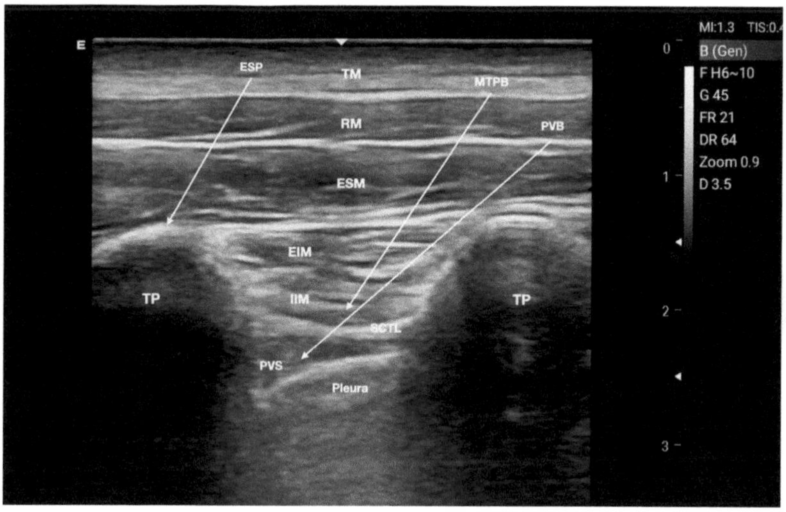

Fig. 8.34 Comparison between the midpoint transverse process block, erector spinae block, and paravertebral block. The midpoint transverse process block is performed by injecting local anesthetic into the muscular layer close and posteriorly to superior costotransverse ligament resulting in downward displacement of the pleura and effective spread of the injectate into the paravertebral space through the multiple fenestrations of the ligament. *TM* trapezius muscle, *RM* rhomboid muscle, *ESM* erector spinae muscle, *TP* transverse process, *PVS* paravertebral space, *SCTL* superior costotransverse ligament, *Pleura* pleura, *IIM* internal intercostal muscle, *EIM* external intercostal muscle, *ESP* erector spinae muscle block target, *MTPB* midpoint transverse process block target, *PVB* paravertebral bock target

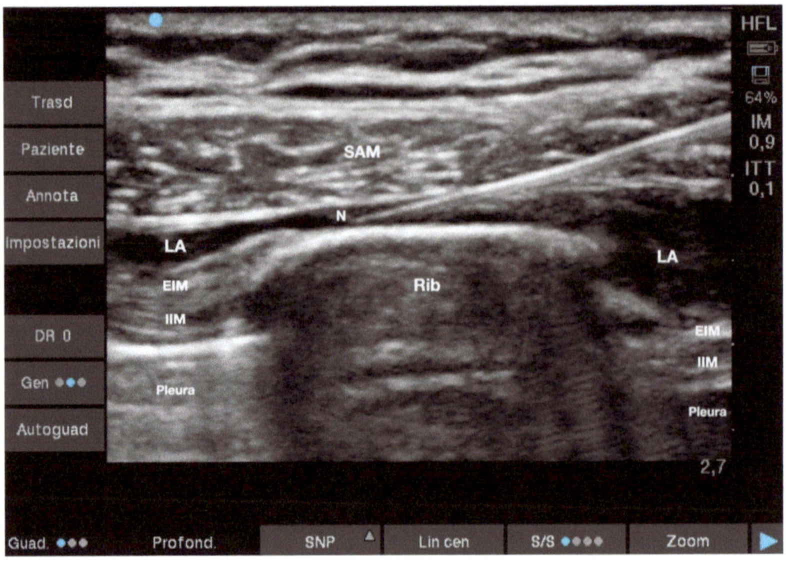

Fig. 8.35 Paraspinal-intercostal plane block. The local anesthetic targets the fascial plane above the ribs and the intercostal muscles. *SAM* serratus anterior muscle, *EIM* external intercostal muscle, *IIM* internal intercostal muscle, *LA* local anesthetic, *Rib* rib, *N* needle, *Pleura* pleura

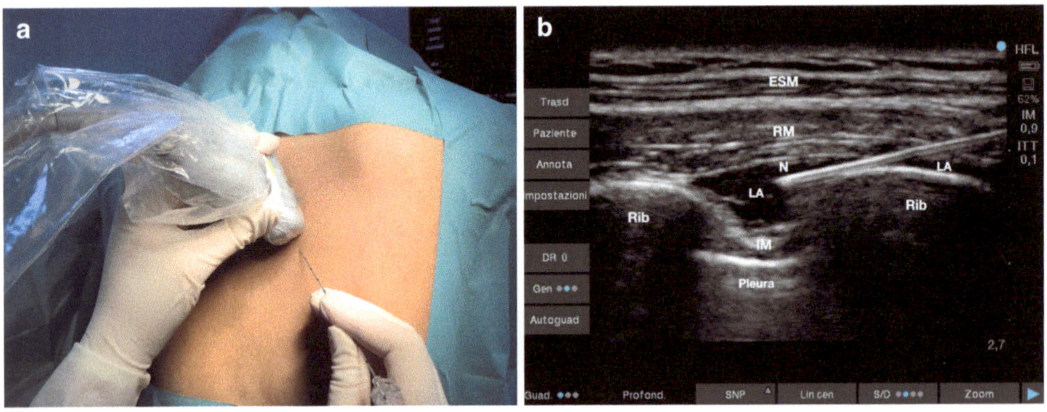

Fig. 8.36 Rhomboid intercostal subserratus plane block. (**a**) Patient and probe position. (**b**) The injection is performed at a very specific site named the anatomical "triangle of auscultation" between the ribs plus the intercostal muscle and the rhomboid major plus erector spinae muscles. *ESM* erector spinae muscle, *RM* rhomboid muscle, *IM* intercostal muscle, *Pleura* pleura, *Rib* rib, *LA* local anesthetic

8.6 Conclusion and Future Directions

Chest wall fascial blocks represent a significant advancement in regional anesthesia. They play a crucial role in managing pain in cardiac surgery due to their safety profile, relative simplicity, and proven efficacy, becoming integral to enhanced recovery multimodal opioid-sparing protocols. This has led to fast-track extubation, reduced incidence of pulmonary complications, and shortened stays in the intensive care unit. Additionally, they offer an attractive alternative to epidural anesthesia in anticoagulated cardiac surgery patients. Further research is focused on utilizing continuous catheter techniques and adjuvants to prolong block duration. Dynamic methods for performing the blocks could also be explored to achieve more homogeneous and widespread local anesthetic spread, potentially reducing injectate volume when blocks are performed for surgical purposes. There is significant potential for growth in this field, with pathways for research remaining to be explored, such as applications in awake cardiac surgery, emergency department settings, and chronic pain management.

References

1. Blanco R. The 'pecs block': a novel technique for providing analgesia after breast surgery. Anaesthesia. 2011;66(9):847–8. https://doi.org/10.1111/j.1365-2044.2011.06838.x.
2. Blanco R, Fajardo M, Parras MT. Ultrasound description of pecs II (modified pecs I): a novel approach to breast surgery. Rev Esp Anestesiol Reanim. 2012;59(9):470–5. https://doi.org/10.1016/j.redar.2012.07.003. Epub 2012 Aug 29.
3. Blanco R, Parras T, McDonnell JG, Prats-Galino A. Serratus plane block: a novel ultrasound-guided thoracic wall nerve block. Anaesthesia. 2013;68(11):1107–13. https://doi.org/10.1111/anae.12344. Epub 2013 Aug 7.
4. Warfield DJ Jr, Barre S, Adhikary SD. Current understanding of the fascial plane blocks for analgesia of the chest wall: techniques and indications update for 2020. Curr Opin Anaesthesiol. 2020;33(5):692–7. https://doi.org/10.1097/ACO.0000000000000909.
5. Balan C, Bubenek-Turconi SI, Tomescu DR, Valeanu L. Ultrasound-guided regional anesthesia-current strategies for enhanced recovery after cardiac surgery. Medicina (Kaunas). 2021;57(4):312. https://doi.org/10.3390/medicina57040312. PMID: 33806175; PMCID: PMC8065933.
6. Smith LM, Barrington MJ. Ultrasound-guided blocks for cardiovascular surgery: which block for which patient? Curr Opin Anaesthesiol. 2020;33(1):64–70. https://doi.org/10.1097/ACO.0000000000000818.
7. Chin KJ, Versyck B, Pawa A. Ultrasound-guided fascial plane blocks of the chest wall: a state-of-the-art review. Anaesthesia. 2021;76(Suppl 1):110–26. https://doi.org/10.1111/anae.15276.
8. Chin KJ, Versyck B, Elsharkawy H, Rojas Gomez MF, Sala-Blanch X, Reina MA. Anatomical basis of fascial plane blocks. Reg Anesth Pain Med. 2021;46(7):581–99. https://doi.org/10.1136/rapm-2021-102506.
9. Kubitz JC, Schubert AM, Schulte-Uentrop L. Enhanced Recovery After Surgery (ERAS®) in der Kardioanästhesie [Enhanced recovery after surgery (ERAS®) in cardiac anesthesia]. Anaesthesiologie. 2022;71(9):663–73. https://doi.org/10.1007/s00101-022-01190-z. Epub 2022 Aug 20.
10. Engelman DT, Ben Ali W, Williams JB, Perrault LP, Reddy VS, Arora RC, et al. Guidelines for perioperative care in cardiac surgery: enhanced recovery after surgery society recommendations. JAMA Surg. 2019;154:755–66.
11. Wong WT, Lai VK, Chee YE, Lee A. Fast-track cardiac care for adult cardiac surgical patients. Cochrane Database Syst Rev. 2016;9:CD003587.
12. Bainbridge D, Cheng D. Current evidence on fast track cardiac recovery management. Eur Heart J Suppl. 2017;19(Suppl A):A3–7.
13. Helwani MA, Copeland C, Ridley CH, Kaiser HA, De Wet CJ. A 3-hour fast-track extubation protocol for early extubation after cardiac surgery. JTCVS Open. 2022;12:299–305. https://doi.org/10.1016/j.xjon.2022.07.006. PMID: 36590715; PMCID: PMC9801240.
14. MacLeod JB, D'Souza K, Aguiar C, Brown CD, Pozeg Z, White C, Arora RC, Légaré JF, Hassan A. Fast tracking in cardiac surgery: is it safe? J Cardiothorac Surg. 2022;17(1):69. https://doi.org/10.1186/s13019-022-01815-9. PMID: 35382846; PMCID: PMC8983083.
15. Hong B, Oh C, Jo Y, Lee S, Park S, Kim YH. Current evidence of ultrasound-guided fascial plane blocks for cardiac surgery: a narrative literature review. Korean J Anesthesiol. 2022;75(6):460–72. https://doi.org/10.4097/kja.22564. Epub 2022 Oct 17. PMID: 36245347; PMCID: PMC9726460.
16. Yu S, Aljure OD. Regional analgesia in cardiac anesthesia: welcoming a new era in perioperative pain management. J Card Surg. 2021;36(8):2824–5. https://doi.org/10.1111/jocs.15667. Epub 2021 Jun 10.
17. Sharma R, Louie A, Thai CP, Dizdarevic A. Chest wall nerve blocks for cardiothoracic, breast surgery, and rib-related pain. Curr Pain Headache Rep. 2022;26(1):43–56. https://doi.org/10.1007/s11916-022-01001-5. Epub 2022 Jan 28.
18. Kelava M, Alfirevic A, Bustamante S, Hargrave J, Marciniak D. Regional anesthesia in cardiac surgery: an overview of fascial plane chest wall blocks. Anesth Analg. 2020;131(1):127–35. https://doi.org/10.1213/ANE.0000000000004682.
19. Mittnacht AJC, Shariat A, Weiner MM, Malhotra A, Miller MA, Mahajan A, Bhatt HV. Regional techniques for cardiac and cardiac-related procedures. J Cardiothorac Vasc Anesth. 2019;33(2):532–46. https://doi.org/10.1053/j.jvca.2018.09.017. Epub 2018 Sep 13.
20. Caruso TJ, Lawrence K, Tsui BCH. Regional anesthesia for cardiac surgery. Curr Opin Anaesthesiol. 2019;32(5):674–82. https://doi.org/10.1097/ACO.0000000000000769.
21. El-Boghdadly K, Wolmarans M, Stengel AD, Albrecht E, Chin KJ, Elsharkawy H, et al. Standardizing nomenclature in regional anesthesia: an ASRA-ESRA Delphi consensus study of abdominal wall, paraspinal, and chest wall blocks. Reg Anesth Pain Med. 2021;46:571–80.
22. Sepolvere G, Coppolino F, Tedesco M, Cristiano L. Ultrasound-guided parasternal blocks: techniques, clinical indications and future prospects. Minerva Anestesiol. 2021;87(12):1338–46. https://doi.org/10.23736/S0375-9393.21.15599-3. Epub 2021 Oct 11.

23. Haskins SC, Memtsoudis SG. Fascial plane blocks for cardiac surgery: new frontiers in analgesia and nomenclature. Anesth Analg. 2020;131(1):125–6. https://doi.org/10.1213/ANE.0000000000004744.
24. Fusco P, Petrucci E, Marinangeli F, Scimia P. Block failure or lack of efficacy? The "double V" sign: a novel sonographic sign for a successful interfascial plane block. Minerva Anestesiol. 2019;85(8):917–8. https://doi.org/10.23736/S0375-9393.19.13457-8.
25. Elsharkawy H, Pawa A, Mariano ER. Interfascial plane blocks: back to basics. Reg Anesth Pain Med. 2018 May;43(4):341–6. https://doi.org/10.1097/AAP.0000000000000750.
26. Scimia P, Gentili L, Fusco P, Tedesco M, Tognu A, Sepolvere G. When a TAP becomes a QL block: a dynamic way to perform the fascial blocks. Minerva Anestesiol. 2022;88(11):976–8. https://doi.org/10.23736/S0375-9393.22.16772-6.
27. Fusco P, Petroni GM, Ciaschi W, Tonelli E, Marinangeli F, Stecco C. Dynamic double V sign: another step to the efficacy of fascial plane block. Minerva Anestesiol. 2022;88(12):1079–81. https://doi.org/10.23736/S0375-9393.22.16773-8.
28. Szamborski M, Janc J, Rosińczuk J, Janc JJ, Leśnik P, Łysenko L. Use of ultrasound-guided interfascial plane blocks in anterior and lateral thoracic wall region as safe method for patient anesthesia and analgesia: review of techniques and approaches during COVID-19 pandemic. Int J Environ Res Public Health. 2022;19(14):8696. https://doi.org/10.3390/ijerph19148696. PMID: 35886547; PMCID: PMC9320164.
29. Sepolvere G, Fusco P, Tedesco M, Scimia P. Bilateral ultrasound-guided parasternal block for postoperative analgesia in cardiac surgery: could it be the safest strategy? Reg Anesth Pain Med. 2020;45(4):316–7. https://doi.org/10.1136/rapm-2019-100872. Epub 2020 Jan 20.
30. Sepolvere G, Tedesco M, Cristiano L. Ultrasound guided parasternal block with dexmedetomidine as effective approach for postoperative analgesia in cardiac surgery. Minerva Anestesiol. 2020;86(7):789–90. https://doi.org/10.23736/S0375-9393.20.14356-6. Epub 2020 Mar 6
31. Droghetti A, Fusco P, Marini M, Harizai F, Scimia P. Ultrasound-guided serratus anterior plane block and parasternal block in cooperative sedation for S-ICD implantation. Pacing Clin Electrophysiol. 2019;42(7):1076–8. https://doi.org/10.1111/pace.13727. Epub 2019 Jun 4
32. King M, Stambulic T, Hassan SMA, Norman PA, Derry K, Payne DM, El Diasty M. Median sternotomy pain after cardiac surgery: to block, or not? A systematic review and meta-analysis. J Card Surg. 2022;37(11):3729–42. https://doi.org/10.1111/jocs.16882. Epub 2022 Sep 13
33. de la Torre PA, García PD, Alvarez SL, Miguel FJ, Pérez MF. A novel ultrasound-guided block: a promising alternative for breast analgesia. Aesthet Surg J. 2014;34:198–200.
34. Fusco P, Scimia P, Petrucci E, Carlo DI, S, Marinangeli F. The ultrasound-guided parasternal block: a novel approach for anesthesia and analgesia in breast cancer surgery. Minerva Anestesiol. 2017;83(2):221–2. https://doi.org/10.23736/S0375-9393.16.11546-9. Epub 2016 Oct 4.
35. Scimia P, Gentili L, Tedesco M, Fusco P, Sepolvere G. A modified approach to a parasternal block: a case report. A A Pract. 2023;17(1):e01644. https://doi.org/10.1213/XAA.0000000000001644.
36. Scimia P, Fusco P. The ultrasound-guided parasternal block: the story continues. Minerva Anestesiol. 2020;86(7):790–1. https://doi.org/10.23736/S0375-9393.20.14535-8. Epub 2020 Mar 6.
37. Sepolvere G, Tedesco M, Cristiano L. Ultrasound parasternal block as a novel approach for cardiac sternal surgery: could it be the safest strategy? J Cardiothorac Vasc Anesth. 2020;34(8):2284–6. https://doi.org/10.1053/j.jvca.2020.03.014. Epub 2020 Mar 19.
38. Costa F, Caruso S, Pascarella G, Nenna A, Grande S, Sarubbi D, Chello M, Agrò FE. Sternotomy debridement in critical patient with difficult predicted airway: can regional anesthesia be the labyrinth exit? Minerva Anestesiol. 2020;86(4):462–3. https://doi.org/10.23736/S0375-9393.19.14133-8. Epub 2019 Dec 9.
39. Dost B, Taflan MG, Kaya C, Gurz S, Tulgar S. Awake sternal fixation using the ultrasound-guided superficial parasternal intercostal plane block in a patient with cervical spine fracture. Cureus. 2022;14(8):e28618. https://doi.org/10.7759/cureus.28618. PMID: 36185906; PMCID: PMC9523735.
40. Ueshima H, Kitamura A. Blocking of multiple anterior branches of intercostal nerves (Th2-6) using a transversus thoracic muscle plane block. Reg Anesth Pain Med. 2015;40:388.
41. Fujii S, Roche M, Jones PM, Vissa D, Bainbridge D, Zhou JR. Transversus thoracis muscle plane block in cardiac surgery: a pilot feasibility study. Reg Anesth Pain Med. 2019;44:556–60.
42. Aydin ME, Ahiskalioglu A, Ates I, Tor IH, Borulu F, Erguney OD, et al. Efficacy of ultrasound-guided transversus thoracic muscle plane block on postoperative opioid consumption after cardiac surgery: a prospective, randomized, double-blind study. J Cardiothorac Vasc Anesth. 2020;34:2996–3003.
43. Zhang Y, Li X, Chen S. Bilateral transversus thoracis muscle plane block provides effective analgesia and enhances recovery after open cardiac surgery. J Card Surg. 2021;36:2818–23.
44. Zhang Y, Min J, Chen S. Sensory assessment and block duration of deep parasternal intercostal plane block in patients undergoing cardiac surgery: a prospective observational study. Pain Ther. 2022;11(3):951–8. https://doi.org/10.1007/s40122-022-00403-y. Epub 2022 Jun 25. PMID: 35751781; PMCID: PMC9314528.
45. Sepolvere G, Tognù A, Tedesco M, Coppolino F, Cristiano L. Avoiding the internal mammary artery

during parasternal blocks: ultrasound identification and technique considerations. J Cardiothorac Vasc Anesth. 2021;35(6):1594–602. https://doi.org/10.1053/j.jvca.2020.11.007. Epub 2020 Nov 16.
46. Liu G, Gao M, Hu Y, Wang B, Lin Y, Guan Y, Chen G, Zhang P, Hu Y, Cai Q, Qin W. Effects of ultrasound-guided transversus thoracic muscle plane block on postoperative pain and side effects: a systematic review and meta-analysis of randomized controlled trials. J Cardiothorac Vasc Anesth. 2023;37(5):788–800. https://doi.org/10.1053/j.jvca.2022.11.001. Epub 2022 Nov 5.
47. Capuano P, Toscano A, Sepolvere G, Tedesco M, Martucci G, Burgio G, Arcadipane A. Parasternal intercostal blocks for cardiac and breast surgery: less is more? J Cardiothorac Vasc Anesth. 2023;37(12):2688–9. https://doi.org/10.1053/j.jvca.2023.09.003. Epub 2023 Sep 6.
48. Padala SRAN, Badhe AS, Parida S, Jha AK. Comparison of preincisional and postincisional parasternal intercostal block on postoperative pain in cardiac surgery. J Card Surg. 2020;35(7):1525–30. https://doi.org/10.1111/jocs.14651. Epub 2020 Jun 24.
49. Zou M, Ruan W, Liu J, Xu J. Preemptive parasternal intercostal nerve block for patients undergoing off-pump coronary artery bypass grafting: a double-blind, randomized, controlled trial. Front Cardiovasc Med. 2023;10:1188518. https://doi.org/10.3389/fcvm.2023.1188518. PMID: 37273884; PMCID: PMC10233104.
50. Sepolvere G, Tedesco M, Fusco P, Scimia P, Donatiello V, Cristiano L. Subxiphoid cardiac drainage pain management: could ultrasound rectus sheath block be the answer? Minerva Anestesiol. 2020;86(9):994–6. https://doi.org/10.23736/S0375-9393.20.14576-0. Epub 2020 May 18.
51. Kang H, Chung YS, Choe JW, Woo YC, Kim SW, Park SJ, et al. Application of lidocaine jelly on chest tubes to reduce pain caused by drainage catheter after coronary artery bypass surgery. J Korean Med Sci. 2014;29:1398–403.
52. Yamamoto T, Seino Y, Matsuda K, Imai H, Bamba K, Sugimoto A, Shiraishi S, Schindler E. Preoperative implementation of transverse thoracic muscle plane block and rectus sheath block combination for pediatric cardiac surgery. J Cardiothorac Vasc Anesth. 2020;34(12):3367–72. https://doi.org/10.1053/j.jvca.2020.07.041. Epub 2020 Jul 16.
53. Everett L, Davis TA, Deshpande SP, Mondal S. Implementation of bilateral rectus sheath blocks in conjunction with transversus thoracis plane and pectointercostal fascial blocks for immediate postoperative analgesia after cardiac surgery. Cureus. 2022;14(7):e26592. https://doi.org/10.7759/cureus.26592. PMID: 35936156; PMCID: PMC9354918.
54. Toscano A, Balzani E, Capuano P, Vaninetti A, Perrucci C, Simonato E, Rinaldi M, Brazzi L. Awake cardiac surgery using the novel pectoralis-intercostal-rectus sheath (PIRS) plane block and subxiphoid approach. J Card Surg. 2022;37(9):2923–6. https://doi.org/10.1111/jocs.16658. Epub 2022 Jun 4.
55. Cibelli M, Brodier EA, Smith FG. Pectoralis-intercostal-rectus sheath (PIRS) plane block with catheters. A new technique to provide analgesia in cardiac surgery. J Cardiothorac Vasc Anesth. 2020;34(3):846–7. https://doi.org/10.1053/j.jvca.2019.09.014. Epub 2019 Sep 18
56. Toscano A, Capuano P, Attisani M, Rinaldi M, Brazzi L. Transversus thoracic plane block and rectus sheath block for left ventricular assist device implantation via full median sternotomy: a case report. J Card Surg. 2022;37(7):2115–9. https://doi.org/10.1111/jocs.16391. Epub 2022 Mar 7.
57. Kumar KN, Kalyane RN, Singh NG, Nagaraja PS, Krishna M, Babu B, Varadaraju R, Sathish N, Manjunatha N. Efficacy of bilateral pectoralis nerve block for ultrafast tracking and postoperative pain management in cardiac surgery. Ann Card Anaesth. 2018;21(3):333–8. https://doi.org/10.4103/aca.ACA_15_18. PMID: 30052231; PMCID: PMC6078028.
58. Magoon R, Kaushal B, Chauhan S, Bhoi D, Bisoi AK, Khan MA. A randomised controlled comparison of serratus anterior plane, pectoral nerves and intercostal nerve block for post-thoracotomy analgesia in adult cardiac surgery. Indian J Anaesth. 2020;64(12):1018–24. https://doi.org/10.4103/ija.IJA_566_20. Epub 2020 Dec 12. PMID: 33542564; PMCID: PMC7852449.
59. Toscano A, Capuano P, Costamagna A, Burzio C, Ellena M, Scala V, Pasero D, Rinaldi M, Brazzi L. The serratus anterior plane study: continuous deep serratus anterior plane block for mitral valve surgery performed in right minithoracotomy. J Cardiothorac Vasc Anesth. 2020;34(11):2975–82. https://doi.org/10.1053/j.jvca.2020.05.021. Epub 2020 May 27.
60. Sepolvere G, Scialdone VR. Single shot serratus anterior plane block for post-thoracotomy pain management in cardiac surgery: could it be enough? Minerva Anestesiol. 2022;88(9):748–9. https://doi.org/10.23736/S0375-9393.22.16467-9. Epub 2022 May 25.
61. He Y, Li Z, Xu M, Du B, Zuo Y. Single-injection serratus anterior plane block for cardiothoracic surgery via thoracotomy in children: a systematic review and meta-analysis of randomised controlled trials. BMJ Paediatr Open. 2023;7(1):e001912. https://doi.org/10.1136/bmjpo-2023-001912. PMID: 37316297; PMCID: PMC10277543.
62. Forero M, Adhikary SD, Lopez H, Tsui C, Chin KJ. The erector spinae plane block: a novel analgesic technique in thoracic neuropathic pain. Reg Anesth Pain Med. 2016;41(5):621–7. https://doi.org/10.1097/AAP.0000000000000451.
63. King M, Stambulic T, Servito M, Mizubuti GB, Payne D, El-Diasty M. Erector spinae plane block as perioperative analgesia for midline sternotomy in cardiac surgery: a systematic review and meta-analysis. J Card

Surg. 2022;37(12):5220–9. https://doi.org/10.1111/jocs.17005. Epub 2022 Oct 11.
64. Dost B, Kaya C, Turunc E, Dokmeci H, Yucel SM, Karakaya D. Erector spinae plane block versus its combination with superficial parasternal intercostal plane block for postoperative pain after cardiac surgery: a prospective, randomized, double-blind study. BMC Anesthesiol. 2022;22(1):295. https://doi.org/10.1186/s12871-022-01832-0. PMID: 36114466; PMCID: PMC9479438.
65. Keshwani M, Dey S, Arora P, Singha SK. A randomized trial to compare the analgesic effect of pecto-intercostal fascial plane block with erector spinae plane block after mid-sternotomy incision for cardiac surgery. Kardiochir Torakochirurgia Pol. 2023;20(3):167–72. https://doi.org/10.5114/kitp.2023.132057. Epub 2023 Oct 30. PMID: 37937164; PMCID: PMC10626400.
66. Cho TH, Kwon HJ, Jehoon O, Cho J, Kim SH, Yang HM. The pathway of injectate spread during thoracic intertransverse process (ITP) block: micro-computed tomography findings and anatomical evaluations. J Clin Anesth. 2022;77:110646.
67. Cho TH, Kim SH, Jehoon O, Kwon HJ, Kim KW, Yang HM. Anatomy of the thoracic paravertebral space: 3D micro-CT findings and their clinical implications for nerve blockade. Reg Anesth Pain Med. 2021;46:699–703.
68. Sepolvere G, Tedesco M, Fusco P, Scimia P, Cristiano L. Fascial plane blocks in cardiac surgery: a future to discover. Minerva Anestesiol. 2021;87(3):382–3. https://doi.org/10.23736/S0375-9393.20.15271-4. Epub 2020 Dec 17.
69. D'Ercole F, Arora H, Kumar PA. Paravertebral block for thoracic surgery. J Cardiothorac Vasc Anesth. 2018;32(2):915–27. https://doi.org/10.1053/j.jvca.2017.10.003. Epub 2017 Oct 4.
70. Naganuma M, Tokita T, Sato Y, Kasai T, Kudo Y, Suzuki N, Masuda S, Nagaya K. Efficacy of preoperative bilateral thoracic paravertebral block in cardiac surgery requiring full heparinization: a propensity-matched study. J Cardiothorac Vasc Anesth. 2022;36(2):477–82. https://doi.org/10.1053/j.jvca.2021.05.001. Epub 2021 May 13.
71. El Shora HA, El Beleehy AA, Abdelwahab AA, Ali GA, Omran TE, Hassan EA, Arafat AA. Bilateral paravertebral block versus thoracic epidural analgesia for pain control post-cardiac surgery: a randomized controlled trial. Thorac Cardiovasc Surg. 2020;68(5):410–6. https://doi.org/10.1055/s--0038-1668496. Epub 2018 Aug 16.
72. Scarfe AJ, Schuhmann-Hingel S, Duncan JK, Ma N, Atukorale YN, Cameron AL. Continuous paravertebral block for post-cardiothoracic surgery analgesia: a systematic review and meta-analysis. Eur J Cardiothorac Surg. 2016;50(6):1010–8. https://doi.org/10.1093/ejcts/ezw168. Epub 2016 May 30.
73. Tahara S, Inoue A, Sakamoto H, Tatara Y, Masuda K, Hattori Y, Nozumi Y, Miyagi M, Sigdel S. A case series of continuous paravertebral block in minimally invasive cardiac surgery. JA Clin Rep. 2017;3(1):45. https://doi.org/10.1186/s40981-017-0119-0. Epub 2017 Aug 29. PMID: 29457089; PMCID: PMC5804641.
74. Okitsu K, Iritakenishi T, Iwasaki M, Imada T, Fujino Y. Risk of hematoma in patients with a bleeding risk undergoing cardiovascular surgery with a paravertebral catheter. J Cardiothorac Vasc Anesth. 2017;31(2):453–7. https://doi.org/10.1053/j.jvca.2016.06.002. Epub 2016 Jun 3.
75. Nisi F, Sella N, Gregorio DI, Lubian M, Giustiniano E, Rosboch GL, Balzani E, Toscano A, Strano G, Rispoli M, Massullo D, Fiorelli S, Santonastaso D, Agnoletti V, Piccioni F. The safety of thoracic paravertebral block and erector spinae plane block in patients treated with anticoagulant or antiplatelet therapy. A narrative review of the evidence. Minerva Anestesiol. 2023;89:914. https://doi.org/10.23736/S0375-9393.23.17288-9. Epub ahead of print.
76. Voscopoulos C, Palaniappan D, Zeballos J, Ko H, Janfaza D, Vlassakov K. The ultrasound-guided retrolaminar block. Can J Anaesth. 2013;60:888–95.
77. Pfeiffer G, Oppitz N, Schöne S, Richter-Heine I, Höhne M, Koltermann C. Analgesie der Achselhöhle durch Paravertebralkatheter in Laminatechnik [Analgesia of the axilla using a paravertebral catheter in the lamina technique]. Anaesthesist. 2006;55(4):423–7. German. https://doi.org/10.1007/s00101-005-0969-0.
78. Nielsen MV, Moriggl B, Hoermann R, Nielsen TD, Bendtsen TF, Børglum J. Are single-injection erector spinae plane block and multiple-injection costotransverse block equivalent to thoracic paravertebral block? Acta Anaesthesiol Scand. 2019;63:1231–8.
79. Ohgoshi Y, Usui Y, Ando A, Takeda Y, Ohtsuka A. Injection at the costotransverse notch facilitates paravertebral spread of the erector spinae plane block: a cadaveric study. J Clin Anesth. 2020;61:109630.
80. Chen X, Yang J, Xia M, Wu H, Wang S, Zhang W. Single-injection midpoint transverse process-to-pleura block versus thoracic paravertebral block for postoperative analgesia after uniportal video-assisted thoracoscopic surgery: a randomized controlled trial. J Cardiothorac Vasc Anesth. 2022;36(8 Pt A):2432–8. https://doi.org/10.1053/j.jvca.2021.12.036. Epub 2022 Jan 2
81. Ökmen K. Efficacy of rhomboid intercostal block for analgesia after thoracotomy. Korean J Pain. 2019;32(2):129–32. https://doi.org/10.3344/kjp.2019.32.2.129. PMID: 31091512; PMCID: PMC6549589.
82. Elsharkawy H, Ince I, Pawa A. Rhomboid intercostal and sub-serratus (RISS) plane block for analgesia after lung transplant. J Clin Anesth. 2019;56:85–7. https://doi.org/10.1016/j.jclinane.2019.01.042. Epub 2019 Jan 28.

9 Anterior and Posterior Abdominal Wall Blocks

Giuseppe Sepolvere, Loredana Cristiano, Andrea Tognù, and Mario Tedesco

9.1 Introduction

The anterior and posterior abdominal wall blocks discussed in this chapter are:

- Transversus abdominis plane (TAP) block - Oblique subcostal transversus abdominis plane (SCTAP) block
- Rectus sheath block (RSB)
- Ilioinguinal and iliohypogastric (II and IH) block
- Erector spinae block (ESP)
- Quadratus lumborum block (QLB)

The indications and complications of abdominal wall blocks for cardio and vascular surgery procedures are reported in Table 9.1. The volume and dosages are listed in Table 9.2.

G. Sepolvere (✉) · L. Cristiano
Department of Anesthesia and Cardiac Surgery Intensive Care Unit, San Michele Hospital, Maddaloni, Caserta, Italy

A. Tognù
Department of Anesthesia, Intensive Care and Pain Therapy, Orthopedic University Hospital Rizzoli, Bologna, Italy
e-mail: andrea.tognu@ior.it

M. Tedesco
Department of Anesthesia and Intensive Care Unit and Pain Therapy, Mater Dei Hospital, Bari, Italy

9.1.1 Transversus Abdominis Plane (TAP) Block

Aortic-bifemoral bypass is a surgery chosen for patients with Leriche syndrome or severe peripheral arteriopathy. This procedure implies a laparotomy supra and infraumbilical. That translates into a severe pain during postoperative period. Therefore, pain management becomes a key pilar for early recovery. Cardiovascular anesthesiologists usually choose low thoracic epidural to control pain. However, the circumstances of some patients make it a non-feasible technique. In those cases, TAP block represents a valid alternative reducing pain, morbidity and the length of stay in hospital. TAP block was first described by Rafi as a blind technique and then developed by the use of ultrasound [1].

The anterior branches of T7–T12 intercostal nerves and the anterior branch of the spinal nerve L1 run between the internal oblique (IOM) and transversus abdominis (TAM) muscles, which represent the anatomical target of TAP block. The procedures may be performed for lower abdominal and infraumbilical surgeries [2–5]. With the patient supine, the probe is placed transversely at midpoint between the lower rib and iliac crest in the midaxillary line in order to visualize the external oblique (EOM), IOM, and TAM. A volume of 20–25 mL of local anesthetic is injected into the fascial plane between the IOM and TAM. Usually, the block is performed bilaterally [6] (Fig. 9.1). Recent studies and meta-analysis demonstrated

G. Sepolvere, S. Silvetti (eds.), *Fast-Track in Cardiac Anesthesia*,
https://doi.org/10.1007/978-3-031-70899-2_9

Table 9.1 Indications and complications of abdominal wall blocks

Block	Indication	Complications
TAP	• Aortobifemoral bypass	• Peritoneal perforation • Visceral injury • Intraperitoneal injection • Local anesthetic systemic toxicity • Hematoma
SCTAP	• Aortobifemoral bypass	• Peritoneal perforation • Visceral injury • Intraperitoneal injection • Local anesthetic systemic toxicity • Hematoma
RSB	• Subxiphoid drainages pain management	• Peritoneal perforation • Visceral injury • Intraperitoneal injection • Local anesthetic systemic toxicity • Hematoma
II and IH	• Transcatheter Aortic Valve Implantation (TAVI)	• Peritoneal perforation • Visceral injury • Intraperitoneal injection • Local anesthetic systemic toxicity • Hematoma
ESP	• Cardiac surgery—minithoracotomy • Visceral pain management after abdominal vascular surgery	• Pneumothorax • Lipotimia • Local anesthetic systemic toxicity
QLB	• Femoral-femoral bypass graft placement	• Peritoneal perforation • Visceral injury • Intraperitoneal injection • Local anesthetic systemic toxicity • Hematoma • Spread to the lumbar plexus or femoral nerve (quadriceps weakness)

Table 9.2 Volume and dosages of abdominal wall blocks

Block	Volume and dosages
TAP	Analgesia: 20–25 mL Levobupivacaine or ropivacaine 0.125–0.25%
SCTAP	Analgesia: 20–25 mL Levobupivacaine or ropivacaine 0.125–0.25%
RSB	Analgesia: 20 mL Levobupivacaine or ropivacaine 0.125–0.25%
II and IH	Analgesia: 10 mL Levobupivacaine or ropivacaine 0.125–0.25%
ESP	Analgesia: 20–25 mL Levobupivacaine or ropivacaine 0.125–0.25%
QLB	Analgesia: 20–25 mL Levobupivacaine or ropivacaine 0.125–0.25%

that local anesthetic volume may spread to the paravertebral space, providing visceral analgesia, if the technique is performed by the hydrodissection of the fascial plane advancing the needle until the quadratus lumborum muscle (QLBM) and confirming the dynamic way to perform a fascial block [7–9] (Figs. 9.2 and 9.3).

9.1.2 Oblique Subcostal Transversus Abdominis Plane (SCTAP) Block

The SCTAP was first described by Hebbard in 2008 and performed for supra-umbilical abdominal surgeries. As with TAP block, the SCTAP is used for the aortic-bifemoral bypass surgery covering the upper abdominal region. The terminal branches of the T6–T9 spinal nerves lie into the fascial plane between the IOM and TAM and represent the target for SCTAP [10]. With the patient supine, the probe is placed obliquely and parallel to the costal edge and then moved laterally until rectus abdominis (RAM), EOM, IOM, and TAM are visualized. A

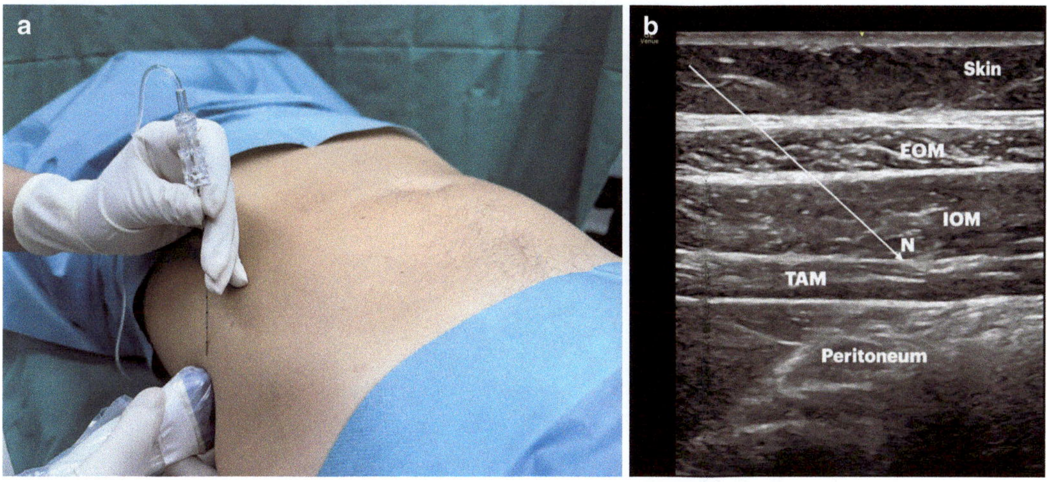

Fig. 9.1 Transversus abdominis plane block. (**a**) Patient and probe position. (**b**) Landmarks and transversus abdominis plane block. The local anesthetic is injected between the internal oblique and transversus abdominis muscle. *Skin* skin, *EOM* external oblique muscle, *IOM* internal oblique muscle, *TAM* transversus abdominis muscle, *Peritoneum* peritoneum, *N* needle

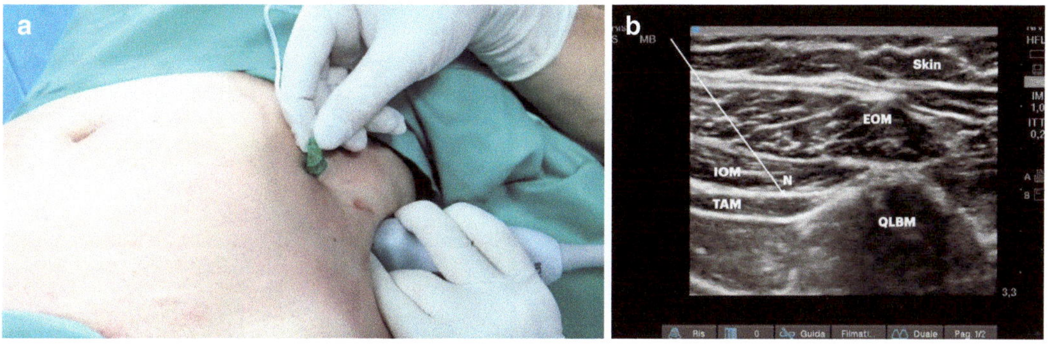

Fig. 9.2 Dynamic transversus abdominis plane block. (**a**) Patient and probe position. (**b**) The local anesthetic is injected between the internal oblique and transversus abdominis muscle through the fascial hydrodissection towards the quadratus lumborum muscle. *Skin* skin, *EOM* external oblique muscle, *IOM* internal oblique muscle, *TAM* transversus abdominis muscle, *QLBM* quadratus lumborum muscle, *Peritoneum* peritoneum, *N* needle, *LA* local anesthetic

volume of 20 mL of local anesthetic is injected into the fascial plane between the IOM and TAM (Fig. 9.4). Both TAP and SCTAP allow a catheter placement for the local anesthetic continuous infusion (Fig. 9.5).

9.1.3 Rectus Abdominis Sheath Block (RSB)

The RSB provides somatic analgesia to the anteromedial abdominal wall and periumbilical area after midline laparotomy abdominal surgery targeting the anterior cutaneous branches from T9 to T12 intercostal nerves. First described as a blind technique in 1899 by Schleich, the introduction of ultrasound made the ultrasound-guided RSB a safe and effective ERAS procedure reducing the opioid requirements and avoiding many complications related to neuraxial techniques and vascular injury. It is used in combination with the parasternal block providing analgesia to the entire anterior chest wall region and to manage pain deriving from subxiphoid

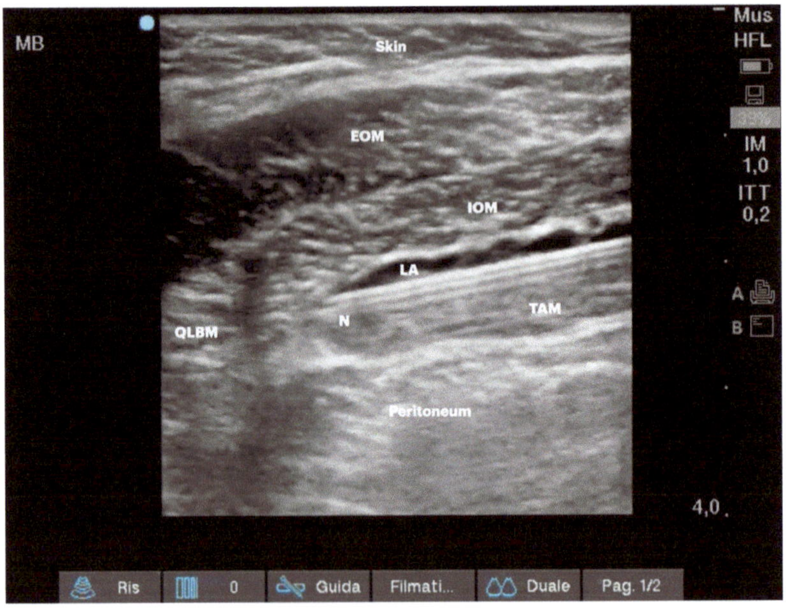

Fig. 9.3 Dynamic transversus abdominis plane block. The local anesthetic is injected between the internal oblique and transversus abdominis muscle through the fascial hydrodissection towards the quadratus lumborum muscle. *EOM* external oblique muscle, *IOM* internal oblique muscle, *TAM* transversus abdominis muscle, *QLBM* quadratus lumborum muscle, *Peritoneum* peritoneum, *N* needle, *LA* local anesthetic, *Skin* skin

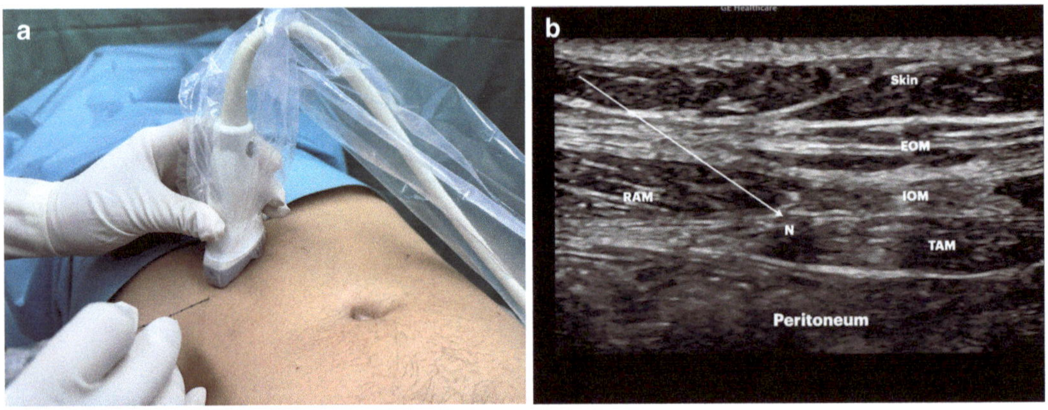

Fig. 9.4 Subcostal transversus abdominis plane block. (**a**) Patient and probe position. (**b**) The local anesthetic is injected between the internal oblique and transversus abdominis muscles. *Skin* skin, *EOM* external oblique muscle, *IOM* internal oblique muscle, *TAM* transversus abdominis muscle, *QLBM* quadratus lumborum muscle, *Peritoneum* peritoneum, *N* needle

drainages. It is described in detail in Chap. 8. With the patient in supine position, a high-frequency linear probe is placed transversely above the umbilical scar until the left and right rectus sheath muscles (LRAM and RRAM), and their sheaths are visualized. Through an in-plane approach and a bilateral injection (lateral to medial first and medial to lateral subsequently), a volume of 15–20 mL of LA for each side is deposited between the RAM and its sheath (Fig. 9.6).

9.1.4 Ilioinguinal (II) and Iliohypogastric (IH) Blocks

Transcatheter aortic valve implantation (TAVI) is becoming a valuable alternative to surgical aortic valve replacement in patients with severe aortic stenosis that are at high surgical risk or deemed inoperable. The optimal anesthesia technique for TAVI is projected towards the conscious sedation in spontaneous breathing through locoregional anesthesia [11]. The II and IH nerve blocks are

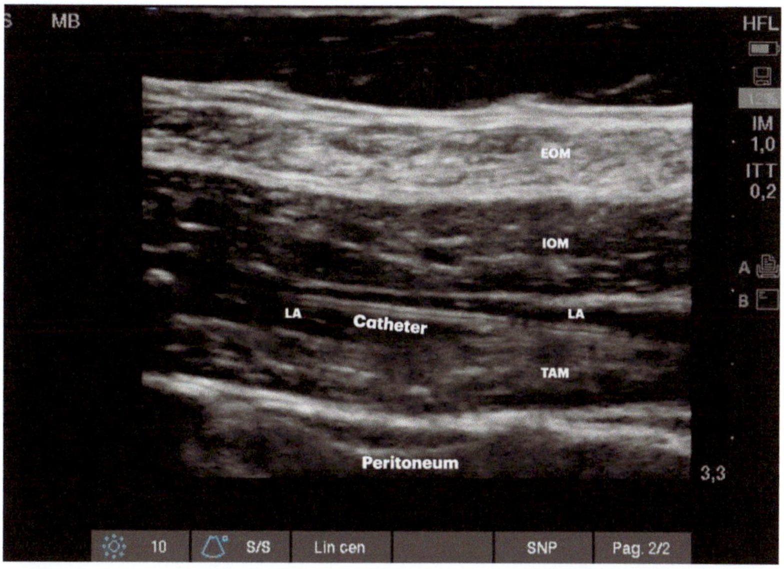

Fig. 9.5 Continuous transversus plane block. The catheter is placed between the internal oblique and transversus abdominis muscles. *EOM* external oblique muscle, *IOM* internal oblique muscle, *TAM* transversus abdominis muscle, *LA* local anesthetic, *Catheter* catheter, *Peritoneum* peritoneum

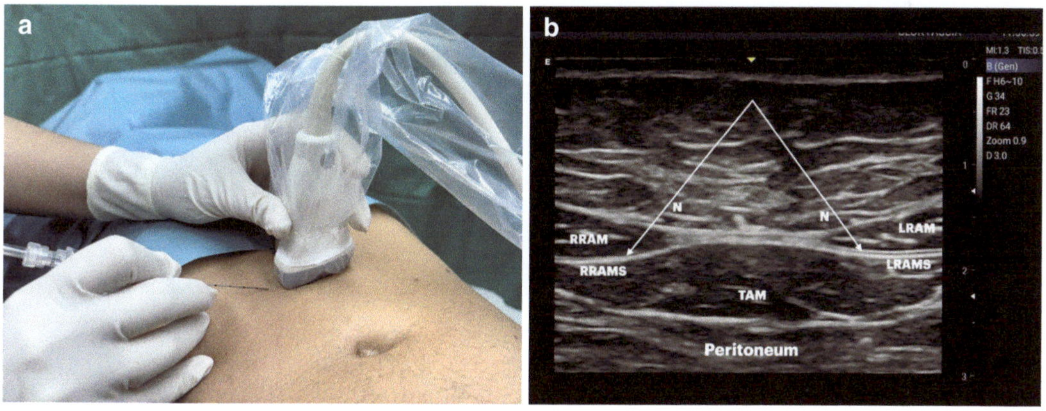

Fig. 9.6 Rectus sheath block. (**a**) Patient and probe position. (**b**) The local anesthetic is injected bilaterally between the body of rectus abdominis muscle and its posterior sheath. *RRAM* right rectus abdominis muscle, *LRAM* left rectus abdominis muscle, *RRAMS* right rectus abdominis muscle sheath, *LRAMS* left rectus abdominis muscle sheath, *TAM* transversus abdominis muscle, *Peritoneum* peritoneum, *N* needle

often used for analgesia of infraumbilical and inguinal surgical procedures allowing the vein and artery femoral devices instertion. The II and IH nerves run between the IOM and TAM at the level of anterior superior iliac spine [12] (ASIS). With the patient in supine position, a high-frequency linear probe is placed transversally between the belly button and ASIS until the EOM, IOM, TAM, deep circumflex iliac artery (DCIA), and ASIS shadows are visualized. A volume of 10 mL of LA is injected between the IOM and TAM where the DCIA lies and represents a vascular landmark for the II and IH technique (Fig. 9.7).

9.1.5 Erector Spinae Plane (ESP) Block

The erector spinae plane (ESP) block was first described by Forero et al. in 2016 as a novel analgesic procedure to manage neuropathic pain resulting from metastatic disease of the ribs and from multiple rib fractures providing an extensive dermatomal sensory block. The ESP block relieves pain in a large area of the posterior, lateral, and anterior chest and lumbar walls also preventing visceral pain. It can be used not only for acute and chronic pain of the

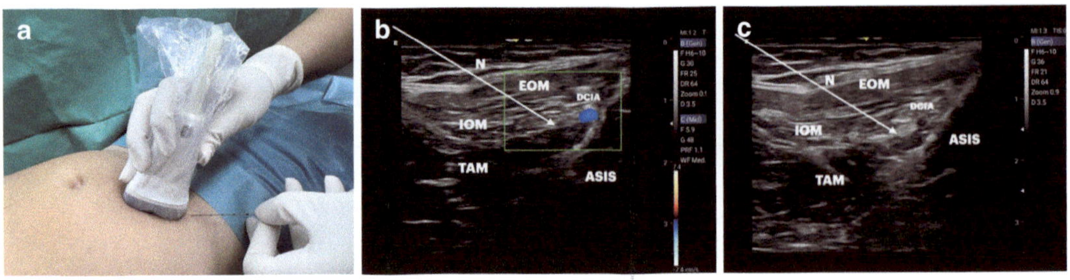

Fig. 9.7 Ilioinguinal and iliohypogastric block. (**a**) Patient and probe position. (**b**, **c**) The local anesthetic is injected between the internal oblique and transversus abdominis muscles in the fascial plane containing the deep circumflex iliac artery. *Skin* skin, *EOM* external oblique muscle, *IOM* internal oblique muscle, *DCIA* deep circumflex iliac artery, *TAM* transversus abdominis muscle, *QLBM* quadratus lumborum muscle, *Peritoneum* peritoneum, *N* needle

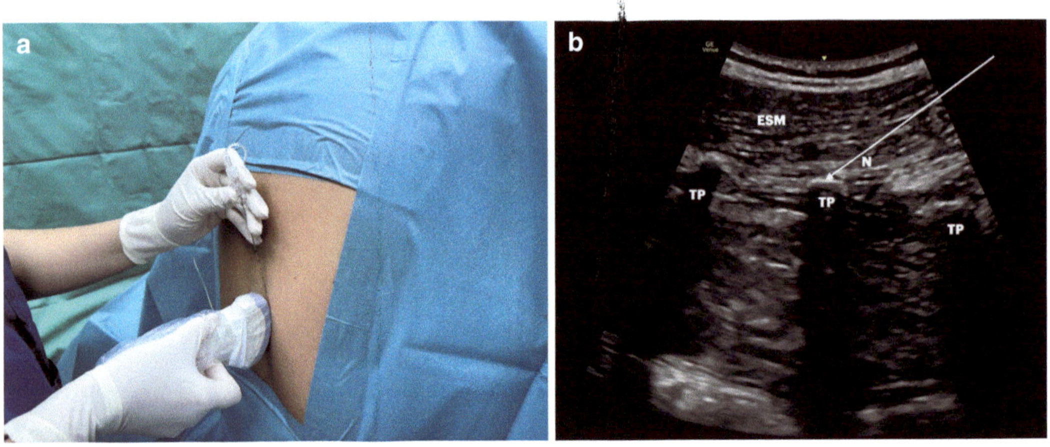

Fig. 9.8 ESP block. (**a**) Patient and probe position. (**b**) The local anesthetic is injected between the erector spinae muscle and the transverse process. *ESM* erector spinae muscle, *TP* transverse process, *N* needle

trunk but also for upper and lower limbs. It is currently performed in wide surgical fields covering several specialties outside anesthesiology including emergency medicine and traumatology and in surgery fields where locoregional anesthesia has played a limited role such as spine surgery and cardiac surgery both for minithoracotomy pain management and visceral pain management from abdominal vascular surgery [13]. The ESP block is described in detail in Chap. 8. The patient may assume the seated, prone, or lateral position. For the abdominal ESP, a low-frequency convex probe is placed approximately 3 cm lateral to the interspinous line at the level of L1–L5 transverse processes. The needle is inserted through an in-plane approach, and a volume of 20 mL of LA is injected into the plane between the edge of the transverse process (TP) and the erector spinae muscle (ESM). At this level, the transverse processes appear as a trident shape (Fig. 9.8).

9.1.6 Quadratus Lumborum Block (QLB)

Atherosclerosis has a complex etiology that leads to arterial obstruction and often results in inadequate perfusion of the distal limbs. Patients with atherosclerosis can have severe complications resulting in femoral obstruction requiring femoral-femoral bypass graft placement. QLB block can be useful performed as analgesic technique for visceral pain management after vascular surgery. First described by Blanco, the QLB aims to anesthetize the thoracolumbar nerves. The local

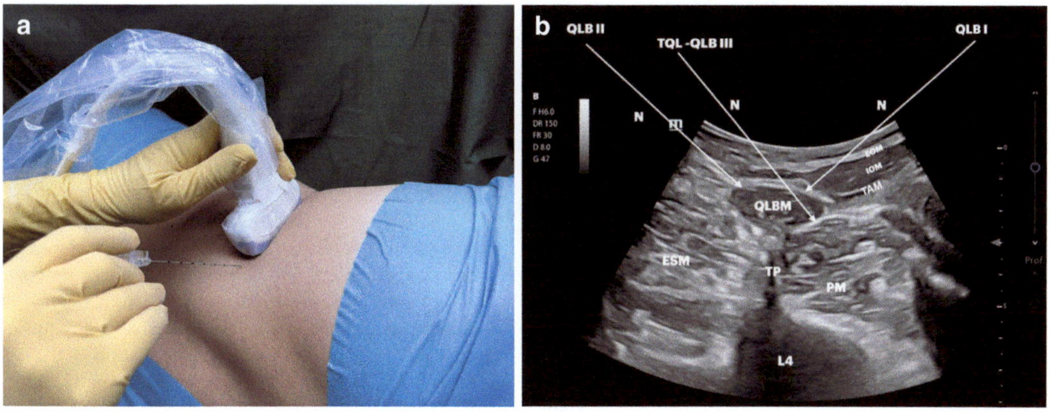

Fig. 9.9 Quadratus lumborum block. (**a**) Patient and probe position. (**b**) The shamrock sign. *QLB I* the local anesthetic is injected anteriorly at the quadratus lumborum muscle, *QLB II* the local anesthetic is injected posteriorly at the quadratus lumborum muscle, *TQL or QLB III* the local anesthetic is injected between the quadratus lumborum and psoas muscles, *QLB I* quadratus lumborum block type I, *QLB II* quadratus lumborum block type II, *TQL-QLB III* trans-quadratus lumborum block or quadratus lumborum block type III, *QLBM* quadratus lumborum muscle, *ESM* erector spinae muscle, *PM* psoas muscle, *TP* transverse process, *L4* L4 vertebral body, *EOM* external oblique muscle, *IOM* internal oblique muscle, *TAM* transversus abdominis muscle, *N* needle

anesthetic is injected adjacent to the quadratus lumborum muscle (QLBM) describing three different approaches [14] (Fig. 9.9):

- QLB I
- QLB II
- Trans-muscular QLB or QLB III [15]

With the patient in a lateral decubitus, a low-frequency convex probe is placed transversally at midpoint between the lower costal edge and the iliac crest at the level of axillary line until the ultrasound shamrock sign is visualized. The shamrock sign is composed by the QLBM superiorly, ESM posteriorly, PM anteriorly surrounding the transverse process, and vertebral body of L4. The anterior-lateral border of QLBM gets in anatomical touch with the EOM, IOM, and TAM and the transversalis fascia (TF):

- QLB I: 20–25 mL of LA is deposited on the anterior-lateral border of the QLBM at its junction with the TF (transversalis fascia).
- QLB II: 20–25 mL LA is injected posteriorly at the QLBM.
- Trans-muscular QLB or QLB III: 20–25 mL of LA is injected into the fascial plane between the QLBM and psoas muscle (PM).

9.2 Conclusion

The knoledgment of new abdominal wall blocks represent an important component of analgesia strategy during vascular surgery and some cardiac procedures.

References

1. Rafi AN. Abdominal field block: a new approach via the lumbar triangle. Anaesthesia. 2001;56(10):1024–6. https://doi.org/10.1046/j.1365-2044.2001.02279-40.x.
2. Carney J, McDonnell JG, Ochana A, Bhinder R, Laffey JG. The transversus abdominis plane block provides effective postoperative analgesia in patients undergoing total abdominal hysterectomy. Anesth Analg. 2008;107(6):2056–60. https://doi.org/10.1213/ane.0b013e3181871313.
3. McDonnell JG, Curley G, Carney J, Benton A, Costello J, Maharaj CH, Laffey JG. The analgesic efficacy of transversus abdominis plane block after cesarean delivery: a randomized controlled trial. Anesth Analg. 2008;106(1):186–91. https://doi.org/10.1213/01.ane.0000290294.64090.f3.
4. McDonnell JG, O'Donnell B, Curley G, Heffernan A, Power C, Laffey JG. The analgesic efficacy of transversus abdominis plane block after abdominal surgery: a prospective randomized controlled trial [Erratum in: Anesth Analg. 2007 May;104(5):1108.]. Anesth Analg. 2007;104(1):193–7. https://doi.org/10.1213/01.ane.0000250223.49963.0f.

5. O'Donnell BD, McDonnell JG, McShane AJ. The transversus abdominis plane (TAP) block in open retropubic prostatectomy [Erratum in: Reg Anesth Pain Med. 2006 May-Jun;31(3):286. McDonnell, John G [added]; McShane, Alan J [added].]. Reg Anesth Pain Med. 2006;31(1):91. https://doi.org/10.1016/j.rapm.2005.10.006.
6. Hebbard P, Fujiwara Y, Shibata Y, Royse C. Ultrasound-guided transversus abdominis plane (TAP) block. Anaesth Intensive Care. 2007;35(4):616–7.
7. Børglum J, Maschmann C, Belhage B, Jensen K. Ultrasound-guided bilateral dual transversus abdominis plane block: a new four-point approach. Acta Anaesthesiol Scand. 2011;55(6):658–63. https://doi.org/10.1111/j.1399-6576.2011.02430.x. Epub 2011 Apr 4.
8. Toshniwal G, Soskin V. Ultrasound-guided transversus abdominis plane block in obese patients. Indian J Anaesth. 2012;56(1):104–5. https://doi.org/10.4103/0019-5049.93368. PMID: 22529445; PMCID: PMC3327059.
9. Scimia P, Gentili L, Fusco P, Tedesco M, Tognu A, Sepolvere G. When a TAP becomes a QL block: a dynamic way to perform the fascial blocks. Minerva Anestesiol. 2022;88(11):976–8. https://doi.org/10.23736/S0375-9393.22.16772-6.
10. Hebbard P. Subcostal transversus abdominis plane block under ultrasound guidance. Anesth Analg. 2008;106(2):674–5; author reply 675. https://doi.org/10.1213/ane.0b013e318161a88f.
11. Zaccarelli M, Testa TS, Buscaglia G, Pratesi G, Crimi G, Balbi M, Gregorio SD, Silvetti S. Anesthetic considerations in combined TAVR and aortic endovascular procedures, a case report. Ann Card Anaesth. 2024;27(2):162–4. https://doi.org/10.4103/aca.aca_97_23.
12. Hannallah RS, Broadman LM, Belman AB, Abramowitz MD, Epstein BS. Comparison of caudal and ilioinguinal/iliohypogastric nerve blocks for control of post-orchiopexy pain in pediatric ambulatory surgery. Anesthesiology. 1987;66(6):832–4. https://doi.org/10.1097/00000542-198706000-00023.
13. Forero M, Adhikary SD, Lopez H, Tsui C, Chin KJ. The erector spinae plane block: a novel analgesic technique in thoracic neuropathic pain. Reg Anesth Pain Med. 2016;41(5):621–7. https://doi.org/10.1097/AAP.0000000000000451.
14. Blanco R, Ansari T, Girgis E. Quadratus lumborum block for postoperative pain after caesarean section: a randomised controlled trial. Eur J Anaesthesiol. 2015;32(11):812–8. https://doi.org/10.1097/EJA.0000000000000299.
15. Børglum J, Moriggl B, Jensen K, Lønnqvist PA, Christensen AF, Sauter A, Bendtsen TF. Ultrasound-guided transmuscular quadratus lumborum blockade. BJA Br J Anaesth. 2013;111:9919. https://doi.org/10.1093/bja/el_9919.

10 Analgesia vs. Anesthesia

Antonio Toscano and Paolo Capuano

10.1 Introduction

Cardiac surgery presents unique challenges due to the complexity of the procedures and the critical nature of the patient's condition. Effective perioperative management is crucial to ensure patient safety and optimal outcomes. Two essential components of this management are analgesia and anesthesia. Although often used interchangeably, analgesia and anesthesia serve distinct purposes in the peri- and postoperative period.

Analgesia refers to the relief from or prevention of pain without necessarily affecting consciousness. The primary goal of analgesia in cardiac surgery is to manage pain effectively, thereby reducing physiological stress, facilitating early mobilization, and improving overall recovery.

Anesthesia, on the other hand, encompasses a broader range of interventions aimed at inducing a state of controlled, temporary loss of sensation or awareness. Anesthesia (local, regional, or general) is used to ensure patient immobility, control of physiological responses, and unawareness during surgical procedures.

In the Enhanced Recovery After Surgery (ERAS) era, some analgesia techniques, which have proved to be very effective, have also been used for anesthetic purposes.

This chapter explores the differences between analgesia and anesthesia in the context of cardiac surgery, highlighting their respective roles, techniques, and implications for patient care, and focuses on the evolution of some analgesic/anesthetic procedures, from their beginnings to their routine use in the context of cardiac surgery.

10.2 The Early Phase: The Opioid-Based Anesthesia

Between the end of the 1960s and the beginning of the 1970s, Lowenstein described the so-called narcotic-based anesthesia [1]. The basis of this technique was the use of high doses of morphine, thus exploiting its sedative as well as analgesic effect with the maintenance of a hemodynamic stability profile without cardiodepression.

The evolution of this technique occurred subsequently with the introduction of fentanyl, which quickly replaced morphine as the opioid of choice for anesthesia in cardiac surgery. Characterized by a better hemodynamic profile and lower histamine release, fentanyl therefore

A. Toscano (✉)
Department of Anesthesia and Critical Care, Città della Salute e della Scienza di Torino, University of Turin, Turin, Italy

P. Capuano
Department of Anesthesia and Intensive Care, Istituto Mediterraneo per i Trapianti e Terapie ad alta Specializzazione (IRCCS-ISMETT), UPMCI (University of Pittsburgh Medical Center Italy), Palermo, Italy

G. Sepolvere, S. Silvetti (eds.), *Fast-Track in Cardiac Anesthesia*,
https://doi.org/10.1007/978-3-031-70899-2_10

became the first choice due to its rapid action in response to the surgical stimulus. The first to describe its use, at a dosage of 25 mg/kg, was Stanley [2].

A further step forward was made in 1979, when sufentanil was introduced.

Characterized by greater potency, hemodynamic stability, and short half-life, a favorable characteristic for earlier extubation of patients, it is still used today in cardiac anesthesia in the context of a balanced general anesthesia [3, 4].

However, the introduction of remifentanil was revolutionary, characterized by high analgesic power and pharmacokinetics capable of guaranteeing a rapid offset and which probably marked the transition from opioid-based anesthesia to balanced anesthesia [5].

10.3 The Transition Phase

As cardiac surgeries became more common towards the end of the twentieth century, there was a shift towards optimizing perioperative care to address these issues.

Several factors contributed to the decline of the "high-dose opioid anesthesia" era. One major factor was the development of intravenous anesthetic agents with rapid offset, which offered better management and faster recovery times [6, 7].

Additionally, there was growing evidence that inhalational agents provided cardioprotection against myocardial ischemia and reperfusion injury, rather than causing the previously suspected coronary steal phenomenon [8–12].

Remifentanil became widely popular because it offered robust analgesia against intraoperative stimuli while maintaining vascular stability with predictable pharmacokinetics. Its suitability for infusions and ability to allow for faster extubation times after cardiac surgery made it a preferred choice over earlier opioids.

Consequently, as cardiac surgeries became more common towards the end of the twentieth century, there was a shift towards optimizing perioperative care to address these issues. The fast-track model of perioperative care was introduced and expanded to include cardiac surgery, aiming to improve patient outcomes and reduce recovery times.

High-dose opioid techniques using morphine or fentanyl, initially popular in cardiac anesthesia due to their ability to provide hemodynamic stability and analgesia, were addressed for significant drawbacks, including respiratory depression and delayed recovery, potentially leading to prolonged ventilation and postoperative complications, with also increasing intensive care unit (ICU) stays and costs.

Over the past decade, there has been a shift towards using lower doses of fentanyl in cardiac surgery to improving recovery times while maintaining effective analgesia. Specifically, using "low" fentanyl doses (12 μg/kg) has been shown to significantly reduce the time to extubation compared to high-dose fentanyl (24 μg/kg). This adjustment in dosing is part of a broader trend aimed at optimizing patient recovery and minimizing the side effects associated with high-dose opioid use [13, 14].

10.4 The Modern Era of Multimodal Analgesia

In the past two decades, there has been a notable shift towards evidence-based multimodal opioid-sparing analgesia following noncardiac surgeries. This approach involves administering different analgesics to achieve effective pain management while reducing opioid usage. The rationale behind this strategy extends beyond just sparing opioids; it also aims to enhance pain relief through both central and peripheral antinociceptive mechanisms.

Indeed, expert panels widely advocate for the adoption of multimodal analgesic approaches to achieve effective pain management in various surgical contexts. This approach involves utilizing a combination of medications and techniques that complement each other, aiming to spare opioids and enhance symptomatic and functional recovery.

The "fast-track" approach laid the foundation for opioid-sparing strategies in cardiac surgical care, emphasizing the importance of multimodal pain management. By leveraging a combination of interventions and minimizing reliance on opioids, these protocols aim to optimize patient recovery, improve pain control, and reduce the risk of long-term opioid dependence and chronic pain.

Multimodal analgesic approaches, including the adjunctive use of non-opioid medications such as acetaminophen and nonsteroidal anti-inflammatory drugs (NSAIDs), have emerged as cornerstone strategies in modern pain management protocols. By combining various analgesic agents and techniques, multimodal analgesia offers superior pain relief, reduces opioid requirements, and promotes enhanced recovery following surgery. These approaches represent a significant advancement in perioperative care, improving patient outcomes and satisfaction while minimizing the risks associated with opioid use.

Acetaminophen, also known as paracetamol, functions by inhibiting the synthesis of prostaglandins within the central nervous system and blocking peripheral pain-impulse generation. This mechanism underlies its widespread use for both pain relief and fever reduction. In the postoperative setting, acetaminophen has been found to reduce the need for opioids, making it valuable for pain management. Randomized trials have indicated that intravenous acetaminophen can effectively reduce opioid consumption, maintain pain control at levels comparable to other analgesics, and potentially mitigate the occurrence of delirium, which may arise from inadequate pain management or adverse effects of opioid medications. Administering IV acetaminophen routinely, particularly in the postoperative period, may contribute to improved pain management and reduce reliance on opioids, thereby potentially enhancing patient outcomes.

NSAIDs work by inhibiting cyclooxygenase (COX) enzymes, thereby reducing the synthesis of prostaglandins responsible for inflammation and pain. While widely used in noncardiac surgery, their utilization in cardiac surgery has been supported by several small prospective studies, generally endorsing their efficacy within multimodal pain management protocols. In 2019, the Food and Drug Administration (FDA) issued a formal warning regarding the use of NSAIDs in patients undergoing coronary revascularization due to their association with thrombotic cardiovascular complications.

Given these considerations, NSAIDs should be cautiously managed in cardiac surgery patients, with attention paid to potential renal and gastrointestinal complications. Their use should be weighed against their benefits within a comprehensive multimodal pain management strategy.

Ketamine is a unique anesthetic drug known for its ability to provide analgesia, hypnosis, and amnesia with minimal respiratory and cardiovascular depression. Its primary mechanism of action involves antagonism of the *N*-methyl-D-aspartate (NMDA) receptor, which is responsible for its distinctive properties such as amnesic and psychosensory effects, analgesia, and neuroprotection. Ketamine also interacts with various other binding sites, including opioid receptors, which contribute to its pharmacological effects.

Despite its potential benefits, ketamine's significant side effects have limited its widespread use in cardiac surgery. Notably, ketamine reliably causes tachycardia, which can be problematic for patients with underlying heart conditions. It can also increase myocardial oxygen consumption and may enhance the arrhythmogenic potential of other medications used during cardiac surgery.

Multimodal pain management after cardiac surgery often involves the use of local anesthetics, and lidocaine is a commonly utilized medication in this regard. Unlike some other local anesthetics, lidocaine is available in topical formulations and can be safely administered intravenously, making it versatile in its therapeutic applications.

It is important to note that lidocaine infusion requires careful dosing to avoid toxicity. While lidocaine offers potential benefits in managing postoperative pain after cardiac surgery, further research is needed to better understand its optimal dosing, administration routes, and overall impact on patient outcomes.

10.5 State of the Art: Anesthesia in Cardiac Surgery

What is the best general anesthesia technique for cardiac surgery? Balanced anesthesia with volatile anesthetics (VA) and opioid, TIVA, or opioid-free anesthesia (OFA)? This question has long been a focus for anesthesiologists.

The superiority of different anesthetic regimens in cardiac surgery is debated. Clinical trials on CABG suggested cardioprotection with VA, leading to a 2011 American College of Cardiology Foundation (ACCF)/American Heart Association (AHA) guidelines recommending VA to reduce perioperative myocardial ischemia and infarction [15]. The 2017 European Association for Cardio-Thoracic Surgery (EACTS) guidelines also recommended VA for additional organ protection and reduced mortality in CABG patients [16]. The MYRIAD trial [17], the largest and most recent, did not find any discrepancy in mortality or cardiac biomarkers between VA and TIVA, leading to questions about their equivalence, resulting in a downgraded class IIa B recommendation from EACTS/European Association of Cardiothoracic Anaesthesiology (EACTA)/European Board of Cardiovascular Perfusion (EBCP). Notably, VA is more commonly used in North America, while intravenous agents are preferred in Europe [18].

Anesthetic conditioning, like ischemic conditioning, protects the heart and other organs against ischemia-reperfusion (IR) injury, reducing mitochondrial damage and enhancing cellular resistance to hypoxia. Volatile anesthetics provide both pre- and postconditioning effects, preparing cardiomyocytes for hypoxic stress and offering significant cardioprotection [19].

The timing and method of VA administration are crucial, with continuous administration during surgery often showing better outcomes than intermittent use. However, the optimal protocol remains unclear, and factors like genetics, age, obesity, and diabetes can affect effectiveness. Conversely, conditions like angina and certain medications can enhance VA's protective effects [19].

Intravenous anesthetics (IV) like propofol also offer cardioprotection through anti-inflammatory and antioxidant actions, though they do not activate the same protective pathways as VA and may interfere with VA benefits.

Opioid-induced cardioprotection, like volatile anesthetics, inhibits mitochondrial transition pores. Additionally, opioid receptor activation in cardiomyocytes triggers a complex signal cascade involving sarcolemmal ATP-sensitive K+ (KATP) channels, reactive oxygen species, protein kinase C, and inducible nitric oxide synthetase, which contributes to cardioprotection by inhibiting apoptotic pathways [19]. No study has been conducted to demonstrate the cardioprotection or the feasibility of an opioid-free anesthesia (OFA) protocol in cardiac surgery to improve patient care.

OFA is based on the fact that a sympathetic reaction evidenced by hemodynamic changes in an anesthetized patient does not systematically reflect pain. In addition, a sleeping patient will not recall pain, while hormonal stress and sympathetic and inflammatory reactions can be controlled by therapeutic classes other than opioids. OFA is an anesthesia strategy that replaces opioids (balanced general anesthesia) with non-opioid drugs (multimodal general anesthesia). Opioids are usually administered during anesthesia for their antinociceptive effects, to control the responses of the autonomic nervous system (ANS) to surgical stress, and for their hypnotic effect. OFA was based on published literature, which demonstrates that each of the effects associated with opioids can be obtained with lidocaine (analgesic, hypnotic, and ANS control), dexamethasone (analgesic), and ketamine (analgesic and hypnotic). Several OFA protocols have also been published: the most commonly used non-opioid agents are lidocaine, dexamethasone, and ketamine, and all have been studied separately in cardiac surgery. Murphy et al. [20] demonstrated that the administration of dexamethasone decreased morphine consumption and ICU length of stay. Lidocaine and ketamine were shown to have analgesic and opioid-sparing effects. More specifically, the use of lidocaine has been associated with a decrease in arrhythmias and a nonconstant improvement in postoperative cognitive functions [21]. Adverse effects, such as elevated blood pressure events or toxicity from high plasma concentrations, may be linked to OFA. Although in noncardiac surgery OFA was demonstrated to be associated with lower postoperative opioid use and better respiratory outcomes [21], to our knowledge, no study has evaluated the effect of OFA on morphine consumption and the postoperative course in cardiac surgery patients.

10.6 Future Perspectives: The Ultra-Fast-Track Era

The second millennium marks the fast-track era in cardiac care, characterized by comprehensive strategies aimed at enhancing recovery and reducing hospital stays. Fast-track cardiac care is a multifaceted approach involving several key components during cardiac anesthesia and the postoperative period. The primary goals are early extubation post-surgery and reducing the length of stay in the ICU and hospital overall.

In the 1990s, the anesthetic management of cardiac surgery commonly involved high-dose opioid strategies and extended mechanical ventilation in the ICU for 12–24 h. The use of opioids was considered advantageous due to their hemodynamic stability and protective anti-ischemic and preconditioning effects [22]. However, it became evident over time that the extensive use of these drugs did not yield beneficial outcomes for patients. Instead, high-dose opioids were associated with numerous adverse effects, such as respiratory depression and bradycardia, which contributed to prolonged extubation times and extended ICU stays [23].

The transition from high-dose opioid anesthetic strategies to ERAS cardiac (ERASc) protocols represents a paradigm shift in cardiac anesthesia. The focus has moved from relying heavily on opioids to adopting balanced, multimodal approaches that enhance recovery and improve patient outcomes. The foundation of the ERASc Society and its recommendations have been instrumental in consolidating this new approach, promoting safer and more effective perioperative care for cardiac surgery patients [24].

ERASc protocols underscore the significance of effective perioperative pain management to ensure better patient outcomes, reduced complications, and enhanced recovery. By advocating for multimodal analgesia and opioid-sparing strategies, along with the use of locoregional analgesia, ERASc aims to provide comprehensive pain relief while minimizing the risks associated with opioid use. These approaches are critical for optimizing the recovery process and improving the overall experience and health of cardiac surgery patients [25, 26].

Cardiac anesthesia has evolved beyond the era of neuraxial blocks, such as epidural and paravertebral blocks, due to their associated risks, including the potential for serious complications like epidural hematoma, pneumothorax, and concerns related to anticoagulation therapy. As a result, the focus has shifted towards newer regional techniques that offer effective pain control with fewer risks, and fascial plane blocks have emerged as a promising alternative in the setting of cardiac surgery [27].

In fact, several evidences are growing and support the efficacy of fascial plane blocks in promoting faster extubation, potentially leading to worldwide implementation of fast-track programs and, in selected patients, of ultra-fast-track strategies.

In a randomized controlled trial, Zhang et al. [28] investigated the effect of bilateral pectointercostal fascial block in 108 patients undergoing open cardiac surgery. They reported that the nerve block provides effective analgesia and accelerates recovery in terms of time of extubation and ICU and hospital length of stay.

In line with these results, in a meta-analysis, Dost et al. [29] analyzed the effects of regional anesthesia on postoperative opioid consumption in patients undergoing open cardiac surgery. They concluded that all the regional anesthesia techniques evaluated significantly reduced postoperative opioid consumption at 24 h and that the erector spinae plane block (ESPB) was the most effective treatment. Moreover, in another meta-analysis, Li et al. [30] evaluated the ultrasound-guided parasternal block (PSB) and found a decrease in opioid consumption and contextually an improvement in clinical outcomes, such as mechanical ventilation time and total length of ICU stay and hospital days.

This transition from neuraxial blocks to fascial plane blocks in cardiac anesthesia reflects a shift towards safer, more effective pain management strategies. Fascial plane blocks offer significant advantages in terms of safety, efficacy, and ease of use, making them a valuable component of multimodal analgesia protocols in cardiac surgery. As research continues to evolve, these techniques are likely to become standard practice, further enhancing patient outcomes and recovery in the cardiac surgical setting.

10.7 Conclusion

In conclusion, the evolution of analgesia and anesthesia in cardiac surgery reflects significant advancements aimed at improving patient outcomes and enhancing recovery processes. From the initial reliance on high-dose opioid-based anesthesia in the 1960s to the modern era of multimodal analgesia and opioid-sparing strategies, there has been a clear shift towards optimizing perioperative care. The adoption of non-opioid drugs like acetaminophen, NSAIDs, and ketamine has proven to reduce opioid consumption, mitigate side effects, and promote faster recovery. Additionally, the emergence of fascial plane blocks offers a safer and more effective alternative to traditional neuraxial blocks, further supporting the goals of ERAS protocols. As the field continues to evolve, future perspectives such as ultrafast-track strategies promise to revolutionize cardiac surgical care, emphasizing early extubation and reduced ICU stays, ultimately enhancing the overall patient experience and outcomes.

References

1. Lowenstein E, Hallowell P, Levine FH, et al. Cardiovascular response to large doses of intravenous morphine in man. N Engl J Med. 1969;281:1389–93.
2. Stanley TH, Philbin DM, Coggins CH. Fentanyl-oxygen anaesthesia for coronary artery surgery: cardiovascular and antidiuretic hormone responses. Can Anaesth Soc J. 1979;26:168–72.
3. Howie MB, Smith DF, Reilley TE, et al. Postoperative course after sufentanil or fentanyl anesthesia for coronary artery surgery. J Cardiothorac Vasc Anesth. 1991;5:485–9.
4. Sanford TJ, Smith NT, Dec-Silver H, et al. A comparison of morphine, fentanyl, and sufentanil anesthesia for cardiac surgery: induction, emergence, and extubation. Anesth Analg. 1986;65:259–66.
5. Mhollhoff T, Herregods L, Moerman A, et al. Comparative efficacy and safety of remifentanil and fentanyl in 'fast track' coronary artery bypass graft surgery: a randomized, double blind study. Br J Anaesth. 2001;87:718–26.
6. Khanykin B, Siddiqi R, Jensen PF, et al. Comparison of remifentanil and low-dose fentanyl for fast-track cardiac anesthesia: a prospective randomized study. Heart Surg Forum. 2013;16:E324–8.
7. Maddali MM, Kurian E, Fahr J. Extubation time, hemodynamic stability, and postoperative pain control in patients undergoing coronary artery bypass surgery: an evaluation of fentanyl, remifentanil, and nonsteroidal antiinflammatory drugs with propofol for perioperative and postoperative management. J Clin Anesth. 2006;18:605–10.
8. Murry CE, Jennings RB, Reimer KA. Preconditioning with ischemia: a delay of lethal cell injury in ischemic myocardium. Circulation. 1986;74:1124–36.
9. Schultz JE, Rose E, Yao Z, et al. Evidence for involvement of opioid receptors in ischemic preconditioning in rat hearts. Am J Phys. 1995;268:H2157–61.
10. Wong GTC, Huang Z, Ji S, et al. Remifentanil reduces the release of biochemical markers of myocardial damage after coronary artery bypass surgery: a randomized trial. J Cardiothorac Vasc Anesth. 2010;24:790–6.
11. Zuo Y, Cheng X, Gu E, et al. Effect of aortic root infusion of sufentanil on ischemia-reperfusion injury in patients undergoing mitral valve replacement. J Cardiothorac Vasc Anesth. 2014;28:1474–8.
12. Murphy GS, Szokol JW, Marymont JH, et al. Opioids and cardioprotection: the impact of morphine and fentanyl on recovery of ventricular function after car-

diopulmonary bypass. J Cardiothorac Vasc Anesth. 2006;20:493–502.
13. Myles PS, Hunt JO, Fletcher H, et al. Remifentanil, fentanyl, and cardiac surgery: a double-blinded, randomized, controlled trial of costs and outcomes. Anesth Analg. 2002;95:805–12.
14. Ahonen J, Olkkola KT, Hynynen M, et al. Comparison of alfentanil, fentanyl and sufentanil for total intravenous anaesthesia with propofol in patients undergoing coronary artery bypass surgery. Br J Anaesth. 2000;85:533–40.
15. Sousa-Uva M, Head SJ, Milojevic M, Collet JP, Landoni G, Castella M, Dunning J, Gudbjartsson T, Linker NJ, Sandoval E, Thielmann M, Jeppsson A, Landmesser U. 2017 EACTS guidelines on perioperative medication in adult cardiac surgery. Eur J Cardiothorac Surg. 2018;53(1):5–33. https://doi.org/10.1093/ejcts/ezx314.
16. Landoni G, Lomivorotov VV, Nigro Neto C, Monaco F, Pasyuga VV, Bradic N, Lembo R, Gazivoda G, Likhvantsev VV, Lei C, Lozovskiy A, Di Tomasso N, Bukamal NAR, Silva FS, Bautin AE, Ma J, Crivellari M, Farag AMGA, Uvaliev NS, Carollo C, Pieri M, Kunstýř J, Wang CY, Belletti A, Hajjar LA, Grigoryev EV, Agrò FE, Riha H, El-Tahan MR, Scandroglio AM, Elnakera AM, Baiocchi M, Navalesi P, Shmyrev VA, Severi L, Hegazy MA, Crescenzi G, Ponomarev DN, Brazzi L, Arnoni R, Tarasov DG, Jovic M, Calabrò MG, Bove T, Bellomo R, Zangrillo A, MYRIAD Study Group. Volatile anesthetics versus total intravenous anesthesia for cardiac surgery. N Engl J Med. 2019;380(13):1214–25. https://doi.org/10.1056/NEJMoa1816476. Epub 2019 Mar 19.
17. Barry AE, Chaney MA, London MJ. Anesthetic management during cardiopulmonary bypass: a systematic review. Anesth Analg. 2015;120(4):749–69. https://doi.org/10.1213/ANE.0000000000000612.
18. Ştefan M, Predoi C, Goicea R, Filipescu D. Volatile anaesthesia versus total intravenous anaesthesia for cardiac surgery-a narrative review. J Clin Med. 2022;11(20):6031. https://doi.org/10.3390/jcm11206031. PMID: 36294353; PMCID: PMC9604446.
19. Tanaka K, Kersten JR, Riess ML. Opioid-induced cardioprotection. Curr Pharm Des. 2014;20(36):5696–705. https://doi.org/10.2174/1381612820666140204120311. PMID: 24502571; PMCID: PMC4216587.
20. Murphy GS, Sherwani SS, Szokol JW, Avram MJ, Greenberg SB, Patel KM, Wade LD, Vaughn J, Gray J. Small-dose dexamethasone improves quality of recovery scores after elective cardiac surgery: a randomized, double-blind, placebo-controlled study. J Cardiothorac Vasc Anesth. 2011;25(6):950–60. https://doi.org/10.1053/j.jvca.2011.03.002. Epub 2011 May 11.
21. Guinot PG, Spitz A, Berthoud V, Ellouze O, Missaoui A, Constandache T, Grosjean S, Radhouani M, Anciaux JB, Parthiot JP, Merle JP, Nowobilski N, Nguyen M, Bouhemad B. Effect of opioid-free anaesthesia on post-operative period in cardiac surgery: a retrospective matched case-control study. BMC Anesthesiol. 2019;19(1):136. https://doi.org/10.1186/s12871-019-0802-y. PMID: 31366330; PMCID: PMC6668113.
22. Ishii H. Cardioprotection with opioids—trusted old friends—clinical science. Curr Pharm Des. 2014;20(36):5794–8.
23. Engelman DT, Ali WB, Williams JB, et al. Guidelines for perioperative care in cardiac surgery enhanced recovery after surgery society recommendations. JAMA Surg. 2019;154(8):755–66.
24. Wick EC, Grant MC, Wu CL. Postoperative multimodal analgesia pain management with nonopioid analgesics and techniques: a review. JAMA Surg. 2017;152(7):691–7. https://doi.org/10.1001/jamasurg.2017.0898.
25. Bailey JG, Uppal V. Fascial plane blocks: moving from the expansionist to the reductionist era. Blocs des plans fasciaux : de l'ère expansionniste à l'ère réductionniste. Can J Anaesth. 2022;69(10):1185–90. https://doi.org/10.1007/s12630-022-02309-x.
26. Barr LF, Boss MJ, Mazzeffi MA, Taylor BS, Salenger R. Postoperative multimodal analgesia in cardiac surgery. Crit Care Clin. 2020;36(4):631–51.
27. Toscano A, Capuano P, Galatà M, Tazzi I, Rinaldi M, Brazzi L. Safety of ultrasound-guided serratus anterior and erector spinae fascial plane blocks: a retrospective analysis in patients undergoing cardiac surgery while receiving anticoagulant and antiplatelet drugs. J Cardiothorac Vasc Anesth. 2022;36(2):483–8. https://doi.org/10.1053/j.jvca.2021.05.037. Epub 2021 May 24.
28. Zhang Y, Gong H, Zhan B, Chen S. Effects of bilateral pecto-intercostal fascial block for perioperative pain management in patients undergoing open cardiac surgery: a prospective randomized study. BMC Anesthesiol. 2021;21(1):175. https://doi.org/10.1186/s12871-021-01391-w.
29. Dost B, De Cassai A, Balzani E, Tulgar S, Ahiskalioglu A. Effects of ultrasound-guided regional anesthesia in cardiac surgery: a systematic review and network meta-analysis. BMC Anesthesiol. 2022;22(1):409. https://doi.org/10.1186/s12871-022-01952-7.
30. Li J, et al. Efficacy of ultrasound-guided parasternal block in adult cardiac surgery: a meta-analysis of randomized controlled trials. Minerva Anestesiol. 2022;88(9):719–28.

Chronic Pain and Fascial Blocks

11

Pierfrancesco Fusco, Paolo Scimia,
Francesca De Sanctis, and Gian Marco Petroni

11.1 Introduction

Chronic postsurgical pain (CPSP) represents a clinical condition that in some cases can be more disabling than the underlying pathology. CPSP is defined as chronic pain that develops or increases in intensity after a surgical procedure and persists beyond the healing process, at least 3 months after the surgery [1]. Every year, surgery is performed in over 40 million patients in the European Union. Therefore, the number of patients potentially exposed to CPSP is large, and it represents a major, largely unresolved clinical problem. In Europe, the incidence of moderate-to-severe CPSP was 11.8% and of severe pain (NRS >6) 2.2% [2]. This condition negatively affects the patient's quality of life and slows down postoperative recovery.

P. Fusco
Unit of Anesthesia and Intensive Care, S. Filippo e Nicola Hospital, Avezzano, Italy

P. Scimia
Unit of Anesthesia and Intensive Care, Mazzini Hospital, Teramo, Italy

F. De Sanctis · G. M. Petroni (✉)
Unit of Anesthesia and Intensive Care, S. MAria Hospital, Terni, Italy

11.2 Transition from Acute to Chronic Pain: An Overview of the Literature

The presence of acute pain represents the fundamental requirement for the chronicity of pain. Chemical and mechanical stimulation of peripheral nociceptors causes peripheral sensitization. In fact, acute tissue insults such as heat, cold, and chemical or mechanical injury cause disturbance in homeostasis and stimulate the nociceptors. After an injury, a wide range of inflammatory mediators are released locally either from damaged tissue or by activated mast cells and neutrophils. These mediators are adenosine-5-triphosphate, bradykinin, prostaglandin, sodium, hydrogen, potassium, histamine, and serotonin. After tissue injury, macrophages release proinflammatory substances such as interleukin-1B, interleukin-6, nerve growth factor, and tumor necrosis factor-alpha. Peripheral inflammation at the site of tissue injury activates C-fibers, which release substance P, calcitonin gene-related peptide, neurokinin A, and nitric oxide. The end result is further activation of "silent" C fibers with a reduction of pain threshold and increased excitability [3].

Generated action potential is transmitted from the injury site to the spinal cord via primary afferent sensory fibers with their cell bodies located at the dorsal root ganglion (DRG). Primary afferent C and Ad fibers enter the spinal cord through the dorsal horn and synapse with the secondary affer-

G. Sepolvere, S. Silvetti (eds.), *Fast-Track in Cardiac Anesthesia*,
https://doi.org/10.1007/978-3-031-70899-2_11

ent neurons at Rexed laminae I and II [3]. Ascending pathways or secondary afferent neurons from dorsal horn terminate at the thalamus and cerebral cortex [3]. Spinothalamic tract is an important ascending pathway originating from laminae I, II, and V. Via the thalamus, it ends at the somatosensory cortex. Descending pathways arise from periaqueductal gray matter, rostroventromedial medulla, and adjacent reticular formation secreting either noradrenaline or serotonin. Noradrenaline stimulates a2-adrenoceptors inhibiting the release of neurotransmitters from primary afferent neurons to minimize the nociceptive transmission [3].

Continuous or repetitive nociceptive stimulation leads to a series of pathophysiological changes in pain processing that underlie the transition between acute and chronic pain. Continuous nociception stimulation leads to a number of changes in gene and protein expression in both DRG and dorsal horn neurons. The most prominent change is an increase in the mRNA coding for the production of various receptors and ion channels such as Na and TRPV1 receptors. The repeated nociceptive stimulus causes the activation of NMDA receptors. Activation of NMDA receptors leads to the "windup" phenomenon. Once windup has developed, it induces and potentiates a wide dynamic range (WDR) neuronal response to each stimulus. Subsequent sensory stimulation via Ab fiber (touch) ends up with exaggerated WDR neuronal output. Clinically, this manifests as allodynia. The end result of the windup process is "neuroplasticity," which is a change in neuronal structure with potential enhancement of signal transduction [3].

All these changes cause "central sensitization," which is a state of reduced thresholds to stimulations associated with escalated neuronal activity response in the dorsal horn [3].

11.3 Predisposing Risk Factors for CPSP

A variety of operative, anesthetic, and patient factors have been observed to correlate with the increased risk for development of CPSP:

- Genetic factors: The correlation between genetic factors and the development of CPSP is still uncertain. Studies are still needed to determine whether there is a predisposition to the development of CPSP. Currently, it seems that there are several genes that can be correlated to an increased predisposition such as those of sodium channels [4, 5].
- Psychosocial factors and pain cognition: The psychosocial aspect has an important role in the development of CPSP. Several studies have highlighted the presence of risk factors such as fear of surgery and fear of pain, anxiety, depression, neuroticism, post-traumatic stress disorder (PTSD), past trauma, and catastrophizing [4, 5].
- The presence of preoperative pain is a risk factor for the development of acute and CPSP.
- Type of surgery: The choice of anterior approach in thoracotomies and mastectomies has been shown to minimize rates of CPSP. In thoracotomies and mastectomies, intercostal nerve damage is believed to be a major contributor to chronic neuropathic pain [4, 5].
- Anesthesia technique and drugs: Ketamine may reduce chronic postoperative pain, although the optimum treatment duration and dose for different operations have yet to be identified. The evidence for gabapentin and pregabalin is encouraging but weak; further work is needed before these drugs can be recommended for the prevention of chronic pain [4, 5].

11.4 Chronic Pain After Thoracotomy or Sternotomy

One of the most frequent forms of CPSP is following cardiac surgery or thoracic surgery. Chronic pain after thoracotomy or sternotomy is chronic pain that develops after a surgical incision to the chest wall. It is very common and occurs in approximately 50% of patients who underwent a thoracotomy. Moderate-to-severe pain occurs in 3–18% of patients. The pain is localized to the chest wall and over the sternum, often closely related to the area of surgery and the scar. Commonly, it is aggravated by movement, and often, it is of a neuropathic nature (in around 45% of cases). Such neuropathic pain is often accompanied by sensory changes in the area of the scar. Intercostal nerve injury seems to be one important pathogenic factor. In children and adolescents, the prevalence is much lower with around 2% [6–8].

11.5 Locoregional Anesthesia and the Role of Fascial Plane Block to Prevent and Treat CPSP After Cardiac Surgery or Thoracic Surgery

Persistent pain, postoperative hyperalgesia, and allodynia after surgery are the consequences of neuronal plasticity that are permanent synaptic neuronal changes in the peripheral and central nervous system in response to tissue trauma and nerve injury. The enormous progress in the anesthetic field with the introduction of new techniques of locoregional anesthesia together with studies on the pathophysiology of the fascial system has made a great contribution to the prevention of CPSP and also to its treatment. Regional anesthesia may reduce the risk of persistent (chronic) pain after surgery. Hence, blocking nociception during any part of the perioperative experience may prevent persistent pain after surgery [9].

Over the last two decades, the use of fascial plane blocks in locoregional anesthesia has allowed enormous progress in the management of anesthesia and analgesia, both in the perioperatory and postoperatory periods. Initially, the fascia was considered only a container of local anesthetic, and the target of the block was considered the nerves between the fascial layer. Now thanks to studies on the anatomy and physiology of the fascial system, it is precisely the fascia with its free nerve endings that is considered the target of the fascial plane block.

In fact, it has been highlighted that the fascia is richly innervated and contains free nerve endings, baroreceptors, and mechanoreceptors [5, 9]. Today, it represents the structure of the human body with the greatest number of free nerve endings [6] (Figs. 11.1 and 11.2). Pathological fascia is characterized by innervation changes such as increased density and sensitization of nociceptive nerve fibers. If peripheral sensitization is not interrupted, it could represent the substrate for the development of central sensitization with the development of chronic pain. The fascial plane blocks therefore have a double role, preventing peripheral sensitization and making the nociceptors insensitive to the surgical stimulus, and the second role is the treatment of CPSP by trying to reset the nociceptive transmission from the periphery towards the center. The pathophysiology of CPSP remains complex, and common mechanism is the primary sensitization of the afferent peripheral neurons and later central sensitization. Pain sensitization leads to the sprouting of nerves from damaged nerve endings and

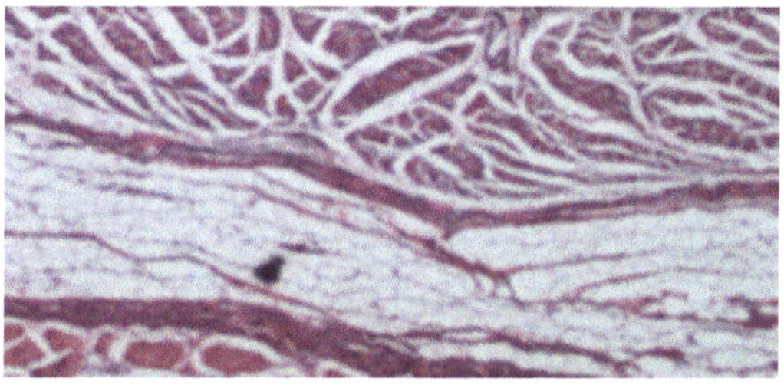

Fig. 11.1 Image owned by Professor Carla Stecco. Kindly granted for this study. Fibrous septa between the fascial layers

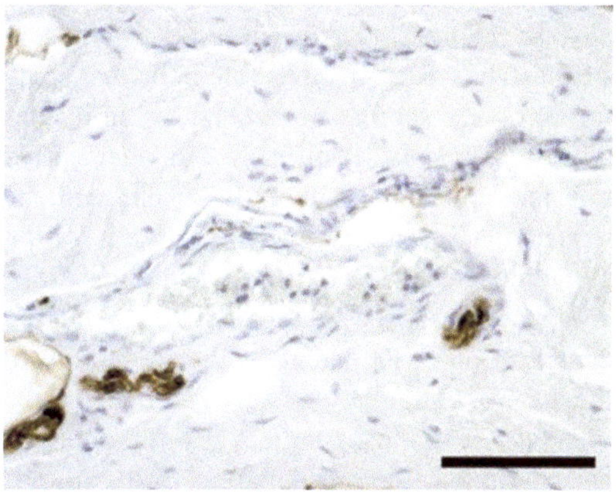

Fig. 11.2 Image owned by Professor Carla Stecco. Kindly granted for this study. Superficial fascia innervation, 100 mu

hyper-excitability leading to synaptic plasticity and windup phenomenon. Therefore, the first role of locoregional anesthesia is to block nociceptive transmission before the surgical incision.

11.6 The Role of Fascial Plane Block in Chronic Pain

Randomized controlled trials have demonstrated a positive effect of regional anesthesia on the prevention of CPSP following cardiac surgery and breast surgery. Furthermore, a Cochrane review has found that epidural anesthesia and paravertebral blocks significantly decrease the incidence of CPSP at 6 months following thoracotomy and breast surgery, respectively. Tissue inflammation and damage resulting from the surgical incision cause structural changes in the fascial system that contribute to the development of CPSP. In fact, there is an increase in the number and density of nociceptors and the aggregation of hyaluronic acid (HA) secreted by fasciocytes. Stecco et al. identified this phenomenon in fascial tissue defining it as "densification": a high viscous state of extracellular matrix due to HA super-aggregation with a decreased water-binding capacity. The presence of HA aggregates creates a stiffness of the fascial layers with continuous mechanical stimulation of the nociceptors [10, 11].

The fascial plane blocks act on chronic pain by restoring the physiological characteristics of the fascia. Thanks to the use of elastosonography, the relationship between fascia and muscle stiffness has been demonstrated. In fact, performing a fascial plane block causes an instant reduction in muscle stiffness and nociceptive transmission. Some authors have also demonstrated that even the injection of hot saline alone reduces muscle stiffness and pain, probably by reducing the aggregation of HA and the densification of the fascia, with a reduction in mechanical stimulation on the nociceptive fibers [12, 13]. Furthermore, various pathological conditions such as inflammatory pathologies cause the formation of connective septa between the fascial layers, contributing to stiffness and pain [14, 15].

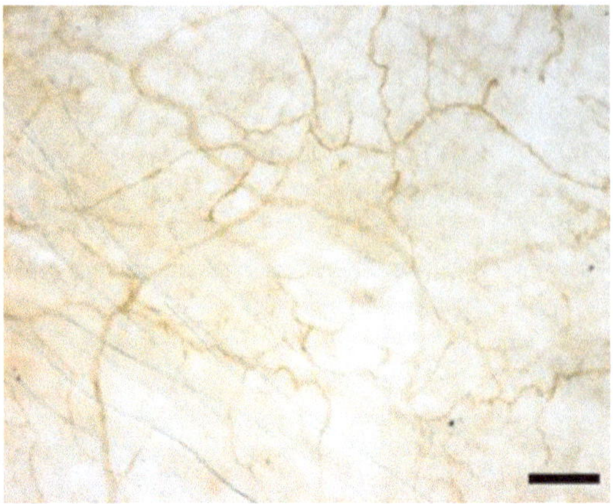

Fig. 11.3 Image owned by Professor Carla Stecco. Kindly granted for this study. Deep fascia innervation, 100 mu

The rationale for the use of fascial plane blocks in the treatment of chronic pain is based on the pathophysiological alterations of the fascial system [16]. In chronic pain, there are many fascial changes, and connective septa can compromise in fascial sliding and an alteration in the synergistic contraction of the connected muscle groups; for these reasons, the fascia could be an important target in the management of chronic pain itself (Fig. 11.3). The fascial plane blocks in fact allow the connective septa between the fascial layers to be broken, and the aggregation of HA to be reduced, with an improvement in the sliding of the different fascial layers [14]. Blocking nociceptive transmission reduces the possibility of developing peripheral and central sensitization.

11.7 Pain Management Medications

The management of chronic pain is based primarily on pharmacological therapy where the most used drugs are opioids, antiepileptics, tricyclic antidepressants, and serotonin reuptake inhibitors as well as fascia blocks [17].

- Antidepressant medications: Both tricyclic antidepressants (TCAs) and selective serotonin and norepinephrine reuptake inhibitors

(SNRIs) inhibit the reuptake of two important neurotransmitters: serotonin and noradrenaline. This inhibition increases the descending inhibitory pathways of the central nervous system related to pain. Additionally, TCAs also act on cholinergic, histamine, beta-2 adrenergic, opioid, and *N*-methyl-D-aspartate (NMDA) receptors and sodium channels [17].

- Antiepileptic medications: Both gabapentin and pregabalin are ligands to the αδ subunit of the voltage-dependent calcium channels, which overexpress in patients with neuropathic pain. By reducing this calcium-dependent release of excitatory neurotransmitters, these drugs decrease neuronal excitability [17].
- **Opioids** are available in diverse dosage forms to use for several routes of administration: oral, transdermal, intramuscular, intravenous, subcutaneous infusion, rectal, epidural, intrathecal, intranasal, and transmucosal [17].

11.8 Minimally Invasive Management of Chronic Pain

Among the minimally invasive methods for managing chronic pain, the most used are:

- Continuous and pulsed radio frequency
- Spinal cord stimulation
- Peripheral nerve stimulation

11.9 Conclusion

Even in the management of chronic pain and therefore in the execution of fascial plane blocks in the perioperative period, the fascia must be considered a target. Blocking nociceptive transmission reduces the possibility of developing peripheral and central sensitization.

References

1. Schug SA, Lavand'homme P, Barke A, Korwisi B, Rief W, Treede RD. The IASP taskforce for the classification of chronic pain. The IASP classification of chronic pain for ICD-11: chronic postsurgical or posttraumatic pain. Pain. 2019;160(1):45–52. https://doi.org/10.1097/j.pain.0000000000001413.
2. Fletcher D, Stamer UM, Pogatzki-Zahn E, Zaslansky R, Tanase NV, Perruchoud C, Kranke P, Komann M, Lehman T, Meissner W. euCPSP group for the Clinical Trial Network group of the European Society of Anaesthesiology. Chronic postsurgical pain in Europe: an observational study. Eur J Anaesthesiol. 2015;32(10):725–34. https://doi.org/10.1097/EJA.0000000000000319.
3. Feizerfan A, Sheh G. Transition from acute to chronic pain. Contin Educ Anaesth Crit Care Pain. 2015;15(2):98–102. https://doi.org/10.1093/bjaceaccp/mku044.
4. Katz J, Seltzer Z. Transition from acute to chronic postsurgical pain: risk factors and protective factors. Expert Rev Neurother. 2009;9(5):723–44. https://doi.org/10.1586/ern.09.20.
5. Fregoso G, Wang A, Tseng K, Wang J. Transition from acute to chronic pain: evaluating risk for chronic postsurgical pain. Pain Physician. 2019;22(5):479–88.
6. Lahtinen P, Kokki H, Hynynen M. Pain after cardiac surgery: a prospective cohort study of 1-year incidence and intensity. Anesthesiology. 2006;105(4):794–800. https://doi.org/10.1097/00000542-200610000-00026.
7. Charlton E, Atkins KJ, Evered L, Silbert B, Scott DA. The long-term incidence of chronic post-surgical pain after coronary artery bypass surgery—a prospective observational study. Eur J Pain. 2024;28(4):599–607. https://doi.org/10.1002/ejp.2203. Epub 2023 Nov 15.
8. Pak DJ, Yong RJ, Kaye AD, Urman RD. Chronification of pain: mechanisms, current understanding, and clinical implications. Curr Pain Headache Rep. 2018;22(2):9. https://doi.org/10.1007/s11916-018-0666-8.
9. Katz J, Clarke H, Seltzer Z. Review article: Preventive analgesia: quo vadimus? [Erratum in: Anesth Analg. 2011 Dec;113(6):1475.]. Anesth Analg. 2011;113(5):1242–53. https://doi.org/10.1213/ANE.0b013e31822c9a59. Epub 2011 Sep 30.
10. Pavan PG, Stecco A, Stern R, Stecco C. Painful connections: densification versus fibrosis of fascia. Curr Pain Headache Rep. 2014;18(8):441. https://doi.org/10.1007/s11916-014-0441-4.
11. Stecco A, Cowman M, Pirri N, Raghavan P, Pirri C. Densification: hyaluronan aggregation in different human organs. Bioengineering (Basel). 2022;9:159.
12. Fusco P, Stecco C, Maggiani C, Ciaschi W. Erector spine plane block with warm saline solution for treating chronic myofascial pain. Minerva Anestesiol. 2023. [Epub ahead of print].;90:217.
13. Fusco P, Stecco C, Petroni GM, Ciaschi W, Marinangeli F. ESP block and chronic pain: the dark side of the moon. Minerva Anestesiol. 2022;88(6):528–9. https://doi.org/10.23736/S0375-9393.22.16282-6. Epub 2022 Mar 23.

14. Fusco P, Nazzaro E, Petroni G, Stecco C, Ciaschi W, Marinangeli F. Fascial plane blocks and chronic pain: another step towards the future. J Clin Anesth. 2023;84:111010.
15. Stecco C, Macchi V, Porzionato A, Duparc F, De Caro R. The fascia: the forgotten structure. Ital J Anat Embryol. 2011;116(3):127–38.
16. Kondrup F, Gaudreault N, Venne G. The deep fascia and its role in chronic pain and pathological conditions: a review. Clin Anat. 2022;35(5):649–59. https://doi.org/10.1002/ca.23882. Epub 2022 Apr 27.
17. Queremel Milani DA, Davis DD. Pain management medications. In: StatPearls [Internet]. Treasure Island (FL): StatPearls Publishing; 2024. https://www.ncbi.nlm.nih.gov/books/NBK560692/.

12 Nociception Monitoring

Michele Martinelli, Valentina Trinchero, and Simona Silvetti

12.1 Introduction

The International Association for the Study of Pain (IASP) defines pain as 'an unpleasant sensory and emotional experience associated with actual or potential tissue damage or described in terms of such damage' [1]. The right to freedom from pain has long been recognized as a fundamental human right [2]. Differently, the nociception is not a subjective sensation as pain, but it is the physiological encoding and processing of noxious stimuli. Importantly, both pain and nociception can exist independently of each other [2]. In awake patients, pain evaluation is commonly assessed by clinical pain rating scales [3, 4], and the most common are:

- Visual analogue scale (VAS): This tool is commonly used to assess pain intensity. Patients rate their pain on a scale from 0 (no pain) to 10 (worst possible pain), providing a quantifiable measure that guides analgesic interventions.
- Numeric rating scale (NRS): Similar to the VAS, this scale allows patients to rate their pain from 0 to 10. It is simple and effective, particularly useful in the post-operative setting where patients may have difficulty with more complex scales.
- McGill Pain Questionnaire: This tool is used for a more detailed assessment and categorizes pain into various dimensions, providing a comprehensive overview that is useful for tailoring pain management strategies.

Unfortunately, the applicability of these systems is limited in anaesthesia and intensive care units (ICUs) where patients may be unconscious, delirious, or paediatric. Pain monitoring historically relies on the clinical evaluation and expertise of healthcare providers, who interpret clinical signs and surrogate measures (i.e. heart rate, blood pressure, tearing, pupillary response, or sweating). All these signs are also influenced by factors unrelated to pain, such as hypoxia, hypercapnia, hyperthermia, and medications. Nowadays, in anaesthetized subjects, pain cannot be directly measured, while nociception or the physiological response to nociceptive stimuli can be gauged. Patients' characteristic and different procedures compound the challenge of titrating analgesia effectively. Furthermore, the analgesia management is subjective, varying between anaesthetists, leading to wide variability in drug administration.

M. Martinelli · V. Trinchero
Department of Surgical Sciences and Integrated Diagnostics, School of Medical and Pharmaceutic Sciences, University of Genoa, Genoa, Italy

S. Silvetti (✉)
Department of Cardiac Anesthesia and Intensive Care, Cardiovascular Network, IRCCS Ospedale Policlinico San Martino, Genoa, Italy

G. Sepolvere, S. Silvetti (eds.), *Fast-Track in Cardiac Anesthesia*,
https://doi.org/10.1007/978-3-031-70899-2_12

Given these complexities, there is a clear need for the implementation of pain monitoring instruments in clinical practice to guide providers in perioperative analgesic therapy management toward a standard care.

12.2 Nociception Monitoring

Nociception monitoring is based on parameters that dynamically respond to the organism's nociceptive reactions. These parameters predominantly manifest as sympathetic nervous system activity, following stress-inducing events such as surgical procedures. These include alterations in heart rate and its variability, heightened peripheral vasoconstriction, galvanic skin conductance, and pupillary dilation. Additionally, certain electroencephalographic and electromyographic patterns, alongside thresholds of peripheral reflexes, are subject to evaluation. Monitoring systems commercially deployed are structured upon the utilization of one or more parameters, thereby stratified into single-parameter, two-parameter, and multi-parameter methodologies.

12.2.1 Single-Parameter Scores

12.2.1.1 Analgesia Nociception Index (ANI)

ANI is a simple non-invasive monitoring tool used to assess parasympathetic tone, pain, and discomfort. It relies on data from the electrocardiogram (ECG) obtained through two electrodes placed on the patient's chest. By analysing the time intervals between heartbeats (known as R-R intervals), ANI can gauge changes in the heart rate variability (HRV), which is influenced by both sympathetic and parasympathetic activity.

The variations of HRV in the high-frequency (HF) range primarily reflect parasympathetic activity, while those in the low-frequency (LF) range reflect both sympathetic and parasympathetic activities. A decrease in HF HRV or an increase in LF HRV typically indicates a decrease in parasympathetic tone, which has been associated with pain or discomfort. Based on these observations, ANI assigns a numerical value ranging from 0 to 100 where value above 50 suggests sufficient pain relief (high parasympathetic tone), while a value below 50 suggests the presence of pain (high sympathetic tone) [5]. A systematic review and meta-analysis of 30 studies illustrated the usefulness of ANI monitoring in predicting pain levels both during and after the surgical procedure and showed correlations with haemodynamic variables and a decrease in intraoperative opioid use [6].

Some studies [7–9] examined how ANI values changed in response to different stimuli, including variations in opioid concentrations and the administration of analgesic agents like opioid boluses. These studies collectively revealed that ANI values accurately reflect the body's responses to these stimuli. Susano et al. [7] noted a decrease in ANI values during a noxious stimulus (tetanic stimulation), and consequently, ANI values increase boosting remifentanil infusion. They observed, likewise to Gruenewald et al. [8], that as the concentration of remifentanil increased, the difference in ANI values before and after tetanic stimulation became statistically insignificant. Similarly, Ledowski et al. [9] found a notable increase in average ANI values after fentanyl bolus administration. These findings provide robust evidence that ANI monitoring reflects the equilibrium between nociceptive stimulation and analgesic levels, supporting its effectiveness as a tool for assessing intraoperative nociception.

Additionally, certain studies suggest that ANI values not only reflect nociception during surgery but also post-operative pain. Boselli et al. [10] discovered a significant negative relationship between ANI levels immediately before extubation and pain scores upon arrival in the post-anaesthesia care unit (PACU), indicating ANI's potential in evaluating post-operative pain.

Furthermore, ANI monitoring can serve as a diagnostic adjunct, facilitating the differentiation between real hypertension and pain causing hypertension, thereby curbing unnecessary opioid administration precipitated solely by haemodynamic indices.

Despite the potential advantages of ANI monitoring, its utility has some limitations: severe arrhythmias, atrial fibrillation, implanted pacemakers, cardiopulmonary bypass, and administration of antimuscarinic drugs [11].

Consequently, while ANI monitoring may not be suitable for intraoperative pain surveillance during cardiac procedures, its utility may be more pronounced in selected clinical contexts during the post-operative phase within intensive care settings.

12.2.1.2 Skin Conductance System

Skin conductance (SC) systems are based on the ortho-sympathetic response of spinal reflex, leading to increased secretion of sweat glands on the palms and soles. Skin activation of sympathetic nervous system fills sweat glands, reducing skin resistance and consequently increasing skin conductance until the sweat is reabsorbed, resulting in decrease in conductance. This event results in an SC peak. The magnitude of this peak corresponds to the intensity of sympathetic nerve activity, with small bursts yielding small peaks and large bursts yielding large peaks [12].

The MED-STORM AS 2005 monitor utilizes three self-adhesive electrodes labelled C (current), R (reference), and M (measurement), applied to the palmar or plantar skin. By employing a feedback configuration between the C and R electrodes, it applies a consistent alternating voltage across the R and M electrodes, recording the return current from the M electrode to directly measure skin conductance [13].

Research by Storm and colleagues has shown that the frequency of fluctuations in mean skin conductance per second (NFSC) significantly correlates with intraoperative noxious stimuli [14].

More specifically, both the number and amplitude of these fluctuations positively correlate with amine levels and blood pressure. In their study, they demonstrated that during tracheal intubation, and moreover during known surgical painful stimuli, NFSC reflected the stress response similarly to norepinephrine levels [15]. Furthermore, Ledowski et al. [12] support NFSC as a potential surrogate marker for assessing post-operative stress responses. They found that changes in post-operative pain levels, reported by patients on NRS, corresponded with NFSC changes, effectively distinguishing between mild and moderate/severe pain with high sensitivity and acceptable specificity.

Several studies validate NFSC efficacy in evaluating pain across different age groups and clinical settings, including the post-operative period and the ICU [16–18].

However, Sugimine et al. [19], in accordance with Treister et al. [20], suggest that while both NFSC and skin conductance level (SCL) can distinguish between 'high pain' and 'no pain' equally, SCL may be more accurate in differentiating pain intensity. Their primary focus was on determining if SC could discriminate between physical pain stimuli and other sympathetic stimuli, and they concluded that, while both NFSC and SCL increase during mechanical stimulation, only SCL increases during heat stimulation, indicating its superior utility in detecting physical pain.

SC may have some limitations particularly central and peripheral modulators of the autonomic nervous system, such as neuromuscular reversal agents or alpha-2-agonists, that could impact SC measurement [12]. The device is also contraindicated in patients with electrically sensitive life support systems like implantable pacemakers or defibrillators [13].

12.2.1.3 Pupillometric Assessment of Nociception

Pupillometry (Fig. 12.1) is a non-invasive technique utilizing infrared light, employed to assess iris muscle response across various clinical scenarios.

Pupillary diameter is regulated by the autonomic nervous system: sympathetic output induces pupillary dilation, known as mydriasis, and parasympathetic output determines pupillary constriction, termed miosis.

The parasympathetic innervation reaches the iris sphincter muscle through the oculomotor nerve (III cranial nerve) and short ciliary nerves, while the sympathetic innervation attains the iris

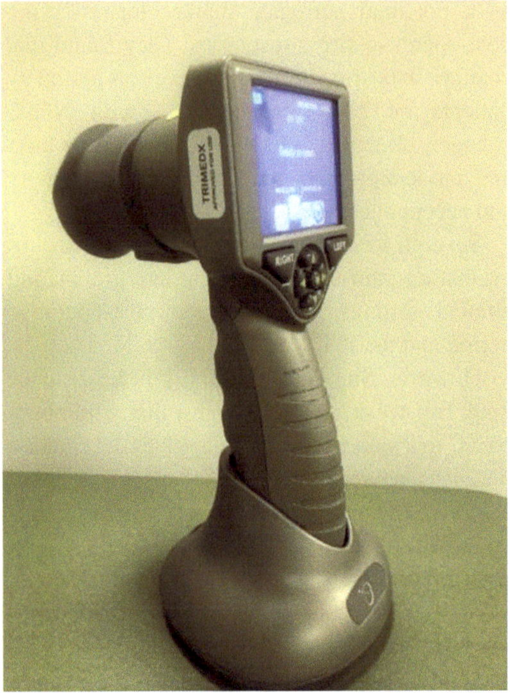

Fig. 12.1 Pupillometry. (Reproduced from Packiasabapathy et al. [21] with permission)

dilator muscle via long ciliary nerves that originate from the cervical sympathetic ganglion [21].

During anaesthesia, sedative medications depress sympathetic activity amplifying the influence of the parasympathetic nervous system on the Edinger–Westphal (EW) nucleus. The EW neurons act as pacemaker cells that affect the sphincter pupillae muscle fibres. Consequently, general anaesthesia leads to miosis [22].

More specifically, opioids exert a direct influence on pupillary diameter by diminishing inhibitory control over the EW nucleus, enhancing the activity of the efferent parasympathetic pathway connecting the EW nucleus to the pupil [23]. This leads to a contraction of the circular sphincter of the iris and to a reduction in the extent of the light reflex amplitude due to a limitation in the mechanical range of pupil [24]. Other agents such as propofol, sevoflurane, and desflurane independently decrease pupil size, attenuate the extent of the light reflex (irrespective of opioid administration), and do not depress pupillary reflex dilation in response to pain [21], while ketamine and nitrous oxide diminish the pupillary light reflex [25]. Dexmedetomidine and neuromuscular blocking agents do not significantly affect pupil size or pupillary reflexes [21, 26, 27].

When an applied noxious stimulus is sufficient to activate nociceptors via A or C fibres in an anaesthetized individual, pupil dilation occurs due to inhibition of EW neurons, resulting in relaxation of the sphincter muscle [22].

Its primary utility lies in neurologic evaluation, particularly in patients unable to communicate verbally due to altered states of consciousness induced by sedatives, analgesics, or specific clinical conditions. In anaesthesia setting, research indicates that the employing of pupillometry to guide analgesic administration can lead to an optimized pain management, reducing the opioid consumption during and after surgery, thereby minimizing opioid-related adverse effects [23]. In cardiac surgery, pupillometry has demonstrated utility in reducing opioid and noradrenaline dosages in the perioperative period, and it can also be utilized during cardiopulmonary bypass, where traditional methods of ECG and pulse contour-based analgesia monitoring are precluded by cardioplegia [28, 29].

Some condition could compromise the utilization of pupillometry for pain management, as the susceptibility of pupillary measures to ambient light, facial or ocular injuries, medications, and age-related miosis. Moreover, pupillometry is also constrained in providing continuous monitoring of nociception and analgesia, proving particularly challenging in surgical settings that require prone position, where access to the eyes is restricted. Furthermore, a range of pathological conditions, including Horner syndrome, Argyll Robertson pupil, Adie's pupil, and pupillary adhesions secondary to uveitis/endophthalmitis, have the potential to impair pupillary reflexes. Hence, baseline pupillometry prior to anaesthesia administration is essential to identify and mitigate these conditions, preventing misinterpretation of pupillary responses [21].

12.2.2 Two-Parameter Scores

12.2.2.1 Entropy

The spectral entropy monitor (Fig. 12.2) (manufactured by GE Healthcare, USA) is a dual-index electroencephalogram (EEG)-based monitoring system: the state entropy (SE), characterizing the depth of hypnosis, and the response entropy (RE), assessing the patient's reaction to noxious stimuli.

In essence, spectral entropy is calculated over the range of 0.8–32 Hz to define SE, focusing on the EEG-dominant spectrum, and from 0.8 to 47 Hz to define RE, covering both EEG-dominant and EMG-dominant frequencies. These entropy measurements are then converted into two distinct unitless scores: SE ranges from 0 (indicating deep anaesthesia) to 91 (representing wakefulness), while RE ranges from 0 to 100. The rationale behind extending the frequency bands to higher frequencies is rooted in the prevalence of electromyography (EMG) activities, particularly in the 32–47 Hz range, especially in frontal areas. Electromyography activity escalates when noxious stimulation is not effectively counteracted by adequate analgesia, leading to a motor response; meanwhile, spontaneous EEG predominantly reflects the level of hypnosis. Consequently, RE, incorporating EMG activity, was anticipated to capture both hypnosis (via EEG components below 32 Hz, akin to SE) and analgesia (via EMG components above 32 Hz) [30]. The difference between RE and SE, termed the RE-SE gap, was hypothesized to specifically indicate insufficient analgesia. This holds true for non-paralyzed patients and those with incomplete blockade. Notably, frontal muscles, being relatively resistant to neuromuscular blocking agents (NMBAs), may exhibit EMG response preceding a motor response or train-of-four (TOF) detection. For instance, a skin incision often triggers a notable increase in RE, SE, and RE-SE gap [31].

In patients administered rocuronium, EMG arousal is suppressed, leaving only EEG arousal detectable. The majority of EEG arousals typically manifest as mixed high-amplitude slow activity transitioning into lower frequency, low-amplitude activity, categorized as either *b arousal* (characterized by an increase in activity over 8 Hz and a decrease in activity under 4 Hz, exhibiting a typical b pattern) or *d arousal*, also termed 'paradoxical' or 'reverse' arousal (marked by an increase in activity under 4 Hz with the rhythmic d pattern and a decrease in activity over 8 Hz).

Recognizing these patterns is crucial for anaesthesiologists to adjust sedation and analgesia levels effectively. EMG and *b arousals* trigger an increase in entropy values, prompting anaesthesiologists to deepen anaesthesia. However, EMG contamination of EEG signals can lead to the inadvertent administration of excessive anaesthetic agents. There is also a suggestion of a direct impact of neuromuscular blocking agents (NMBAs) on anaesthesia depth. A debated 'afferent muscle spindle' theory posits that NMBAs diminish muscle tone and proprioceptive inputs to the reticulo-thalamic activating system, thus reducing arousal levels. While some studies support this theory, others dispute it.

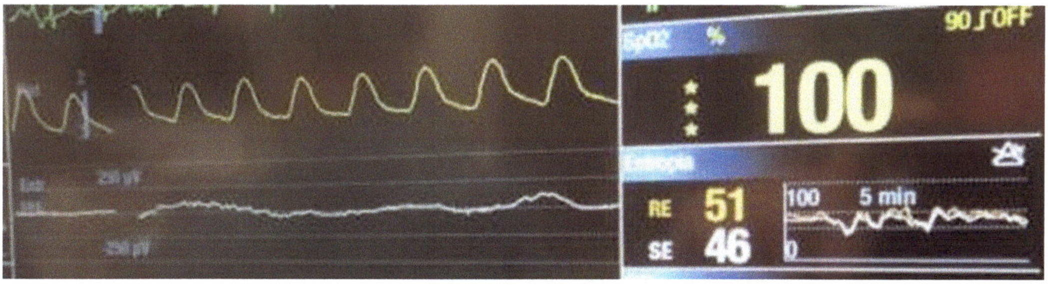

Fig. 12.2 Entropy

Misinterpretation of *d arousal* and subsequent SE value decreases may lead to a reduction in anaesthetic concentration, heightening the risk of intraoperative awareness. It is proposed that d arousal occurs when surgical stimuli are encountered amid inadequate analgesia.

In patients receiving rocuronium, a painful stimulus can trigger a significant rise in RE, often succeeded by an elevation in SE, resulting in no change in RE-SE. This underscores the importance of carefully monitoring and interpreting arousal patterns to ensure optimal anaesthesia management [31]. This phenomenon is further exemplified in Musialowicz's study [32], where they observed that the RE and RE-SE responses to surgical stimulation persisted even when muscle relaxation was achieved at a surgical level. Notably, RE and SE-RE values were notably elevated following skin incision and sternotomy. These findings strongly suggest that RE effectively mirrors nociception in response to painful stimuli, even in paralyzed patients undergoing cardiac surgery.

In another study focusing on cerebral monitoring during anaesthesia for coronary artery bypass graft surgery, researchers concluded that RE and SE appear to be the more reliable cerebral monitoring tools. They demonstrate superior resistance against both electrical and mechanical artefacts and significantly less interference from EMG patterns, whether with or without cardiopulmonary bypass [33].

Furthermore, Jiahai et al. demonstrated that entropy monitoring holds significant promise in optimizing off-pump coronary artery bypass surgery in several ways: firstly, it facilitates the monitoring of anaesthesia depth, potentially preventing intraoperative awareness; secondly, it enables the reduction of anaesthetic dosage. Finally, it aids in mitigating adverse effects of medications, such as haemodynamic instability and cardiac depression. Through these mechanisms, entropy monitoring emerges as a valuable tool in enhancing patient safety and surgical outcomes in these procedures [34].

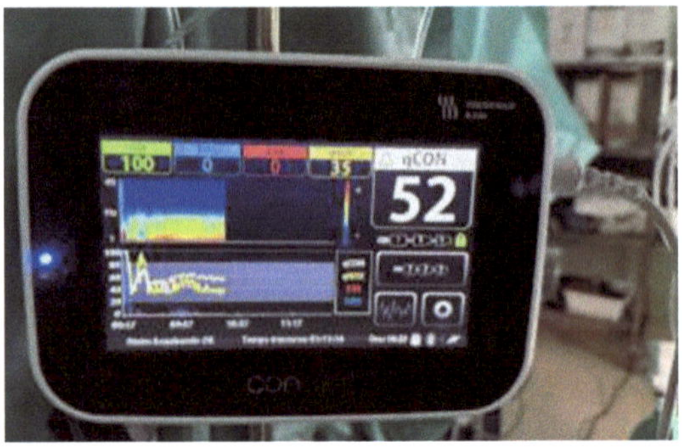

Fig. 12.3 Conox

12.2.2.2 Conox

The Conox monitor (Fig. 12.3) (Fresenius Kabi AG, Germany) represents an advancement in EEG-based monitoring, integrating two pivotal indices: the qCON index gauges the patient's level of consciousness, and the qNOX index is specifically tailored to evaluate responses to noxious stimuli [35]. The qCON index is a combination of various EEG frequency bands processed through a quadratic model. This model produces an output tailored to hypnosis-related variables, including the effect-site concentration of propofol and clinical scales like the Observer's Assessment of Alertness/Sedation or the Ramsay scale. The qNOX index integrates autonomic nervous system activity measured from brain signals with a direct assessment of pain/nociception levels. It selects and fits spectral features correlated with the pharmacological parameters of analgesic drugs, such as the effect-site concentration of remifentanil. It predicts the patient's response to painful stimuli, such as laryngeal mask airway insertion, laryngoscopy, and tracheal intubation, which are clinical scenarios where the tool has been extensively evaluated. Despite qNOX being constructed to target analgesic-related variables and qCON focusing on hypnotic variables, these two components of balanced anaesthesia are closely intertwined, and discrepancies between both indices may arise in situations of improper balance. Thus, while each index has the same target value focus, they are intricately linked and should be interpreted in conjunction to provide a comprehensive assessment of the patient's state under anaesthesia. The qNOX index quantifies nociception on a scale ranging from 0 to 100, and in general anaesthesia, the identified values typically fall within the range of 40–60. Values exceeding 60 indicate a heightened probability of response to external noxious stimuli, whereas a value below 40 suggests a reduced likelihood of response [36].

The utilization of the Conox monitoring tool has yielded notable benefits, including a substantial reduction in opioid dosages without compromising the quality of general anaesthesia, along with a commendable 25% decrease in the incidence of post-operative nausea and vomiting (PONV) [37].

The distinct feature of this monitoring tool lies in its ability to evaluate the central nervous system independently of autonomic activation measurements, such as changes in blood pressure, heart rate, and pupil dilation. Consequently, its applicability has been scrutinized in the context of cardiac surgery, where cardiovascular status and medication exert a significant influence due to the concurrent use of medications like beta-blockers, sympathomimetics, calcium blockers, vagolytics, and vasodilators. Additionally, haemodynamic instability stemming from factors such as hypovolaemia, vasoplegia, and low cardiac output further underscores the complexity of this surgical setting. However, a study [38] examining Conox in cardiac surgery setting in patients receiving lower doses of sufentanil showed higher incidences of haemodynamic and hormonal signs associated with nociceptive stimulation, despite no corresponding changes observed in the qNOX index between groups. The authors hypothesized that the qNOX index may be influenced by the concurrent use of muscle relaxants, which are indispensable in cardiac surgery. As such, they concluded recommending further investigations involving larger patient cohorts to establish the validity of monitoring the qNOX index and its relationship with the simultaneous administration of muscle relaxants. Another study [39] in cardiac surgery explored the impact of hypothermia during cardiopulmonary bypass on EEG indices assessing analgesia in patients undergoing on-pump coronary artery bypass grafting. The study findings revealed a robust positive correlation between the qNOX index and temperature across all patients, and authors concluded that it could shed light on the potential role of temperature modulation in influencing nociception assessment via EEG indices.

The potential of the qNOX to utilize pre-arousal data obtained at the conclusion of surgery to predict acute post-operative pain in ICU has also been explored. This investigation was grounded in the notion that establishing a connection between pre-arousal nociception and post-arousal pain could offer some level of quantitative validation for a nociception monitor. However, despite these efforts, researchers were unable to demonstrate a predictive value for the qNOX score measured at the end of surgery concerning the severity of acute post-operative pain upon admission to the ICU [40].

Conox emerges as an intriguing alternative to many other monitoring tools for the assessment of nociception, primarily due to its independence from measures of peripheral autonomic activity. This feature potentially enhances the robustness of the score against the influence of cardiovascular medications and comorbidities, offering a promising avenue for improved pain management strategies.

12.2.2.3 Surgical Plethysmographic Index (SPI)

The surgical plethysmographic index (SPI) (Fig. 12.4) is a valuable monitoring tool in the context of general anaesthesia, offering insights into the balance between nociceptor activation and analgesia. Derived from photoplethysmographic signals of the finger arteriole, SPI values are calculated through a specific equation: $SPI = 100 - (0.33 \times HBI + 0.67 \times PPGA)$, where HBI represents the heartbeat interval and PPGA signifies the photoplethysmographic waveform amplitude [41]. SPI values range from 0 to 100. Higher scores indicate elevated stress levels, while an SPI range between 20 and 50 is utilized to guide adequate analgesia administration during the anaesthesia [41].

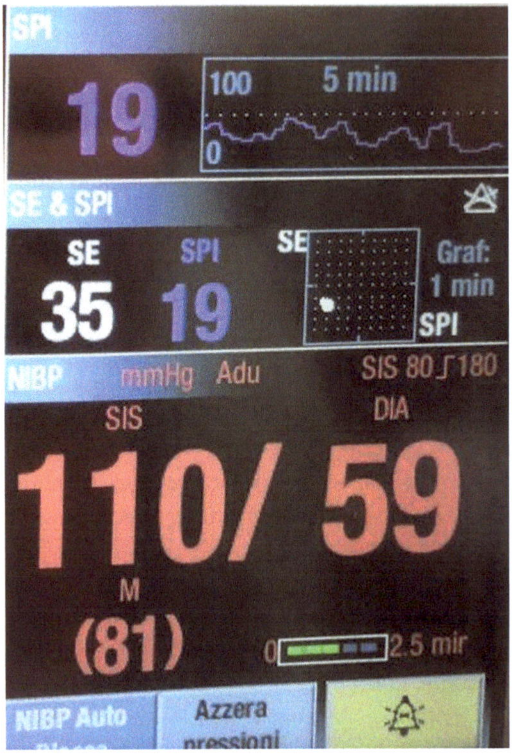

Fig. 12.4 Surgical Plethysmographic Index (SPI)

SPI values measured pre-arousal or in response to surgical stimuli exhibit a close correlation with subsequent pain intensity and opioid usage. Park et al. [42] noted a significant link between higher SPI values pre-arousal and increased pain scores in the ICU. They identified an SPI threshold of 60, indicative of moderate-to-severe pain with an NRS score ≥5. Furthermore, patients surpassing an SPI of 60 pre-arousal required higher fentanyl doses during the subsequent 48-h post-operative period. Conversely, Ledowski et al. [43] proposed a cut-off near 30 for optimal sensitivity/specificity in predicting moderate-to-severe ICU pain, albeit with modest overall predictive accuracy. Variations in consciousness levels at surgery's conclusion likely contribute to these discrepancies, as SPI values are notably influenced by arousal status.

SPI values obtained during the pre-awareness phase (under anaesthesia) reliably predict post-operative pain and analgesic requirements in the immediate post-operative period. Variability in patients' consciousness levels pre-arousal may explain differing study outcomes. Studies examining SPI levels at surgery's conclusion and immediate post-operative moderate-to-severe pain revealed elevated SPI values in patients experiencing significant pain. A higher SPI at surgery's conclusion exhibited potential to predict such pain with moderate sensitivity (0.71) and specificity (0.58), suggesting SPI's utility as a post-operative pain predictor in adult patients undergoing general anaesthesia [44].

Some considerations must be made when applying SPI monitoring in elderly and paediatric populations. In older adults, SPI may be overestimated due to a decrease in PPGA resulting from sympathetic stimulation, which diminishes with age. This potential increase in SPI value may be mitigated by the relatively unchanged heartbeat interval (HBI) response in older patients, as the cardiovascular response tends to be blunted. A study [41] showed that SPI-guided remifentanil administration during laparoscopic colorectal cancer surgery in elderly patients under general anaesthesia resulted in significantly higher remifentanil dosage administration compared to conventional analgesia practices, leading however to lower occurrences of intraoperative hypertension and tachycardia events without compromising post-operative pain management and recovery in the ICU. On the other hand, in paediatric patients, who typically exhibit lower vascular tone and higher vascular distensibility compared to adults, SPI values may be underestimated. Paediatric patients are less likely to demonstrate notable decreases in PPGA from sympathetic stimulation, which can lead to an inaccurate SPI estimation. Several studies have been conducted evaluating SPI applicability in children undergone anaesthesia, resulting in a less validity of the tool in this specific population [45].

Several limitations can impact the reliability of the SPI across different clinical scenarios. First, anaesthesia regimen: variations in anaesthesia protocols can influence SPI guidance efficacy. For instance, propofol-induced vasoplegia, characterized by decreased peripheral vascular resistance at high concentrations, may alter vascular wall distensibility. This phenomenon may lead to increased sensitivity to sympathetic stimulation, as observed in elderly patients. Additionally, studies have shown that dexmedetomidine administration reduced intraoperative SPI and NRS scores compared to saline control. Furthermore, deep neuromuscular blockade has been associated with reduced remifentanil requirements and shorter ICU stays during SPI-guided analgesia, indicative of its potential to alleviate post-operative pain. Second, vascular properties and medications: age-related changes in vascular properties, such as arterial stiffness and elasticity, can affect SPI readings, as PPGA depends on vascular distensibility and intravascular pulse pressure. Concurrent use of cardiovascular medications, particularly vasoactive agents like ephedrine, phenylephrine, and nicardipine, may also influence SPI values by modifying PPGA and heartbeat interval. Chronic hypertension treatment has been associated with reduced SPI responsiveness. Factors such as atropine administration, presence of pacemakers, and arrhythmias can further confound SPI measurements. Third, fluid status: SPI may decrease with worsening hypovolemia, but remains unaffected by fluid challenges in normovolemic conditions. Acute blood loss episodes pose challenges to nociception monitoring, as evidenced by significant increases in ANI during intraoperative blood loss or noradrenaline coadministration, while SPI remains unaffected. Fourth, positioning: SPI levels can fluctuate with changes in patient positioning. A 30° head-up tilt increases SPI, whereas a head-down tilt decreases it, with effects lasting at least 45 min. Prone positioning has also been shown to induce a notable increase in SPI. Last, peripheral nerve block: administration of peripheral nerve blocks during general anaesthesia has been associated with reduced remifentanil doses and pain scores. SPI monitoring can help confirm the regional analgesic effect during surgery [44].

12.2.3 Multiparameter Score

12.2.3.1 Nociception Level (NOL) Index

The PMD-200 system with Nociception Level (NOL) index (Fig. 12.5) technology (Medasense

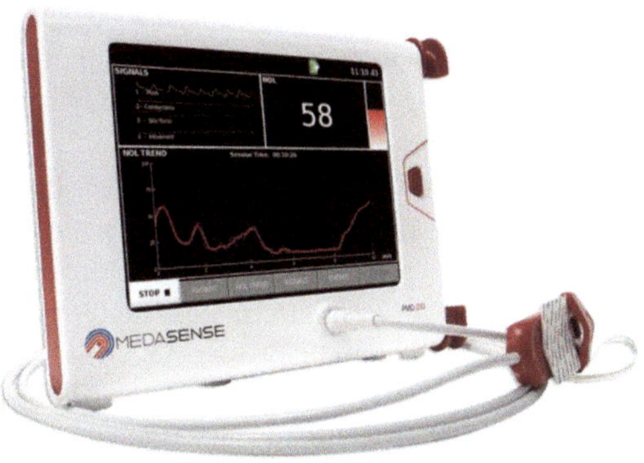

Fig. 12.5 PMD-200 system with Nociception Level (NOL) index

Biometrics Ltd, Ramat Gan, Israel) comprises a display and computing unit, a reusable non-invasive finger probe, and a single-use sensor. The finger sensor incorporates four distinct sensors: photoplethysmograph (PPG), galvanic skin response (GSR), peripheral temperature (Temp), and accelerometer (ACC). Through analysis of PPG and GSR signals, the system evaluates multiple physiological parameters related to nociception (e.g. pulse rate, pulse rate variability, pulse wave amplitude, skin conductance level, peripheral temperature, movement) and their derivatives, which correlate with the sympathetic nervous system's response to noxious stimuli. Temp and ACC signals serve as safeguards for signal acquisition. Utilizing a non-linear random forest regression technique, the system estimates nociception or related pain levels to generate a single index: the NOL index [46].

The NOL index, ranging from 0 to 100, is categorized into three ranges: 0–10, 10–25, and 25–100, corresponding to excessive anti-nociception, appropriately suppressed response to pain, and insufficient pain coverage, respectively. These ranges facilitate clinical management of analgesic drugs.

Clinical evidence suggests the following guidelines during surgical procedures under general anaesthesia: NOL above 25 for over 1 min may signify the need for additional analgesic therapy, with higher values indicating a stronger response to nociception; NOL between 0 and 25 indicates a properly suppressed physiological response to noxious stimuli, implying adequate analgesia; and NOL below 10 for over 1 min, specifically during painful stimulation, may suggest excessive anti-nociception.

The sensitivity of the NOL index has been assessed across a diverse spectrum of patients, categorized by age (18–65 years old, over 65 years old), sex (female, male), body mass index (normal, overweight, obese), ASA physical status (ASA I, II, III), anaesthesia drugs (propofol, sevoflurane, desflurane), and opioids (fentanyl, remifentanil). The findings consistently demonstrate that NOL delivers precise evaluations of nociception across various patient profiles and anaesthetic contexts [47]. Notably, it has been studied in patients chronically treated with beta-blockers, demonstrating its applicability in this subgroup as well [48]. Furthermore, in addition to its wide applicability, the use of the NOL index has been associated with a significant 1.6-point reduction in post-operative pain scores [49]. Additionally, subjects who received opioid treatment based on their nociceptive state during surgery experienced, on average, a 50% decrease in stress hormone concentrations during and after the procedure [49].

Several studies have sought to assess the utility of intraoperative NOL values in predicting post-operative pain. Ledowski et al. [50] found that NOL at the time of the initial skin incision, but not NOL throughout or at the end of the surgery, was significantly associated with the level of acute post-operative pain. Morrison et al. [51] utilized data from the NOLGYN study, a randomized controlled trial investigating the impact of NOL-guided intraoperative fentanyl administration on overall fentanyl consumption compared to standard care for gynaecological laparoscopic surgery. The study revealed that NOL post-intubation, median NOL during surgery, percentage of surgical time spent with NOL >25, and percentage of surgical time spent with NOL <10 were significantly linked to acute post-operative pain. Recently, Bornemann-Cimenti et al. [52] conducted a systematic review and meta-analysis focusing on nociception level index-guided analgesia compared to standard care. They found a statistically significant reduction in post-operative pain intensity and opioid consumption within the first 60–120 min after surgery with nociception level index-guided anaesthesia. However, they noted that the reduction in opioid use was not clinically significant for patients. No significant differences were observed in the duration of PACU stay or incidence of post-operative nausea and vomiting in the post-anaesthesia care unit with the use of NOL.

The NOL index has also been evaluated for pain assessment in post-operative awake patients following cardiac surgery, both during non-nociceptive and nociceptive procedures in the ICU. This study performed by Gélinas et al. [53] aimed to detect a moderate positive correlation between the NOL index and self-reported pain during nociceptive procedures, revealing positive mild correlations between the two NOL threshold values and pain intensity levels ≥1 and ≥5. The authors concluded that NOL effectively discriminated between nociceptive and non-nociceptive procedures, as well as between different pain levels (no pain, mild pain, moderate-to-severe pain).

12.3 Benefits of Pain Monitoring

Pain monitoring in anaesthesia and ICU is crucial for ensuring optimal pain management and improving patient outcomes. It is widely shown that surgery triggers a significant stress response, which is characterized by the activation of the hypothalamic-pituitary-adrenal axis. This leads to an increase in cortisol levels, resulting in a cascade of physiological changes that can have detrimental effects on the body such as increased heart rate, blood pressure, respiratory rate, decreased immune function, and increased inflammation. Correct pain management plays a crucial role in reducing the stress response associated with surgery, and by effectively managing pain, healthcare providers can modulate the activation of the hypothalamic-pituitary-adrenal axis and the subsequent collateral effects. One of the primary benefits of pain monitoring is better titration of opioids, which helps to avoid both under- and over-dosage, resulting in a better tailored analgesia to the patient's needs. This is particularly important in high-risk patients, such as the frail, elderly, and obese, who are more susceptible to adverse effects of opioids like respiratory failure, bradycardia, and toxic effects. It seems that it could also lead to a reduction in pain medication requirements in the ICU, resulting in fewer complications and a lower risk of adverse effects, such as respiratory depression, PONV, and delirium, but more studies are needed. Additionally, it seems to help to prevent postoperative hyperalgesia, a condition characterized by increased sensitivity to pain after surgery. Furthermore, in the intraoperative and ICU settings, it promotes greater haemodynamic stability, which is critical in patients who are already vulnerable due to their medical conditions. Moreover, significant benefit of pain monitoring is the confirmation of the effectiveness of multimodal analgesia and regional anaesthesia, techniques that have been shown to provide better pain relief and reduced opioid requirements compared to traditional methods. In addition, by monitoring intraoperative pain levels, healthcare providers can also adjust their analgesic strategies accordingly, ensuring that patients receive the most effective and safest pain management possible. In the ICU setting, pain monitoring is essential for ensuring that patients receive safe and effective analgesia, particularly in high-risk patients who may be more susceptible to complications.

12.4 Conclusion

In conclusion, it results that nowadays pain monitoring in anaesthesia and ICUs is crucial for achieving optimal pain management and improving patient outcomes. By better titrating opioids, reducing pain medication requirements, promoting haemodynamic stability, and confirming the effectiveness of multimodal analgesia and regional anaesthesia, healthcare providers can ensure that patients receive safe, tailored, and effective pain management, ultimately leading to better recovery and reduced complications.

References

1. Raja SN, Carr DB, Cohen M, Finnerup NB, Flor H, Gibson S, Keefe FJ, Mogil JS, Ringkamp M, Sluka KA, Song XJ, Stevens B, Sullivan MD, Tutelman PR, Ushida T, Vader K. The revised International Association for the Study of Pain definition of pain: concepts, challenges, and compromises. Pain. 2020;161(9):1976–82. https://doi.org/10.1097/j.pain.0000000000001939.
2. Loeser JD, Treede RD. The Kyoto protocol of IASP basic pain terminology. Pain. 2008;137(3):473–7.
3. Williamson A, Hoggart B. Pain: a review of three commonly used pain rating scales. J Clin Nurs. 2005;14(7):798–804.
4. Hawker GA, Mian S, Kendzerska T, French M. Measures of adult pain: Visual Analog Scale for Pain (VAS Pain), Numeric Rating Scale for Pain (NRS Pain), McGill Pain Questionnaire (MPQ), Short-Form McGill Pain Questionnaire (SF-MPQ), Chronic Pain Grade Scale (CPGS), Short Form-36 Bodily Pain Scale (SF-36 BPS), and Measure of Intermittent and Constant Osteoarthritis Pain (ICOAP). Arthritis Care Res (Hoboken). 2011;63(Suppl 11):S240–52.
5. Hum B, Christophides A, Jin Z, Elias M, Taneja K, Bergese SD. The validity and applications of the analgesia nociception index: a narrative review. Front Surg. 2023;10:1234246.
6. Kim MK, Choi GJ, Oh KS, Lee SP, Kang H. Pain assessment using the Analgesia Nociception Index (ANI) in patients undergoing general anesthesia: a systematic review and meta-analysis. J Pers Med. 2023;13:1461.
7. Susano MJ, Vide S, Ferreira AD, Amorim P. Effects of varying remifentanil concentrations on Analgesia Nociception Index® under propofol: an observational study. J Clin Monit Comput. 2021;35(1):199–205.
8. Gruenewald M, Ilies C, Herz J, Schoenherr T, Fudickar A, Höcker J, Bein B. Influence of nociceptive stimulation on Analgesia Nociception Index (ANI) during propofol-remifentanil anaesthesia. Br J Anaesth. 2013;110(6):1024–30.
9. Ledowski T, Averhoff L, Tiong WS, Lee C. Analgesia Nociception Index (ANI) to predict intraoperative haemodynamic changes: results of a pilot investigation. Acta Anaesthesiol Scand. 2014;58:74–9.
10. Boselli E, Bouvet L, Bégou G, et al. Prediction of immediate postoperative pain using the analgesia/nociception index: a prospective observational study. Br J Anaesth. 2014;112(4):715–21.
11. Daccache G, Jeanne M, Fletcher D. The Analgesia Nociception Index: tailoring opioid administration. Anesth Analg. 2017;125(1):15–7.
12. Ledowski T, Bromilow J, Paech MJ, Storm H, Hacking R, Schug SA. Monitoring of skin conductance to assess postoperative pain intensity. Br J Anaesth. 2006;97(6):862–5.
13. Storm H. Changes in skin conductance as a tool to monitor nociceptive stimulation and pain. Curr Opin Anaesthesiol. 2008;21(6):796–804.

14. Storm H, Shafiei M, Myre K, Raeder J. Palmar skin conductance compared to a developed stress score and to noxious and awakening stimuli on patients in anaesthesia. Acta Anaesthesiol Scand. 2005;49(6):798–803.
15. Storm H, Myre K, Rostrup M, Stokland O, Lien MD, Raeder JC. Skin conductance correlates with perioperative stress. Acta Anaesthesiol Scand. 2002;46(7):887–95.
16. Ledowski T, Albus S, Stein J, Macdonald B. Skin conductance for monitoring of acute pain in adult postoperative patients: influence of electrode surface area and sampling time. J Clin Monit Comput. 2011;25(6):371–6.
17. Valkenburg AJ, Niehof SP, van Dijk M, Verhaar EJ, Tibboel D. Skin conductance peaks could result from changes in vital parameters unrelated to pain. Pediatr Res. 2012;71(4 Pt 1):375–9.
18. Czaplik M, Hübner C, Köny M, et al. Acute pain therapy in postanesthesia care unit directed by skin conductance: a randomized controlled trial. PLoS One. 2012;7(7):e41758.
19. Sugimine S, Saito S, Takazawa T. Normalized skin conductance level could differentiate physical pain stimuli from other sympathetic stimuli. Sci Rep. 2020;10(1):10950.
20. Treister R, Kliger M, Zuckerman G, Aryeh IG, Eisenberg E. Differentiating between heat pain intensities: the combined effect of multiple autonomic parameters. Pain. 2012;153(9):1807–14.
21. Packiasabapathy S, Rangasamy V, Sadhasivam S. Pupillometry in perioperative medicine: a narrative review. Can J Anaesth. 2021;68(4):566–78.
22. Wildemeersch D, Peeters N, Saldien V, Vercauteren M, Hans G. Pain assessment by pupil dilation reflex in response to noxious stimulation in anaesthetized adults. Acta Anaesthesiol Scand. 2018;62(8):1050–6.
23. Sabourdin N, Barrois J, Louvet N, et al. Pupillometry-guided intraoperative remifentanil administration versus standard practice influences opioid use: a randomized study. Anesthesiology. 2017;127(2):284–92.
24. Shirozu K, Setoguchi H, Tokuda K, et al. The effects of anesthetic agents on pupillary function during general anesthesia using the automated infrared quantitative pupillometer. J Clin Monit Comput. 2017;31(2):291–6.
25. Eilers H, Larson MD. The effect of ketamine and nitrous oxide on the human pupillary light reflex during general anesthesia. Auton Neurosci. 2010;152(1–2):108–14.
26. Larson MD, Talke PO. Effect of dexmedetomidine, an alpha2-adrenoceptor agonist, on human pupillary reflexes during general anaesthesia. Br J Clin Pharmacol. 2001;51(1):27–33.
27. Gray AT, Krejci ST, Larson MD. Neuromuscular blocking drugs do not alter the pupillary light reflex of anesthetized humans. Arch Neurol. 1997;54(5):579–84.
28. Bartholmes F, Malewicz NM, Ebel M, Zahn PK, Meyer-Frießem CH. Pupillometric monitoring of nociception in cardiac anesthesia. Dtsch Arztebl Int. 2020;117(49):833–40.
29. Berthoud V, Nguyen M, Appriou A, et al. Pupillometry pain index decreases intraoperative sufentanil administration in cardiac surgery: a prospective randomized study. Sci Rep. 2020;10(1):21056.
30. Weil G, Passot S, Servin F, Billard V. Does spectral entropy reflect the response to intubation or incision during propofol-remifentanil anesthesia? Anesth Analg. 2008;106(1):152–9, table of contents.
31. Aho AJ, Lyytikäinen LP, Yli-Hankala A, Kamata K, Jäntti V. Explaining entropy responses after a noxious stimulus, with or without neuromuscular blocking agents, by means of the raw electroencephalographic and electromyographic characteristics. Br J Anaesth. 2011;106(1):69–76.
32. Musialowicz T, Lahtinen P, Pitkänen O, Kurola J, Parviainen I. Comparison of spectral entropy and BIS VISTA™ monitor during general anesthesia for cardiac surgery. J Clin Monit Comput. 2011;25(2):95–103.
33. Baulig W, Seifert B, Schmid ER, Schwarz U. Comparison of spectral entropy and bispectral index electroencephalography in coronary artery bypass graft surgery. J Cardiothorac Vasc Anesth. 2010;24(4):544–9.
34. Jiahai M, Xueyan W, Yonggang X, et al. Spectral entropy monitoring reduces anesthetic dosage for patients undergoing off-pump coronary artery bypass graft surgery. J Cardiothorac Vasc Anesth. 2012;26(5):818–21.
35. Martinez-Vazquez P, Jensen EW. Different perspectives for monitoring nociception during general anesthesia. Korean J Anesthesiol. 2022;75(2):112–23.
36. Jensen EW, Valencia JF, López A, Anglada T, Agustí M, Ramos Y, Serra R, Jospin M, Pineda P, Gambus P. Monitoring hypnotic effect and nociception with two EEG-derived indices, qCON and qNOX, during general anaesthesia. Acta Anaesthesiol Scand. 2014;58(8):933–41.
37. Sorsunov SV, Simdyankin K, Gritsan E. Intraoperative control of the depth of anesthesia and analgesia using a non-invasive monitor Conox in laparoscopic cholecystectomy. Russ J Anesthesiol Reanimatol. 2024;(1):51–6.
38. Rogozov V, Vanek T, Maly M, Rocek J, Kacer P. The nociceptive response during adult cardiac surgery measured by the qNOX index: a feasibility study. Biomed Pap Med Fac Univ Palacky Olomouc Czech Repub. 2024;168(1):62–7.
39. Wang X, Zhang J, Feng K, et al. The effect of hypothermia during cardiopulmonary bypass on three electro-encephalographic indices assessing analgesia and hypnosis during anesthesia: consciousness index,

nociception index, and bispectral index. Perfusion. 2020;35(2):154–62.
40. Ledowski T, Schmitz-Rode I. Predicting acute postoperative pain by the Qnox score at the end of surgery: a prospective observational study. Br J Anaesth. 2020;124(2):222–6.
41. Won YJ, Oh SK, Lim BG, Kim YS, Lee DY, Lee JH. Effect of surgical pleth index-guided remifentanil administration on perioperative outcomes in elderly patients: a prospective randomized controlled trial. BMC Anesthesiol. 2023;23(1):57.
42. Park M, Kim BJ, Kim GS. Prediction of postoperative pain and analgesic requirements using surgical pleth index: a observational study. J Clin Monit Comput. 2020;34(3):583–7.
43. Ledowski T, Burke J, Hruby J. Surgical pleth index: prediction of postoperative pain and influence of arousal. Br J Anaesth. 2016;117(3):371–4.
44. Oh SK, Won YJ, Lim BG. Surgical pleth index monitoring in perioperative pain management: usefulness and limitations. Korean J Anesthesiol. 2024;77(1):31–45.
45. Lim BG. Nociception monitoring tools using autonomic tone changes for intraoperative analgesic guidance in pediatric patients. Anesth Pain Med. 2019;14(4):380–92.
46. Edry R, Recea V, Dikust Y, Sessler DI. Preliminary intraoperative validation of the nociception level index: a noninvasive nociception monitor. Anesthesiology. 2016;125(1):193–203.
47. Ruetzler K, Montalvo M, Rotem OM, et al. Generalizability of nociception level as a measure of intraoperative nociceptive stimulation: a retrospective analysis. Acta Anaesthesiol Scand. 2023;67(9):1187–93.
48. Bergeron C, Brulotte V, Pelen F, et al. Impact of chronic treatment by β1-adrenergic antagonists on Nociceptive-Level (NOL) index variation after a standardized noxious stimulus under general anesthesia: a cohort study. J Clin Monit Comput. 2022;36(1):109–20.
49. Meijer F, Honing M, Roor T, et al. Reduced postoperative pain using nociception level-guided fentanyl dosing during sevoflurane anaesthesia: a randomised controlled trial. Br J Anaesth. 2020;125(6):1070–8.
50. Ledowski T, Schlueter P, Hall N. Nociception Level index: do intra-operative values allow the prediction of acute postoperative pain? J Clin Monit Comput. 2022;36(2):349–54.
51. Morisson L, Nadeau-Vallée M, Espitalier F, et al. Prediction of acute postoperative pain based on intraoperative Nociception Level (NOL) index values: the impact of machine learning-based analysis. J Clin Monit Comput. 2023;37(1):337–44.
52. Bornemann-Cimenti H, Lang-Illievich K, Kovalevska K, Brenna CTA, Klivinyi C. Effect of Nociception Level index-guided intra-operative analgesia on early postoperative pain and opioid consumption: a systematic review and meta-analysis. Anaesthesia. 2023;78(12):1493–501.
53. Gélinas C, Shahiri TS, Richard-Lalonde M, et al. Exploration of a multi-parameter technology for pain assessment in postoperative patients after cardiac surgery in the intensive care unit: the Nociception Level Index (NOL)™. J Pain Res. 2021;14:3723–31.

Part III

Minimally Invasive Cardiac Procedures and Fast Track

Evolution of Cardiac Surgery 13

Guohao Chang, Alessandro Caldarola, and Ottavio Alfieri

13.1 Introduction

In 1881, Theodor Billroth, at the Vienna Medical Society, stated that "no surgeon who wished to preserve the respect of his colleagues would ever attempt to suture a wound of the heart." Any surgical attempts made on the heart were therefore considered to some extent unethical.

However, successful repair of potentially fatal heart wounds was carried out by Henry C. Dalton in 1891, Daniel Hale Williams in 1893, Axel Cappelen in 1895, Ludwig Rehn in 1896, and Antonio Parrozzani in 1897.

During World War II, Dwight Harken proved conclusively that not only heart wounds could be sutured, but even intracavitary foreign bodies could be removed from the heart.

In the first half of the last century, cardiac surgery consisted of procedures performed with the heart beating, like closed mitral commissurotomy, and a number of operations for palliation or correction of congenital cardiovascular anomalies.

Following the adoption of the extracorporeal circulation in 1953, cardiac surgery evolved rapidly passing through various phases.

During the *pioneering phase* (1953–1970), almost all cardiac pathologies have been addressed. In the following years, until the end of the last century, the surgical treatment of heart disease progressed steadily and consistently, with new knowledge acquisition and implementation of increasingly precise, refined, and effective methods and techniques. At the same time, all the procedures have been validated with scientific methods, the incremental risk factors have been identified, the natural history of the diseases has been defined, and the operative indications have been clarified. This historical period, corresponding to about 30 years, can be considered the *phase of consolidation* of the cardiac surgical discipline.

In the new millennium, cardiac surgery has undergone a strong evolutionary process, entering a *phase of transformation* aimed at less invasiveness, making use of all the advances in technology including robotics and transcatheter and percutaneous techniques.

This process requires a convinced and intense multidisciplinary collaboration in the spirit of the "heart team" and in the perspective of "patient-centered care."

G. Chang
Department of Cardiac, Thoracic and Vascular Surgery, National University Heart Center, Singapore (NUHCS), Singapore, Singapore
e-mail: guohao_chang@nuhs.edu.sg

A. Caldarola (✉)
Alfieri Heart Foundation, Milan, Italy
e-mail: caldarola.alessandro@alfierifoundation.com

O. Alfieri
Alfieri Heart Foundation, Milan, Italy

Cardiac Surgery Department, San Raffaele University Hospital, Milan, Italy
e-mail: alfieri.ottavio@hsr.it

G. Sepolvere, S. Silvetti (eds.), *Fast-Track in Cardiac Anesthesia*,
https://doi.org/10.1007/978-3-031-70899-2_13

In this chapter, the most significant aspects of the pioneering phase of cardiac surgery will be briefly presented, while more space will be reserved to the phase of consolidation along with a special focus on the phase of transformation which is still in progress. Finally, future prospects will be outlined.

13.2 The Pioneering Phase

In the first half of the last century, due to advances in anesthesiology and particularly due to the introduction of orotracheal intubation, it was possible to perform open-chest operations and therefore to treat surgically some congenital and acquired heart diseases.

Ligation of the duct of Botallo was first performed by Robert Gross in 1938 [1], and correction of aortic coarctation by Clarence Crafoord in 1944 [2].

In the same year, thanks to the joint work of Helen Taussig and Alfred Blalock, the anastomosis between the subclavian artery and the pulmonary artery was developed for palliation of cyanotic congenital heart diseases with reduced pulmonary blood flow with great benefit for a large number of children, mostly affected by tetralogy of Fallot [3].

At the end of the 1940s, closed-heart mitral commissurotomy, an operation intended to alleviate the suffering of thousands of patients affected by mitral stenosis, was introduced into the surgical armamentarium by Charles Bailey [4], Dwight Harken [4], and Russel Brock [5].

In 1953, after years of laboratory experiments, John Gibbon performed the first open-heart operation with extracorporeal circulation [6], and the enormous potential of cardiac surgery in the treatment of heart diseases immediately became evident.

Initially, on the basis of the anatomical and pathophysiological knowledge already existing at that time, it was possible to correct the vast majority of congenital heart defects.

Among the pioneers of this type of surgery were Walton Lillehei in Minneapolis [7] and John Kirklin at the Mayo Clinic [8].

Later, in the early 1960s, due to the availability of mechanical artificial heart valves, it was possible to treat valvular disease with valve replacement.

A pioneer in this field was Albert Starr, who created the first valve prosthesis in collaboration with Lowell Edwards, and performed the first heart valve replacement operation [9].

In those years, using the extracorporeal circulation, also various forms of pathology of the aorta and large vessels were successfully treated. Michael DeBakey and Denton Cooley in Houston were the first to perform thoracic aortic replacement using vascular prostheses made of Dacron tissue [10].

In 1967, thanks to the introduction of selective coronary angiography into clinical practice by Mason Sones [11], René Favaloro was able to perform the first coronary artery bypass graft (CABG) operation for the treatment of myocardial ischemia [12]. Myocardial revascularization by CABG is still the most commonly performed cardiac surgical procedure in the world.

In December 1967, in Cape Town, South Africa, the first heart transplant was performed on a human being by Christian Barnard [13]. The event had an extraordinary worldwide media resonance and aroused great enthusiasm in the cardiac surgical community of that time. The results of the heart transplant were initially quite disappointing due to the difficulty in controlling the rejection. Only in the following years, mainly thanks to the research conducted by Norman Shumway at Stanford, could rejection be adequately managed, and cardiac transplantation became the treatment of choice for end-stage heart failure.

The pioneering phase of cardiac surgery ended with the implantation of the total artificial heart performed for the first time by Denton Cooley in 1969, with the aim of keeping a dying patient alive until a compatible heart was found for cardiac transplantation [14].

This experience, carried out more than half a century ago, paved the way for the great chapter of mechanical circulatory support, which is so important today in the treatment of advanced heart failure.

13.3 The Consolidation Phase

During the pioneering phase, the results of cardiac surgery were suboptimal in terms of operative mortality and rate of immediate and late complications.

It was the inevitable price to pay in a context of lack of knowledge in various areas, lack of consolidated experience, diagnostic imperfections, inadequate surgical techniques, and primordial technologies.

Obviously at this point in time, heart surgeons definitely turned all their efforts to improve outcomes and critically analyze the experience gained during the pioneering phase, using rigorous and sophisticated statistical methods.

The causes of surgical failures were investigated, identifying factors that increased operative risk.

The operated patients were then followed over time, their quality of life was objectively assessed, and adverse events in the follow-up were documented, establishing the probability of their occurrence over time in relation to different individual conditions.

The methodologies of retrospective analysis, introduced since the early 1970s by John Kirklin and Eugene Blackstone [15], were enormously contributing to make the results of cardiac surgery remarkably improved and more predictable.

The pathophysiological aspects of all congenital and acquired heart diseases were also investigated, and the natural history of the diseases was defined. As a consequence, the perioperative care improved, and operative indications as well as the timing of surgical interventions were optimized.

At the same time, the techniques of extracorporeal circulation and blood oxygenation have progressed, as well as the methods of myocardial preservation during aortic cross-clamping and cardiac arrest. In the latter area, the most significant contributions have been made by the experimental and clinical work of Michael Bretschneider in Germany, David Hearse and Mark Bainbridge in England, and Gerald Buckberg in the United States.

After the pioneering phase, surgical techniques have also been refined, with the aim of reducing the operative risk as much as possible and offering an optimal quality of life in the long term.

The following is a brief presentation of the most relevant aspects of the evolution of cardiac surgery in the last 30 years of the last century.

13.3.1 Congenital Heart Diseases

In pediatric cardiac surgery, a progressive trend towards reducing palliative interventions and carrying out complete correction of the congenital anomalies at an early age has been observed.

The immediate elimination of the hemodynamic disorder with its unfavorable consequences was a goal pursued with determination to offer young patients a life that was as normal as possible.

In order to achieve better long-term results, in patients with transposition of the great arteries (TGA), atrial flow reversal procedures have been replaced with radical anatomical reconstruction (arterial switch operation) [16].

Heart diseases considered inoperable and rapidly lethal have also been addressed, such as the hypoplastic left-heart syndrome. In infants with this disease, Norwood's intervention allowed immediate survival and paved the way for surgical solutions (mostly based on the Fontan's principle) that offered further prolongation of life [17].

Like the hypoplastic left-heart syndrome, there are other congenital heart diseases that present insurmountable anatomical limits (e.g., univentricular hearts) in the face of which cardiac surgery does not have the possibility of radical correction with the restoration of a four-chambered heart.

In many of these situations, the Fontan procedure, initially introduced for tricuspid atresia, has been a cost-effective option to enable an acceptable quality of life in the medium to long term [18].

Heart and heart-lung transplantation have been offered for congenital cardiac defects considered inoperable with conventional surgical procedures [19].

A special expertise was also needed for patients with congenital heart disease in adulthood (GUCH). A large proportion of these patients have already undergone surgery in pediatric age and present with various clinical problems that require special experience and deserve a multidisciplinary therapeutic approach [20].

13.3.2 Coronary Artery Disease

Coronary artery bypass grafting surgery has rapidly spread into clinical practice as a treatment for atherosclerotic coronary artery disease (CAD). Based on several prospective randomized trials, surgical myocardial revascularization has been shown to be superior to medical therapy especially in cases of multivessel disease and particularly in the presence of left ventricular dysfunction [21].

Since the patency of saphenous vein has been shown to be significantly lower than the patency of the internal mammary artery used as a revascularizing conduit [22], cardiac surgeons have been committed to increasingly favoring the arterial conduits, and in particular to invariably using the internal mammary artery to revascularize the anterior descending coronary artery [23].

In the 1990s, in order to reduce the trauma of surgery, the beating-heart myocardial revascularization technique was introduced, eliminating extracorporeal circulation and cardioplegic arrest of the heart [24]. Beating-heart coronary surgery, after an initial enthusiasm, has been abandoned by many surgeons due to the demonstrated lower patency of the conduits and is now mostly reserved for patients with serious associated pathologies and more compromised general conditions [24].

Minimally invasive approaches also found some space in selected cases. Particularly, isolated implantation of the left mammary artery on the anterior descending coronary artery could be conveniently performed with a beating heart through a small left anterior thoracotomy [25]. In the presence of multivessel disease, on the other hand, minimally invasive approaches have not found widespread application due to the complexity of the procedures, technical difficulties, and excessively long operating times.

In 1977, Andreas Gruentzig successfully dilated a severely stenotic coronary artery using a balloon catheter [26]. This extraordinary event was of great historical significance and consistently diminished the role of surgery in the treatment of ischemic myocardial disease.

The debate on the optimal treatment of CAD in relation to the number, distribution, extent, and characteristics of obstructive lesions has engaged cardiologists and cardiac surgeons for many years and is still ongoing.

Percutaneous coronary interventions have benefited over the years from various technological advances (bare metal stents, drug-eluting stents, absorbable stents) and represent by far the most prevalent therapeutic modality today.

Several prospective randomized trials comparing surgical therapy and percutaneous treatment have been performed to better define the indications in different circumstances.

Surgery still plays a role in the treatment of CAD and is essentially preferable in multivessel disease and left main trunk disease, as long as the operative risk is not high and there is a long life expectancy [21, 27].

Percutaneous techniques are to be preferred in acute coronary syndromes and particularly in myocardial infarction (primary angioplasty) [21].

Mechanical complications of myocardial infarction (rupture of the free wall of the heart, perforation of the interventricular septum, rupture of a papillary muscle resulting in massive mitral insufficiency) are infrequent but almost always fatal. In these dramatic situations, surgery was the only chance of survival [28].

The experience gained over time led to improved operating protocols and to the development of increasingly effective surgical techniques.

The surgical treatment of the left ventricular post-infarct aneurysm, which in the pioneering phase consisted of the removal of the fibrous sac and the closure of the breach with a linear suture [29], has been conceptually modified. In order to obtain a more efficient contraction of the heart, it has been considered essential to reconstruct the left ventricular cavity while maintaining its ellipsoidal morphology and preserving the physiological arrangement of the muscle fibers [30].

13.3.3 Valvular Heart Disease

Heart valve replacement in orthotopic position has been possible with the advent of extracorporeal circulation, and it has been carried out for several years almost exclusively implanting mechanical prostheses, with caged-ball or tilting-disc configuration [31].

The need for anticoagulant therapy along with the occurrence of thromboembolic and/or hemorrhagic complications soon led some surgeons to look for alternatives, such as biological tissue valves.

First, the possibility of using homologous aortic valves taken from cadavers was explored [32].

In addition to the advantage of avoiding anticoagulant drugs, homologous aortic valves allowed a central blood flow, associated with lower transvalvular gradients.

The extensive application of biological valves was possible only after the introduction into clinical practice of heterologous valves (first porcine, then constructed with bovine pericardium) fixed by an appropriate chemical process and mounted on a stent (bioprostheses) [33]. The limitation of bioprostheses is represented by structural degeneration, which occurs more rapidly in young patients [34].

Over the years, biological valves have been significantly improved, both in terms of hemodynamics and durability. As a result, the use of bioprostheses has increased steadily and consistently in recent decades, and the age threshold for their use has progressively lowered [35].

Valve replacement in children, due to the lack of sufficiently small prostheses, is definitely a challenge for cardiac surgeons.

As far as the aortic valve is concerned, the surgical procedure described by Donald Ross represented a solution that has proven to be valid and long-lasting [36].

The procedure essentially consists of replacing the pathological aortic valve with the patient's own pulmonary valve and reconstructing the outflow of the right ventricle with a valved conduit.

The principles of mitral valve repair, introduced by Alain Carpentier at the end of the 60s, had in the following decades a widespread application and an important positive impact on survival and quality of life of many patients with mitral insufficiency [37–39].

The preservation of the native mitral apparatus allowed avoidance of anticoagulant therapy with its complications, along with preservation of the structural continuity between valve and ventricle and of the physiological rheological conditions. Carpentier also proposed an anatomical-functional classification of mitral insufficiency that facilitated the standardization and therefore the universal diffusion of valve repair techniques [37].

In regard to conservative mitral surgery, it is worth mentioning the contributions of many other surgeons, including Carlos Duran and Robert Frater, who have effectively expanded the spectrum of reconstructive techniques [40, 41].

The preservation of the aortic valve was also a goal to be pursued in selected cases. In the presence of an aneurysm of the first portion of the ascending aorta, Magdi Yacoub proposed the aortic root remodeling surgery [42], while Tirone David introduced the technique of aortic valve reimplantation [43]. The results of these procedures on the function of the aortic valve have been very satisfactory even in the long term [44].

In the absence of aneurysmal dilatation, aortic repair for valvular insufficiency has been performed less frequently, although in expert hands and in well-defined anatomical contexts, it has been shown to be effective [45].

13.3.4 Congestive Heart Failure

After the introduction of myocardial biopsy for the early diagnosis of rejection in the early 70s [46] and especially following the use of cyclosporine as an immunosuppressive drug in the early 80s [47], cardiac transplantation has progressively consolidated as the therapy of choice for end-stage heart failure. Over the years, the results of the transplant have significantly improved, offering acceptable life expectancy, both in terms of duration and quality.

Of substantial importance in this regard were the improved criteria for the selection of recipients and donors, as well as the more effective preservation of the organ to be transplanted.

In addition, the modalities aimed at optimizing the compatibility between donor and recipient have been better defined, and a more articulated use of antirejection drugs has been applied.

Progress has also been made in many aspects of the complex organization, coordination, and transport of organs. Finally, the use of various mechanical circulatory assistance systems as a "bridge to transplantation" made it possible to save many patients for whom the organ to be transplanted was not immediately available.

Survival in heart transplant patients stabilized at 90% after the first year and 70% after the fifth year [48]. The most common causes of death documented in the first year after surgery were rejection and infections [48]. Later, deaths were recorded for various causes, particularly including coronary vasculopathy and malignancies secondary to immunosuppressive therapy [49].

The role of cardiac transplantation in the treatment of heart failure is severely limited by the small number of donors available and the rigorous selection criteria of candidates.

Since the 80s, looking at an alternative to heart transplantation, some cardiac surgeons have directed their research towards the creation of devices for prolonged mechanical circulatory support [50, 51]. Technological evolution has led to increasingly advanced devices in terms of safety and efficacy. Total artificial hearts and circulatory support devices to the left ventricle were created.

The evolution was from bulky para-corporeal to intra-corporeal systems, and from the use of a pulsatile flow generated by pneumatic pumps to the delivery of continuous flow by electrically powered centrifugal rotary pumps.

Initially, the purpose of mechanical assistance was to keep patients with advanced (end-stage) heart failure alive until a donor was found. More recently, mechanical assistance devices, significantly improved and more reliable, have also been implemented for permanent support ("destination therapy") or for "bridge to recovery" in the presence of potential reverse remodeling.

The systematic clinical use of mechanical circulatory support devices originated at the end of the last century has shown great potential since its initial experiences and is expected to play an increased role in the treatment of heart failure in the future [52].

13.3.5 Aortic Diseases

The most common acquired pathologies of the aorta are dissection and aneurysms. Both of these situations are potentially life-threatening and are effectively treated with surgery.

The surgical risk, initially very high, has been progressively lowered over the years, thanks to the understanding of the pathophysiology, the early diagnosis, the refinement of imaging modalities, the improvement of perioperative management, and the standardization of surgical techniques [53–55].

Regarding acute aortic dissection, the high surgical mortality was mainly attributed to the often very compromised general condition, the state of shock, and the multiorgan damage already present at the time of surgery.

In addition, tissue fragility could create technical difficulties that were sometimes insurmountable. The most significant contributions to the treatment of aortic dissection were made by Michael DeBakey, who developed an anatomical-surgical classification of proven practical utility, formulated the criteria for indicating the intervention, and established the objectives of surgical treatment [56].

Thoracic and thoracoabdominal aortic aneurysms represent a surgical challenge associated with high operative mortality and potentially devastating postoperative complications.

By implementing appropriate surgical strategies, however, the results of the interventions have progressively improved over the years. Selective anterograde cerebral perfusion techniques, introduced separately by Teruhisa Kazui and Jean Bachet in the second half of 1990, allowed replacement of the aortic arch without the need to deep hypothermia and circulatory arrest reducing neurological complications and post-extracorporeal coagulopathy [57, 58]. The surgical treatment of thoracoabdominal aneurysms has benefited greatly from the technical innovations introduced by Stanley Crawford, consisting of connecting visceral arteries and selected intercostal and lumbar arteries to the implanted vascular prosthesis [59].

13.4 The Transformation Phase

In the new millennium, the explosion of technology led to a radical change in the spectrum of therapeutic options for heart disease [60]. More specifically, the space reserved for minimally invasive, percutaneous, and hybrid approaches has been expanded, while conventional cardiac surgery through midline sternotomy has been drastically reduced.

In the new millennium, the epidemiology of the population to be treated for cardiac pathologies underwent a substantial change, and at the present time, the mean age of the patients is remarkably higher as well as the prevalence of severe comorbidities, ventricular dysfunction, and arrhythmias (especially atrial fibrillation). In this scenario, the need to reduce the invasiveness of the procedures, while maintaining their safety and effectiveness, is unquestionable.

As a matter of fact, minimally invasive approaches are associated with a lower rate of postoperative complications, a shorter hospital stay, and a faster functional recovery.

Nowadays, almost all patients with acute coronary syndromes are treated by interventional cardiologists in the catheterization laboratories. Coronary surgery is almost exclusively carried out in chronic ischemic heart disease and limited to situations well defined in prospective randomized trial [21, 61–64].

A large number of congenital heart diseases can be corrected by transcatheter procedures.

The treatment of heart valve diseases has been revolutionized by the introduction of transcatheter aortic valve implantation (TAVI) in the clinical practice in 2002 [65] and by the percutaneous correction of mitral insufficiency with a clip replicating the surgical edge-to-edge repair in 2003 [66].

The devices for these procedures have refined and diversified over time, and the expansion of the percutaneous treatment to an increasing number of patients became possible.

The non-inferiority of TAVI compared to surgical aortic valve replacement in high-, intermediate-, and low-risk elderly patients has been demonstrated in a large number of prospective randomized trials [67, 68].

The role of percutaneous correction of functional mitral insufficiency with a clip has been investigated in patients with heart failure, and the profile of the candidates for the procedure has been sufficiently defined [69, 70]. Surgery remains the preferred option in degenerative mitral insufficiency if the surgical risk is not excessive. Mitral regurgitation is also occasionally treated with devices that mimic the surgical annuloplasty [71] or the implantation of artificial cords for the correction of prolapse of valve leaflets [72, 73]. The percutaneous approach can be conveniently employed in other situations, such as periprosthetic leaks or degeneration of a previously implanted bioprostheses [74, 75].

More recently, transcatheter procedures have also shown efficacy in the treatment of tricuspid insufficiency and represent an excellent alternative to surgery in selected cases [76].

In addition to structural heart defects, many arrhythmias, which used to be treated in the operating room by means of specially designed operations, are now effectively treated percutaneously [77].

Similarly, an increasing number of aortic pathologies may benefit from endovascular procedures or hybrid strategies [78].

The transformation of cardiac surgery is not limited to the modality of approach (definitely less invasive) but is involving the practice of the profession as a whole.

In this regard, special consideration has to be given to the "Heart Team" and to the guidelines.

The "Heart Team" plays a central role in the decision-making process leading to the choice of therapy for a given patient. It includes various specialists with different skills and complementary knowledge cooperating to provide an objective assessment of the clinical picture and an evaluation of the risks associated with all possible therapeutic options.

The choice of treatment is made with the aim of offering the best possible solution, also considering the wishes and expectations of the patient himself.

Therefore, the "Heart Team" represents an essential tool for "patient-centered care" and personalized treatment.

The multidisciplinary discussion also represents an extraordinary opportunity to develop new ideas and original treatment strategies, as well as a unique opportunity for advanced teaching.

In day-to-day clinical practice, there are many cases that do not present particular decision-making difficulties and therefore do not need to be discussed within the "Heart Team."

On the other hand, in the presence of complex heart diseases and/or clinically relevant comorbidities, the evaluation of the "Heart Team" becomes essential to choose the best alternative within the spectrum of the available therapeutic options.

Furthermore, many procedures are nowadays carried out in hybrid operating rooms where close multidisciplinary collaboration is mandatory.

Finally, it should not be forgotten that shared collegial decisions and actions constitute a robust protection in any medicolegal dispute.

A privileged aspect of the medical practice today is the availability of the guidelines developed by professional societies and offering to physicians all the existing knowledge on each pathology. Recommendations are given by recognized experts and are based on available scientific evidence or consensus in the task force.

Since the guidelines cannot cover all situations that arise in clinical practice, the physician must always maintain the capacity to exercise his or her power of judgment and discernment.

A limitation of the guidelines is that on certain topics, they can quickly become obsolete, given the rapid production of knowledge by the scientific community at our time.

13.5 Future Perspectives

Future generations of cardiac surgeons will have to adapt psychologically to the various aspects of the transformation phase.

First of all, it will be necessary to have an aptitude to teamwork, offering one's contribution with generosity and humility, feeling an integral part of a multidisciplinary group with a common mission and shared intentions.

Personal ambition should not be to be the best, but to become better every day. Only in this way will it be possible to avoid harmful attitudes of preeminence or self-centeredness, without sacrificing motivation and gratification.

Teamwork requires open-mindedness, respect for others, listening skills, and willingness to discuss.

In terms of specific skills, it is likely that in the future, each cardiac surgeon will have his or her own personal and peculiar profile mainly built based on the experience gained in the role held within the multidisciplinary team.

This creates a scenario of superspecialists dedicated to specific diseases and well-defined clinical problems.

Cardiac surgery is presumably expected to differentiate into three main lines:

- Conventional interventions of great complexity (pathology of the thoracic aorta, endocarditis, mechanical complications of myocardial infarction, reoperations)

- Minimally invasive interventions, including percutaneous procedures and robotic-assisted procedures
- Interventions for advanced heart failure (heart transplantation and mechanical circulatory assistance)

Each of these three areas of activity requires in-depth knowledge, solid experience, specific interdisciplinary collaborations, special aptitudes, and talents. Therefore, it is difficult for the same specialist to devote himself to all areas of cardiac surgery.

The cardiac surgeon of tomorrow, with focused clinical interests, will not be able to avoid the commitment to continuous training, as well as to scientific research and innovation. There can be no clinical activity of excellence if there is no critical analysis of the data collected and if the mind does not concentrate on exploring new ways and finding original solutions. Creativity has always characterized the discipline of cardiac surgery, as well demonstrated by the extraordinary history of the pioneering phase and the continuous progress made subsequently.

13.6 Summary

The roots of cardiac surgery date back to the first half of the last century. Subsequently, thanks to the development of the heart-lung machine, which made it possible to operate inside the heart cavities under direct vision, the enormous potential of this discipline in the treatment of cardiovascular diseases became evident.

In the years that followed, until the end of the last century, the surgical treatment of heart disease progressed steadily and consistently. Since the beginning of the millennium, cardiac surgery has undergone a strong evolutionary process with the advent of minimally invasive and transcatheter techniques.

These procedures have transformed the landscape of cardiac care, providing new hope even to individuals who were once considered at high risk or inoperable.

References

1. Taylor EJ. Opening the heart; the operation. The New York Times. New York: McGraw-Hill Book Company; 1958. p. 277.
2. Kvitting JP, Olin CL. Clarence Crafoord: a giant in cardiothoracic surgery, the first to repair aortic coarctation. Ann Thorac Surg. 2009;87:342–6.
3. Cooley DA. The first Blalock-Taussig shunt. J Thorac Cardiovasc Surg. 2010;140:750–1.
4. Gonzalez-Lavin L, Charles P. Bailey and Dwight E. Harken—the dawn of the modern era of mitral valve surgery. Ann Thorac Surg. 1992;53:916–9.
5. Brock R. The technique of mitral valvotomy. Ann R Coll Surg Engl. 1956;19:1–22.
6. Hill JD. John H. Gibbon, Jr. Part I. The development of the first successful heart-lung machine. Ann Thorac Surg. 1982;34:337–41.
7. Gott VL. C. Walton Lillehei (1918–1999). J Thorac Cardiovasc Surg. 1999;118:774–5.
8. Cooley DA. In memoriam John W. Kirklin 1917–2004. Tex Heart Inst J. 2004;31:113.
9. Starr A, Edwards ML. Mitral replacement: clinical experience with a ball-valve prosthesis. Ann Surg. 1961;154:726–40.
10. De Bakey ME, Cooley DA. Successful resection of aneurysm of thoracic aorta and replacement by graft. JAMA J Am Med Assoc. 1953;152:673–6.
11. Bourassa MG. The history of cardiac catheterization. Can J Cardiol. 2005;21:1011–4.
12. Bakaeen FG, Blackstone EH, Pettersson GB, Gillinov AM, Svensson LG. The father of coronary artery bypass grafting: René Favaloro and the 50th anniversary of coronary artery bypass grafting. J Thorac Cardiovasc Surg. 2018;155:2324–8.
13. Barnard CN. The operation. A human cardiac transplant: an interim report of a successful operation performed at Groote Schuur Hospital, Cape Town. S Afr Med J. 1967;41:1271–4.
14. Cooley DA. The total artificial heart as a bridge to cardiac transplantation: personal recollections. Tex Heart Inst J. 2001;28:200–2.
15. Sabik JF III. 2013 Scientific Achievement Award recipient: Eugene H. Blackstone, MD. J Thorac Cardiovasc Surg. 2013;146:1003–5.
16. Lecompte Y, Zannini L, Hazan E, et al. Anatomic correction of transposition of the great arteries. J Thorac Cardiovasc Surg. 1981;82:629–31.
17. Norwood WI, Lang P, Casteneda AR, Campbell DN. Experience with operations for hypoplastic left heart syndrome. J Thorac Cardiovasc Surg. 1981;82:511–9.
18. D'Udekem Y, Iyengar AJ, Cochrane AD, et al. The Fontan procedure: contemporary techniques have improved longterm outcomes. Circulation. 2007;116(11 Suppl):I157–64.
19. Dipchand AI. Current state of pediatric cardiac transplantation. Ann Cardiothorac Surg. 2018;7:31–55.

20. Baumgartner H, Bonhoeffer P, De Groot NMS, et al., Task Force on the Management of Grown-up Congenital Heart Disease of the European Society of Cardiology (ESC); Association for European Paediatric Cardiology (AEPC); ESC Committee for Practice Guidelines (CPG). ESC Guidelines for the management of grownup congenital heart disease (new version 2010). Eur Heart J. 2010;31: 2915–57.
21. Neumann FJ, Sousa-Uva M, Ahlsson A, et al. 2018 ESC/EACTS Guidelines on myocardial revascularization. Eur Heart J. 2019;40:87–165.
22. Boylan MJ, Lytle BW, Loop FD, et al. Surgical treatment of isolated left anterior descending coronary stenosis. Comparison of left internal mammary artery and venous autograft at 18 to 20 years of follow-up. J Thorac Cardiovasc Surg. 1994;107:657–62.
23. Schmitto JD, Rajab TK, Cohn LH. Prevalence and variability of internal mammary graft use in contemporary multivessel coronary artery bypass graft. Curr Opin Cardiol. 2010;25:609–12.
24. Gaudino M, Angelini GD, Antoniades C, et al. Off-pump coronary artery bypass grafting: 30 years of debate. J Am Heart Assoc. 2018;7:e009934.
25. Kettering K, Dapunt O, Baer FM. Minimally invasive direct coronary artery bypass grafting: a systematic review. J Cardiovasc Surg. 2004;45:255–64.
26. Meier B, Bachmann D, Lüscher T. 25 Years of coronary angioplasty: almost a fairy tale. Lancet. 2003;361:527.
27. Gaudino M, Bakaeen FG, Benedetto U, et al. Arterial grafts for coronary bypass: a critical review after the publication of ART and RADIAL. Circulation. 2019;140:1273–84.
28. Gong FF, Vaitenas I, Malaisrie SC, Maganti K. Mechanical complications of acute myocardial infarction: a review. JAMA Cardiol. 2021;6: 341–9.
29. Vural KM, Şener E, Özatik MA, Taşdemir O, Bayazit K. Left ventricular aneurysm repair: an assessment of surgical treatment modalities. Eur J Cardiothorac Surg. 1998;13:49–56.
30. Menicanti L, Di Donato M. Left ventricular aneurysm/reshaping techniques. Multimed Man Cardiothorac Surg. 2005;2005:mmcts.2004.000596.
31. Donatelli R, Palminiello A, Colombi P. Multiple valve substitutions. Minerva Cardioangiol. 1968;16:1029–46.
32. El-Hamamsy I, Eryigit Z, Stevens LM, et al. Long-term outcomes after autograft versus homograft aortic root replacement in adults with aortic valve disease: a randomised controlled trial. Lancet. 2010;376:524–31.
33. Vesely I. The evolution of bioprosthetic heart valve design and its impact on durability. Cardiovasc Pathol. 2003;12:277–86.
34. Kostyunin AE, Yuzhalin AE, Rezvova MA, Ovcharenko EA, Glushkova TV, Kutikhin AG. Degeneration of bioprosthetic heart valves: update 2020. J Am Heart Assoc. 2020;9:e018506.
35. Baumgartner H, Falk V, Bax JJ, et al. 2017 ESC/EACTS Guidelines for the management of valvular heart disease. Eur Heart J. 2017;38:2739–91.
36. Etnel JRG, Grashuis P, Huygens SA, et al. The Ross procedure: a systematic review, meta-analysis, and microsimulation. Circ Cardiovasc Qual Outcomes. 2018;11:e004748.
37. Carpentier A. Cardiac valve surgery—the "French correction". J Thorac Cardiovasc Surg. 1983;86:323–37.
38. Perier P, Hohenberger W, Lakew F, et al. Toward a new paradigm for the reconstruction of posterior leaflet prolapse: midterm results of the "respect rather than resect" approach. Ann Thorac Surg. 2008;86:718–25.
39. Alfieri O, Maisano F, De Bonis M, et al. The double-orifice technique in mitral valve repair: a simple solution for complex problems. J Thorac Cardiovasc Surg. 2001;122:674–81.
40. Duran CM. Surgical techniques for the repair of anterior mitral leaflet prolapse. J Card Surg. 1999;14:471–81.
41. Frater RW, Berghuis J, Brown ALJ, Ellis FHJ. The experimental and clinical use of autogenous pericardium for the replacement and extension of mitral and tricuspid value cusps and chordae. J Cardiovasc Surg. 1965;6:214–28.
42. Sarsam MA, Yacoub M. Remodeling of the aortic valve anulus. J Thorac Cardiovasc Surg. 1993;105:435–8.
43. David TE, Feindel CM. An aortic valve-sparing operation for patients with aortic incompetence and aneurysm of the ascending aorta. J Thorac Cardiovasc Surg. 1992;103:617–22.
44. David TE, Feindel CM, David CM, Manlhiot C. A quarter of a century of experience with aortic valve-sparing operations. J Thorac Cardiovasc Surg. 2014;148:872–80.
45. Schneider U, Miyahara S, Giebels C, Karliova I, Schäfers HJ. Isolated aortic valve repair-how to do it and long-term results: suture annuloplasty. Ann Cardiothorac Surg. 2019;8:422–5.
46. Caves PK, Stinson EB, Graham AF, Billingham ME, Grehl TM, Shumway NE. Percutaneous transvenous endomyocardial biopsy. JAMA. 1973;225:288–91.
47. Colombo D, Ammirati E. Cyclosporine in transplantation—a history of converging timelines. J Biol Regul Homeost Agents. 2011;25:493–504.
48. Kittleson MM, Kobashigawa JA. Cardiac transplantation: current outcomes and contemporary controversies. JACC Heart Fail. 2017;5:857–68.
49. Kirklin JK, Naftel DC, Bourge RC, et al. Evolving trends in risk profiles and causes of death after heart transplantation: a ten-year multi-institutional study. J Thorac Cardiovasc Surg. 2003;125:881–90.
50. DeBakey ME. Development of mechanical heart devices. Ann Thorac Surg. 2005;79:S2228–31.
51. Rose EA, Gelijns AC, Moskowitz AJ, et al., Randomized Evaluation of Mechanical Assistance for the Treatment of Congestive Heart Failure (REMATCH) Study Group. Long-term use of a left ventricular assist device for end-stage heart failure. N Engl J Med. 2001;345:1435–43.

52. Han JJ, Acker MA, Atluri P. Left ventricular assist devices. Circulation. 2018;138:2841–51.
53. Abe T, Yamamoto H, Miyata H, et al. Patient trends and outcomes of surgery for type A acute aortic dissection in Japan: an analysis of more than 10 000 patients from the Japan Cardiovascular Surgery Database. Eur J Cardiothorac Surg. 2020;57:660–7.
54. Evangelista A, Isselbacher EM, Bossone E, et al., IRAD Investigators. Insights from the International Registry of Acute Aortic Dissection: a 20-year experience of collaborative clinical research. Circulation. 2018;137:1846–60.
55. Achneck HE, Rizzo JA, Tranquilli M, Elefteriades JA. Safety of thoracic aortic surgery in the present era. Ann Thorac Surg. 2007;84:1180–5.
56. DeBakey ME, Henly WS, Cooley DA, Morris GCJ, Crawford ES, Beall ACJ. Surgical management of dissecting aneurysms of the aorta. J Thorac Cardiovasc Surg. 1965;49:130–49.
57. Kazui T, Yamashita K, Washiyama N, et al. Usefulness of antegrade selective cerebral perfusion during aortic arch operations. Ann Thorac Surg. 2002;74:S1806–9.
58. Pacini D, Leone A, Di Marco L, et al. Antegrade selective cerebral perfusion in thoracic aorta surgery: safety of moderate hypothermia. Eur J Cardiothorac Surg. 2007;31:618–22.
59. Crawford ES, Crawford JL, Safi HJ, et al. Thoracoabdominal aortic aneurysms: preoperative and intraoperative factors determining immediate and long-term results of operations in 605 patients. J Vasc Surg. 1986;3:389–404.
60. Del Forno B, De Bonis M, Agricola E, et al. Mitral valve regurgitation: a disease with a wide spectrum of therapeutic options. Nat Rev Cardiol. 2020;17:807–27.
61. Serruys PW, Morice MC, Kappetein AP, et al., SYNTAX Investigators. Percutaneous coronary intervention versus coronary-artery bypass grafting for severe coronary artery disease. N Engl J Med. 2009;360:961–72.
62. Farkouh ME, Domanski M, Sleeper LA, et al., FREEDOM Trial Investigators. Strategies for multivessel revascularization in patients with diabetes. N Engl J Med. 2012;367:2375–84.
63. Stone GW, Kappetein AP, Sabik JF, et al., EXCEL Trial Investigators. Five year outcomes after PCI or CABG for left main coronary disease. N Engl J Med. 2019;381:1820–30.
64. Holm NR, Mäkikallio T, Lindsay MM, et al., NOBLE Investigators. Percutaneous coronary angioplasty versus coronary artery bypass grafting in the treatment of unprotected left main stenosis: updated 5-year outcomes from the randomised, non-inferiority NOBLE trial. Lancet. 2020;395:191–9.
65. Cribier A, Eltchaninoff H, Bash A, et al. Percutaneous transcatheter implantation of an aortic valve prosthesis for calcific aortic stenosis: first human case description. Circulation. 2002;106:3006–8.
66. Condado JA, Acquatella H, Rodriguez L, Whitlow P, Vélez-Gimo M, St Goar FG. Percutaneous edge-to-edge mitral valve repair: 2-year follow-up in the first human case. Catheter Cardiovasc Interv. 2006;67:323–5.
67. Thyregod HGH, Ihlemann N, Jørgensen TH, et al. Five-year clinical and echocardiographic outcomes from the Nordic Aortic Valve Intervention (NOTION) randomized clinical trial in lower surgical risk patients. Circulation. 2019;139:2714–23.
68. Mack MJ, Leon MB, Thourani VH, et al., PARTNER 3 Investigators. Transcatheter aortic-valve replacement with a balloon-expandable valve in low-risk patients. N Engl J Med. 2019;380:1695–705.
69. Stone GW, Lindenfeld J, Abraham WT, et al., COAPT Investigators. Transcatheter mitral-valve repair in patients with heart failure. N Engl J Med. 2018;379:2307–18.
70. Obadia JF, Messika-Zeitoun D, Leurent G, et al., MITRA-FR Investigators. Percutaneous repair or medical treatment for secondary mitral regurgitation. N Engl J Med. 2018;379:2297–306.
71. Messika-Zeitoun D, Nickenig G, Latib A, et al. Transcatheter mitral valve repair for functional mitral regurgitation using the Cardioband system: 1 year outcomes. Eur Heart J. 2019;40:466–72.
72. Colli A, Besola L, Bizzotto E, et al. Mechanisms of recurrent regurgitation after transapical off-pump mitral valve repair with neochord implantation. Eur J Cardiothorac Surg. 2019;56:479–87.
73. Gerosa G, Besola L, Beiras-Fernandez A, et al. The neochord procedure after failed surgical mitral valve repair. Semin Thorac Cardiovasc Surg. 2021;33:35–44.
74. Yoon SH, Whisenant BK, Bleiziffer S, et al. Outcomes of transcatheter mitral valve replacement for degenerated bioprostheses, failed annuloplasty rings, and mitral annular calcification. Eur Heart J. 2019;40:441–51.
75. Cruz-Gonzalez I, Rama-Merchan JC, Rodríguez-Collado J, et al. Transcatheter closure of paravalvular leaks: state of the art. Neth Heart J. 2017;25:116–24.
76. Taramasso M, Benfari G, van der Bijl P, et al. Transcatheter versus medical treatment of patients with symptomatic severe tricuspid regurgitation. J Am Coll Cardiol. 2019;74:2998–3008.
77. Rottner L, Bellmann B, Lin T, et al. Catheter ablation of atrial fibrillation: state of the art and future perspectives. Cardiol Ther. 2020;9:45–58.
78. Carino D, Singh M, Molardi A, et al. Non-A non-B aortic dissection: a systematic review and meta-analysis. Eur J Cardiothorac Surg. 2019;55:653–9.

14 Minithoracotomy

Antonio Toscano, Davide Ricci, and Giacomo Bianchi

14.1 Introduction

Minimally invasive cardiac surgery (MICS), and in particular minithoracotomy, is appealing to many patients, partly because it offers benefits over traditional surgery, including less postoperative pain, shorter hospital stay, and a quicker return to normal life with lower risk of wound infection, bleeding, respiratory complications, and atrial fibrillation [1]. Younger patients are particularly interested in the better cosmetic outcomes [2]. Minithoracotomy involves a small incision in the chest, reducing surgical trauma and accelerating postoperative recovery compared to traditional sternotomy. Cardiac surgeries that can be performed through minithoracotomy include mitral valve surgery, aortic valve surgery, tricuspid valve repair, surgical ablation for atrial fibrillation, and atrial septal defect repair. In some selected cases, coronary artery bypass grafting (CABG) can be performed through minithoracotomy, although this procedure is more commonly done using traditional sternotomy or minimally invasive techniques such as minimally invasive direct coronary artery bypass (MIDCAB).

The choice of minithoracotomy as a surgical approach depends on various factors, including the patient's clinical condition, the surgeon's experience, and the complexity of the required procedure. However, MICS via minithoracotomy has disadvantages, including complications, considerable surgical and anesthesiologic training, and need for careful selection of patients. In this section, we will focus specifically on mitral valve surgery, one of the most common and significant applications of the minimally invasive minithoracotomy technique.

14.2 Minimally Invasive Mitral Valve Surgery

Since the mid-to-late 1990s, when pioneering surgeons Alain Carpentier and Randolph Chitwood first introduced minimally invasive mitral valve surgery (MIMVS), the techniques have advanced to encompass minithoracotomy, port-access thoracoscopic surgery, partial sternotomy, and robotic methods [3]. According to

A. Toscano (✉)
Department of Anesthesia and Critical Care, Città della Salute e della Scienza di Torino, University of Turin, Turin, Italy

D. Ricci
Department of Integrated Surgical and Diagnostic Sciences, University of Genova, Genoa, Italy

Division of Cardiac Surgery, IRCCS University Hospital San Martino-IST, Genoa, Italy
e-mail: davide.ricci1@unige.it

G. Bianchi
Division of Cardiac Surgery, Ospedale del Cuore, Fondazione Toscana Gabriele Monasterio, Massa, Italy
e-mail: gbianchi@ftgm.it

G. Sepolvere, S. Silvetti (eds.), *Fast-Track in Cardiac Anesthesia*,
https://doi.org/10.1007/978-3-031-70899-2_14

the Society of Thoracic Surgeons (STS) database, 23% of isolated mitral valve surgeries from 2011 to 2016 were performed using minimally invasive techniques [4]. Although the adoption of MIMVS has been motivated by perceived patient-centered advantages, such as better cosmetic outcomes, reduced short-term morbidity, and quicker recovery to normal function, the debate over its safety and effectiveness compared to traditional sternotomy continues.

The goal of MIMVS was to minimize morbidity, postoperative pain, and blood loss; enhance cosmetic outcomes; shorten hospital stays; and lower costs compared to the traditional median sternotomy method used for the past 50 years [5, 6]. Additionally, it was thought that smaller incisions, avoiding diaphragm interference and reducing tissue dissection, could lead to better outcomes, especially in terms of respiratory function [7].

Studies have validated the previously unproven belief that minimally invasive surgery has no downsides: procedure times are not longer, risks are comparable or lower, transfusions are less frequent, respiratory function is improved, early postoperative pain is reduced, hospital stays are comparable or shorter, long-term survival is similar, and return of mitral regurgitation (MR) is rare and comparable. Although there was no significant difference in overall survival, hospital and 30-day survival rates exceeded 99% in both groups, indicating that detecting differences in early postoperative risk would require a large patient sample. Consequently, early and late surgical outcomes were not compromised.

The reduced perioperative bleeding and fewer transfusions are likely due to the less extensive mediastinal dissection in minimally invasive surgery. Reduced pain is likely due to less surgical dissection, minimal spreading of the sternum, and no increased tension on the posterior rib head and costovertebral ligaments, as the chest wall is not opened extensively. Improved pulmonary function can be attributed to the absence of diaphragm interference or dissection, and less chest wall pain might lead to deeper breathing due to reduced chest splinting.

14.2.1 Patient Selection

Generally, MIMVS can be conducted on most patients with mitral valve disease. MICS can also be performed on patients needing double- or triple-valve surgery [8], but this topic is beyond the scope of this chapter and will not be discussed here. For patients with severe peripheral vascular disease, where peripheral cannulation for cardiopulmonary bypass is not possible, axillary cannulation can be used. In obese patients with mitral disease, we found that minimally invasive mitral surgery is beneficial, resulting in faster recovery, earlier ambulation, shorter hospital stays, and better visualization of the mitral apparatus. For patients with prior heart surgery, MIMVS can be done using a ventricular fibrillation approach. Standard preoperative cardiac screening is conducted before surgery, and we typically do not perform CT scans on all patients unless peripheral vascular disease is suspected.

14.2.2 Minimally Invasive Mitral Valve Surgery's Technique

The anesthesia protocol will be detailed in a specific section of this chapter. Defibrillation pads should be positioned on the patient's right shoulder and left chest. A single-lumen endotracheal tube is used, as ventilation can be paused once cardiopulmonary bypass begins; as an alternative, a double-lumen tube can be used for single-lung ventilation. An intraoperative transesophageal echocardiogram is employed to assess the mitral valve pathology and anatomy, crucial for planning mitral valve repair. We also use 3-D echo reconstruction. The patient is positioned with a sheet roll under the right chest and the right arm at a 45° angle to the side of the bed (Fig. 14.1). The chest, abdomen, and pelvis are prepped and draped in the standard surgical manner. Cannulas for cardiopulmonary bypass are usually placed in the femoral artery and vein (Fig. 14.2). For patients with small or calcified femoral arteries or iliac disease, the axillary artery may be used for cannulation. The

Fig. 14.1 Access point

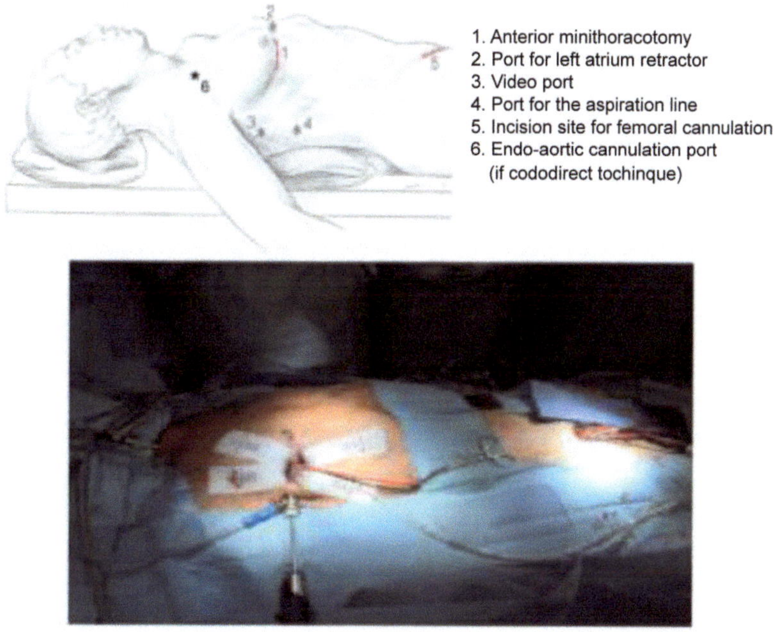

Seldinger technique, guided by transesophageal echocardiogram, is used for femoral artery and vein cannulation. It is crucial to verify the wire's position in the superior vena cava before inserting the venous cannula into the right atrium via the femoral vein. If the transesophageal echocardiogram cannot provide adequate images, fluoroscopy could be used for visualizing the wire and cannula. Limited dissection and exposure of the anterior aspect of the femoral vessels are performed before cannulation to avoid lymphatic injury and lymphocele formation postoperatively. Under TEE guidance, a multistaged femoral venous cannula sized 23–25 Fr and a femoral arterial cannula sized 17–21 Fr should be used (in case of endoaortic balloon clamping, a specific 21–23 Fr Y cannula is necessary—Fig. 14.2), depending on the body surface area (BSA): 17 Fr for BSA <2.0 kg/m^2, 19 Fr for BSA >2.0–2.6 kg/m^2, and 21 Fr for BSA >2.6 kg/m^2 (Fig. 14.3). The tip of the femoral venous cannula should be placed in the superior vena cava to ensure adequate drainage. In many cases, an additional cannula can be added percutaneously (echo guided with Seldinger technique) inserted into the right jugular vein in order to optimize the venous drainage

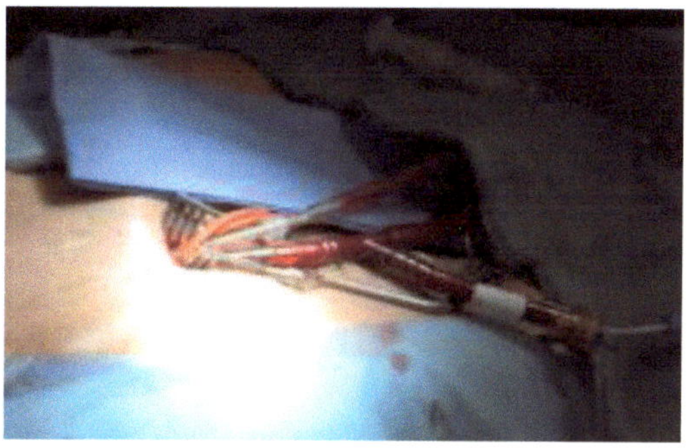

Fig. 14.2 Femoral vessel cannulation (in this case, a Y cannula for both perfusion and endoclamping is used but a high-flow arterious cannula can be adopted in case of transthoracic clamping)

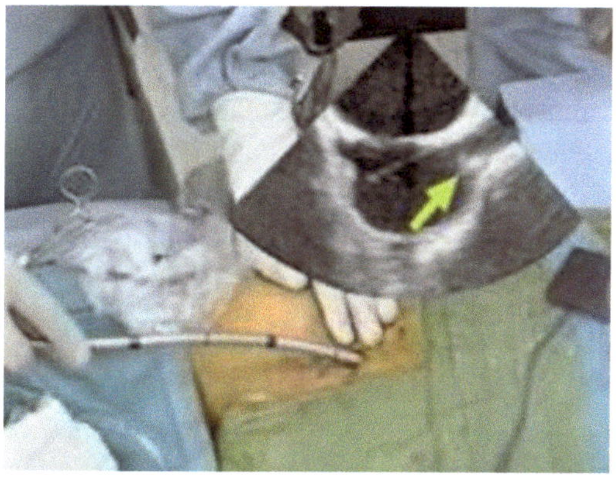

Fig. 14.3 Cannulation under TEE guidance

(Fig. 14.4). This venous configuration is suggested especially in case of endoaortic balloon clamping. A 4–5 cm incision is made in the fourth or fifth intercostal space, lateral to the anterior axillary line. CO_2 inflation in the pleural cavity is mandatory at a 2–3 L/min flow.

For female patients, the incision is made laterally at the mammary crease and dissected up to the third or fourth intercostal space. A plastic drape can be used to retract the breast superiorly and medially if needed. An intercostal rib retractor and soft tissue retractor are used for exposure (Fig. 14.5). Extensive rib spreading is unnecessary and should be avoided to minimize rib fractures and postoperative pain.

Cardiopulmonary bypass is initiated, and mechanical ventilation is paused. If needed, a vacuum within the cardiopulmonary circuit can enhance blood return. The pericardium is opened longitudinally approximately 3–4 cm above the phrenic nerve (Fig. 14.6). Pericardial retraction sutures are placed and brought out through the skin to improve exposure. We typically avoid using diaphragmatic retraction sutures to prevent potential liver injury; instead, we use inferior pericardial retraction sutures to pull the diaphragm downward. Electrocautery and blunt dissection are employed to create a space between the lower part of the aorta and the upper part of the right pulmonary artery for aortic cross-clamping (the pericardial opening and dissection, as above mentioned, can be limited in case of endoaortic balloon clamping). A purse-string suture is placed in the mid-ascending aorta for the placement of the cardioplegia/root vent cannula (this can be avoided in case of endoaortic balloon clamping, due to the possibility to deliver cardioplegia and venting through the tip of the balloon catheter used for clamping). In cases of a calcified ascending aorta or during redo heart surgery, where aortic cross-clamping and anterograde cardioplegia administration are not feasible, ventricular fibrillation arrest can be used as standard practice. In this case, the use of an endoaortic balloon catheter for clamping (Fig. 14.7) could be the solution in order to avoid ventricular fibrillation. A chest tube incision is made two to three rib spaces below the main incision, and cardiotomy suction is inserted. The Waterston's groove is dissected to expose the left atrium, although extensive dissection is unnecessary compared to the sternotomy approach. A specially designed flexible aortic cross-clamp is then placed in the pre-created space through the same incision.

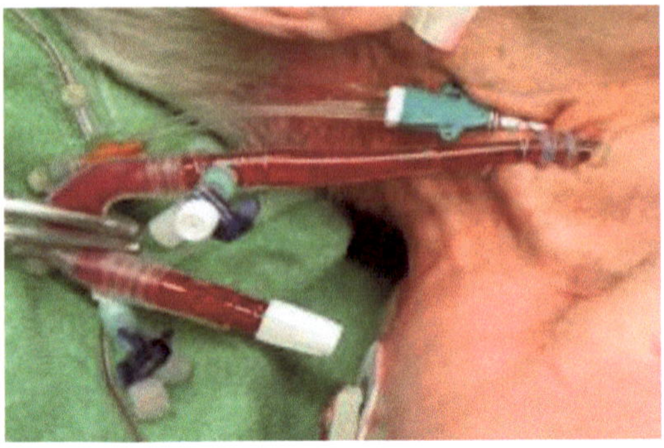

Fig. 14.4 Additional cannula inserted into the right jugular vein in order to optimize the venous drainage

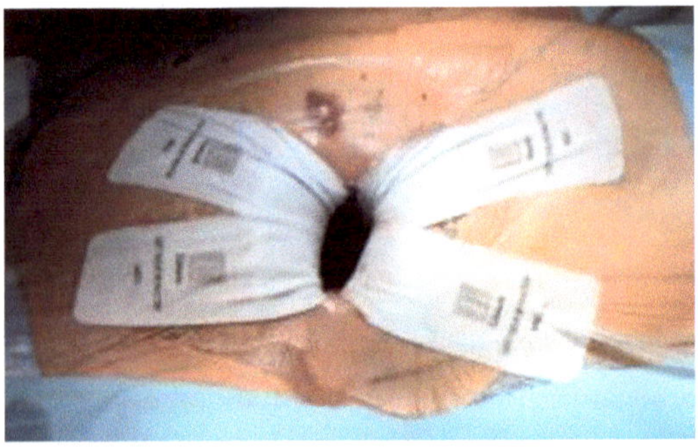

Fig. 14.5 Third or fourth intercostal space incision

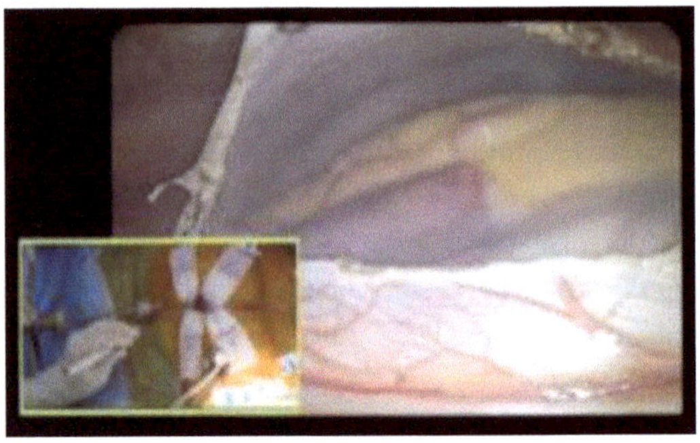

Fig. 14.6 Pericardium opening

Antegrade cardioplegia is administered using Custodiol cardioplegia solution. A left lateral atriotomy is performed through Waterston's groove to access the mitral valve. An atrial lift retractor blade is positioned in the left atrium, and the retractor post is inserted anteriorly into the chest (Fig. 14.8), lateral to the internal mammary artery. A spinal needle can be used initially to guide the post-placement. Care must be taken to avoid injuring the right internal mammary artery, which should be visualized directly or with a thoracoscope.

Proper placement of the left atrial retractor allows for perfect and direct visualization of the mitral valve apparatus. With optimal visualization, the mitral valve can be inspected, followed by either replacement or repair (Fig. 14.9) as needed. For repairs, we typically place annular sutures first to further enhance the view of the mitral apparatus. Under direct vision or better under video assistance, leaflet resections, artificial chord placement, chordal translocation, and mitral annuloplasty can be performed easily. In patients with atrial fibrillation, the left atrium appendage ostium can be closed from within the left atrium using 3-0 or 4-0 Prolene sutures. It is recommended to use at least two layers of closure to prevent future recanalization or reopening of the appendage, an issue we have not encountered with this method.

A maze procedure, involving both radiofrequency ablation and cryoablation, could also be conducted through the same incision in patients with atrial fibrillation. However, this procedure is beyond the scope of this report and will not be detailed here. After completing the mitral repair or replacement, the atriotomy is closed using a 3-0 Prolene suture in a continuous two-layer technique. One or two right ventricular pacing wires are placed at this stage, as it would be challenging to position it after the aortic cross-clamp is removed. The patient is then positioned in the Trendelenburg position, and the aortic cross-clamp is removed. The aortic root vent is utilized for deairing. Cardiopulmonary bypass is gradually discontinued. Protamine is administered, and decannulation is performed according to standard procedure. For patients with femoral arterial cannulation, it is crucial to check distal pulses to confirm patency. At least two chest tubes are placed: one in the pericardial space posteriorly and another in the right pleural space. The groin and chest are closed in the standard manner (Fig. 14.10).

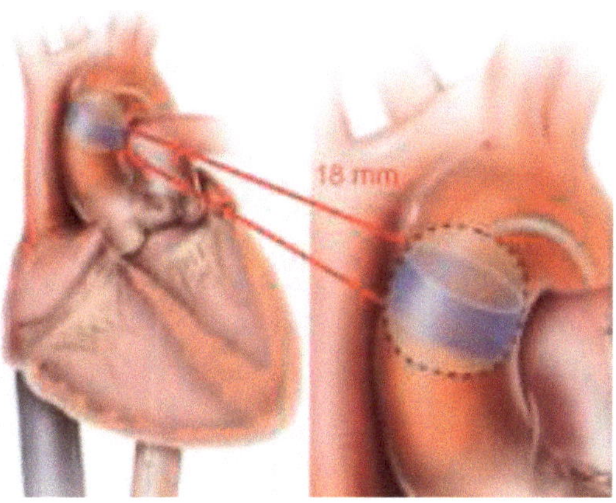

Fig. 14.7 Endoaortic balloon clamping catheter

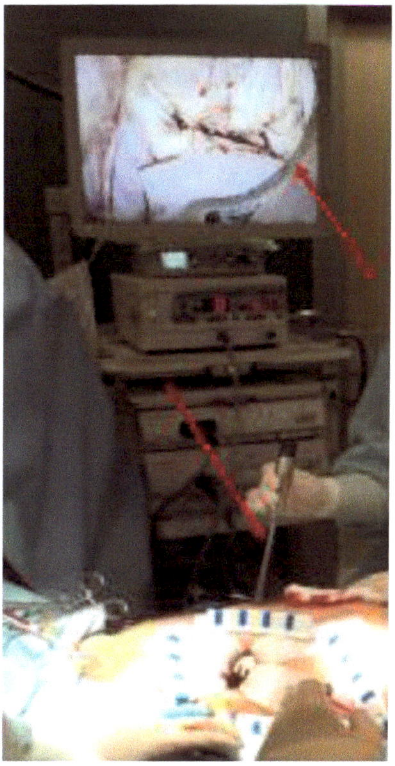

Fig. 14.8 LA retractor

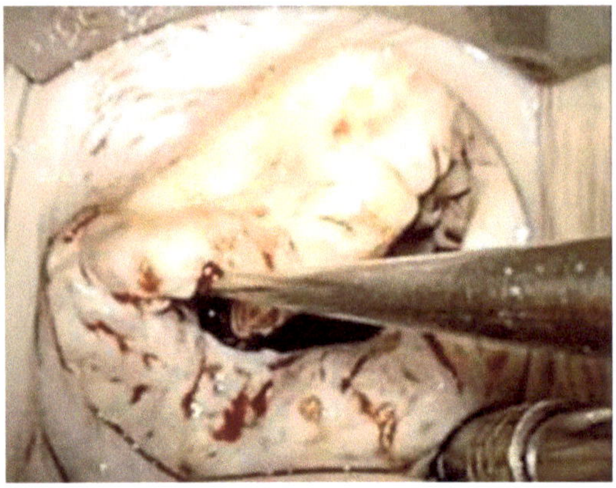

Fig. 14.9 The mitral valve visualization

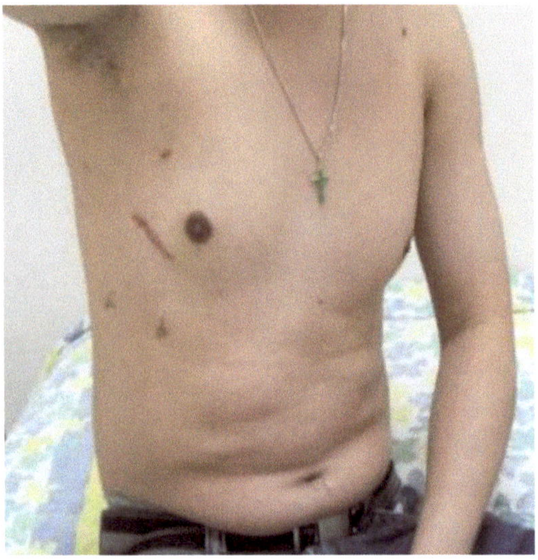

Fig. 14.10 Aesthetic result after minithoracotomy

14.3 Anesthesia for Minimally Invasive Cardiac Surgery via Minithoracotomy

Anesthesia for MICS performed via minithoracotomy requires a highly specialized approach with careful consideration of various clinical factors to ensure the safety and success of the operation. Here are the key aspects to consider.

14.3.1 Preoperative Assessment

The preoperative anesthetic assessment for patients undergoing minimally invasive cardiac surgery through minithoracotomy involves comprehensive evaluation to ensure suitability for the procedure [9]. Key considerations include:

1. **History and examination**: Standard history and examination are conducted, with specific attention to previous thoracic surgeries, chest wall abnormalities, or inflammatory diseases that may complicate the procedure due to adhesion formation.
2. **Cardiac conditions**: Severe aortic regurgitation (AR) is a contraindication to MICS, as it could render cardioplegia delivery ineffective; in fact cardioplegia delivery is challenging due to the lack of antegrade access via the ascending aorta and limited surgical exposure. While MICS typically uses antegrade crystalloid cardioplegia, severe AR requires selective antegrade or retrograde methods, for which no standardized approach exists. Retrograde cardioplegia risks coronary sinus injury, which is hard to repair through a minithoracotomy, and the coronary ostia are often difficult to cannulate securely, increasing the risk of coronary artery injury or inadequate cardioplegia delivery. Transoesophageal echocardiography plays a crucial role in monitoring cardioplegia during minimally invasive surgery via minithoracotomy.
3. **Echocardiographic assessment**: Evaluation focuses on excluding poor ventricular function, aortic valve incompetence, mitral annular calcification, patent foramen ovale (PFO), and persistent left superior vena cava, which can make MICS technically challenging. Transoesophageal Echocardiography is essential for cardiac surgery through minithoracotomy (especially MIMVS) and a contraindication to TEE is often considered a contraindication to a minimal access approach [10].

4. **Vascular assessment**: CT angiography helps assess conditions like aneurysms, atheromas, or previous vascular interventions, crucial for planning peripheral cannulation for cardiopulmonary bypass (CPB).
5. **Respiratory considerations**: MICS via thoracotomy requires one-lung ventilation (OLV) to access the heart adequately. Patients may be positioned supine or semi-laterally, which can increase the risk of hypoxia, especially in those with chronic respiratory diseases. Therefore, it is advisable to conduct pulmonary function tests (PFTs) early in the assessment process. For patients undergoing thoracic surgery, if forced expiratory volume in 1 s (FEV-1) and transfer factor (TLCO) are both greater than 40% of predicted values, the risk of postoperative pulmonary complications is low [11].
6. **Pulmonary hypertension and right ventricular dysfunction**: It is essential to evaluate for pulmonary hypertension and right ventricular dysfunction because using OLV can sometimes lead to complications in these conditions. This includes potentially increasing pulmonary arterial pressure, elevating right ventricular workload, and possibly causing cardiac failure [12].
7. **Musculoskeletal and positioning challenges**: Patients with chest wall deformities, kyphoscoliosis, or orthopedic issues affecting upper limb mobility may pose challenges in positioning for surgery.
8. **Obesity**: Patients with significant obesity present particular challenges for the surgeon and anesthetist. In addition to the difficulty in positioning these patients, it may be difficult to properly site a double-lumen endotracheal tube, they may tolerate OLV less well, and they may require an additional venous drainage cannula to allow adequate flow during CPB.

In summary, a tailored approach to the anesthetic assessment considers these specific factors to optimize patient safety and surgical outcomes in MICS procedures.

14.3.2 Intraoperative Anesthetic Management

Monitoring standards are similar to those used in traditional cardiac surgery. External defibrillator pads must be placed, as internal cardioversion is typically not feasible during MICS. When using an endoballoon, bilateral radial arterial pressure monitoring is required. This is because a loss of perfusion to the right side can indicate distal migration of the balloon, allowing for prompt correction. Additionally, the pressure at the distal tip of the endoballoon is monitored. Often, especially in cases of endoaortic balloon clamping, an additional cannula is inserted percutaneously (echo-guided using the Seldinger technique) into the right jugular vein to optimize venous drainage (Figure 4). This additional cannula can be placed by the anesthesiologist immediately after induction or later on the sterile field by the cardiac surgeon. In both cases, it is inserted percutaneously (echo-guided using the Seldinger technique and dilators of progressively larger sizes). When placed directly by the anesthesiologist, it is connected to a heparinized solution (e.g., UFH 5000 IU in 500 ml of saline solution).

Cerebral oximetry can help detect poor perfusion in one or both sides of the upper body. This issue can arise if the endoballoon migrates or if the heart ejects blood without ventilation, and the CPB return flow is distal to the innominate artery. This condition, known as Harlequin syndrome, occurs when the upper body is perfused with deoxygenated blood while the lower body receives oxygenated blood, potentially leading to life-threatening cerebral hypoxia [9].

The use of one-lung ventilation and lung isolation may result in high impedance of cardiac electrical signals to the skin surface, producing a poor electrocardiograph (ECG) trace. To address this, the standard **ECG** electrode positions may need to be modified.

Anesthetic induction proceeds similarly to any cardiac surgery. The patient is intubated with a **double-lumen endotracheal tube (DLT)**, with its position typically verified using a bronchoscope.

The most commonly used DLT is the left-sided DLT, irrespective of which side requires the isolation because placing a left-sided DLT is less challenging than the right-sided one. This comparative ease is partly due to the short takeoff of the right upper bronchus, which leads to higher chances of dislodgement and impaired ventilation of the right upper bronchus.

Alternatively, a single-lumen tube with a bronchial blocker may be used to isolate the lung. Prophylactic antibiotics are administered, and anesthesia is commonly maintained with an intravenous agent.

The patient is placed with one hemithorax elevated using a gel pad or inflatable bag to facilitate access to the anterior intercostal spaces. The arm is secured away from the surgical site, and care is taken to pad pressure points to prevent brachial plexus tension.

After the correct placement of the tube, a **one-lung ventilation (OLV)** will be started.

A lung-protective approach is designed for patients at high risk of developing acute lung injury (ALI) or progressing to acute respiratory distress syndrome (ARDS). It involves using a low tidal volume strategy, as highlighted by the landmark ARDSnet trials, which demonstrated a reduction in overall mortality. The lung-protective strategy aims to prevent barotrauma, volutrauma, and atelectrauma and includes the following components [13]:

- **Tidal volume**: Initially set at 4–6 mL/kg based on ideal body weight. This is lower than the 6–8 mL/kg typically recommended for mechanical ventilation with both lungs. Adjustments can be made based on airway pressure monitoring to detect alveolar trauma, with inspiratory plateau pressures targeted below 30 cmH_2O in nonobese patients.
- **Respiratory rate (RR)**: Start with a rate of 16 breaths per minute to achieve normocapnia. Blood gas analysis should be conducted approximately 30 min after starting mechanical ventilation, and the RR should be adjusted according to the patient's acid-base status and $PaCO_2$ levels. If $PaCO_2$ exceeds 40 mmHg, increase the RR; if it is below 40, decrease the RR.
- **Inspiratory flow rate**: Set at 60 L/min. This can be increased if the patient shows a need for higher inhalation during the initiation of breaths.
- **Positive end-expiratory pressure (PEEP)**: This is typically set between 5 and 10 cmH_2O, depending on the patient's hemodynamic status, oxygenation needs (FiO_2 requirement), and any presence of obstructive lung disease or auto-PEEP.
- **Inspired oxygen fraction (FiO_2)**: Traditionally, an FiO_2 of 1.0 has been recommended during single-lung ventilation. The reasoning for using a higher FiO_2 is to maintain a safety margin. A higher FiO_2 also promotes vasodilation, potentially increasing blood flow to the ventilated lung. However, oxygenation at FiO_2 of 1.0 can cause atelectasis. Therefore, it is advisable to start with an FiO_2 lower than 1.0, usually 0.8, and increase it if necessary.
- **Oxygenation goal**: Maintain oxygen saturation levels between 88% and 95%.

This strategy ensures that mechanical ventilation is tailored to minimize lung injury while providing adequate respiratory support.

If hypoxia occurs during single-lung ventilation, the following steps should be taken:

1. **Verify tube position**: Ensure that the double-lumen tube, endobronchial tube, or bronchial blocker is correctly positioned, using fiberoptic bronchoscopy if necessary. Clear any secretions by suctioning the lumens.
2. **Increase FiO_2**: Raise the FiO_2 to 1.0.
3. **Perform recruitment maneuvers**: Apply recruitment maneuvers and PEEP to the ventilated lung to address atelectasis and improve oxygenation.
4. **Apply CPAP to the operative lung**: Use CPAP on the non-ventilated lung to reduce shunting and improve oxygenation, though this may complicate the surgery.

5. **Revert to two-lung ventilation**: If severe hypoxemia persists, switch back to two-lung ventilation.
6. **Investigate severe hypoxemia causes**: Check for pneumothorax, especially in COPD patients, and if found, abort the surgery and insert a chest tube immediately.

The transesophageal echocardiogram (TEE) is used at the beginning of the procedure for a thorough examination. This includes confirming the diagnosis and surgical target and evaluating the possible presence and quantification of aortic regurgitation. If an endoballoon is used, the diameters of the ascending aorta and aortic root should also be measured; furthermore, the integrity of the interatrial septum should be assessed.

During cannulation for cardiopulmonary bypass (CPB), TEE aids in guiding the position of the cannulae. The bicaval view is ideal for visualizing venous cannulation, which helps minimize the risk of complications such as malposition in the hepatic vein or perforation of the interatrial septum. Unless a right atriotomy is required, the venous drainage cannula's tip should be positioned in the proximal superior vena cava (SVC). If atrium opening is necessary, the inferior vena cava (IVC) cannula should be placed at the cavoatrial junction, and a separate SVC cannula must be used.

If an endoballoon is utilized, TEE assists in its placement, ensuring that the tip is in the ascending aorta. When the balloon is inflated, it creates an indentation on the aortic wall. TEE can track the flow of cardioplegia into the aortic root and through the coronary ostia, confirming no regurgitation into the left ventricle (LV). It is crucial to monitor the LV during cardioplegia delivery to avoid distortion of aortic valve anatomy and ventricular distention due to valve incompetence. The endoballoon also allows for venting of the aortic root. Lastly, because the anesthetist or surgeon cannot easily visualize the right ventricle as they can during conventional cardiac surgery, TEE provides valuable information regarding volume status and right ventricular (RV) function. This is particularly beneficial during the process of weaning from CPB.

Weaning from cardiopulmonary bypass (CPB) in minimally invasive cardiac surgery via minithoracotomy is largely similar to the process in conventional cardiac surgery. However, there are several reasons why it might be beneficial to temporarily switch to two-lung ventilation during the weaning process:

1. *Improved gas exchange*: Ventilating both lungs enhances gas exchange, promoting normoxia and preventing respiratory acidosis, which supports better cardiac function.
2. *Optimized pulmonary vascular resistance (PVR)*: A collapsed lung increases pulmonary vascular resistance for the right ventricle (RV). Ventilating both lungs reduces PVR, thereby improving RV function.
3. *Enhanced deairing*: Ventilating both lungs helps clear air from the pulmonary veins and assists in deairing the heart. TOE can be used to guide this process, as it is in conventional cardiac surgery.

After successfully separating from CPB, it is often necessary to re-isolate the lung to ensure proper surgical hemostasis.

14.4 Analgesia for Minimally Invasive Cardiac Surgery via Minithoracotomy

Although it is a minimally invasive procedure with a small surgical incision, pain is not to be underestimated, as well as chronic postsurgical pain (CPSP) [14], which is a relatively common complication after cardiothoracic operations with well-known consequences in terms of return to normal activities and quality of life.

Pain after thoracotomy is caused by both nociceptive and neuropathic mechanisms; additionally, pain can be referred from other areas [15].

Nociceptive somatic pain is transmitted by intercostal nerves from the incision, rib retraction, muscle splitting, pleura injury, and chest drain insertion, reaching the spinal cord and brain. **Visceral pain** is carried by the phrenic and vagus nerves from injuries to the bronchi, visceral pleura, and pericardium. Tissue injury releases inflammatory mediators, activating nociceptors and lowering the pain threshold, leading to primary sensitization and increased pain during breathing or coughing. Prolonged nociception can cause central sensitization and chronic pain. Neuropathic pain from intercostal nerve injury leads to reduced sensory input but increased sensitivity, causing conditions like dysesthesia, allodynia, hyperalgesia, and hyperpathia.

In addition, sometimes the **referred pain** to the ipsilateral shoulder is added, caused by the phrenic nerve for lesion of the visceral pleura and pericardium [16]. CPSP, defined as pain developing after surgery and lasting for at least 2 months, has multifactorial etiology including afferent nociceptive input from the skin incision, costochondritis, rib retraction injury, acute intercostal neuralgia, and damage of the pulmonary pleura [17].

Neuraxial anesthesia, mainly thoracic epidural analgesia and deep plexus blocks, has been proposed to achieve a better postoperative pain control [18] particularly in the context of minimally invasive cardiac surgery. Unfortunately, in cardiac surgery patients, anticoagulant and antiplatelet administration increase the risk of epidural hematoma classically related to neuraxial procedures. It follows that the American Society of Regional Anesthesia and Pain Medicine (ASRA) is still recommending a conservative approach to neuraxial techniques and other deep blockades, such as thoracic paravertebral block [19, 20]. Recent evidence suggests that chest wall blocks such as continuous serratus anterior plane block (SAPB) and continuous erector spinae plane block (ESPB) are effective alternatives for postoperative pain control in patients undergoing minimally invasive cardiac surgery via minithoracotomy [21, 22] also in patients receiving antiplatelet and anticoagulant therapy [23]. This has been confirmed by a panel of seven experts of the Regional Anesthesia and Acute Pain Section of the Canadian Anesthesiologists' Society who reviewed the evidence and classified the risk of bleeding complication after thoracic erector spinae plane block and serratus anterior plane block as low and intermediate, respectively [24].

Both the SAPB and the ESPB, included in a multimodal opioid-sparing analgesia protocol, guarantee good analgesia after cardiac surgery in minithoracotomy.

Both blocks were tested as a continuous infusion with perifascial catheter placement or single shot [25, 26].

An observational study conducted on 85 consecutive patients who underwent continuous SAPB and continuous ESPB for MIMVS through right minithoracotomy showed that ESPB, even more than SAPB, appears to be a feasible and effective strategy for the management of postoperative pain, allowing good-quality analgesia with low consumption of opioids, NSAIDs, and antiemetic drugs [27].

In the case of catheter placement, ESPB, both as intermittent bolus [28] and as continuous infusion, is relatively safe and correlated with a reduction in the use of opioids and antiemetics for cardiac surgery through a lateral minithoracotomy and seems to be a safer choice because the catheter is placed away from the surgical site, reducing the risk of displacement.

When performed as a single shot, ESPB should be administered before anesthetic induction with the patient seated or in lateral position, while SAPB is usually performed after induction, thus reducing anesthesiological preparation time.

14.5 Conclusion

Anesthesia for minimally invasive cardiac surgery via minithoracotomy requires a highly specialized approach with meticulous attention to various clinical factors to ensure patient safety and procedural success [29]. The preoperative assessment is comprehensive, focusing on patient history, cardiac and respiratory evaluations, and anatomical considerations. Intraoperative anesthetic management includes advanced monitoring techniques, precise patient positioning, and careful management of ventilation and cardiac function. Effective pain control, both during and after surgery, is achieved through multimodal analgesia strategies, including the use of nerve blocks such as SAPB and ESPB. This tailored anesthetic approach not only enhances surgical outcomes but also improves patient recovery and quality of life post-surgery.

References

1. Parnell A, Prince M. Anaesthesia for minimally invasive cardiac surgery. BJA Educ. 2018;18(10):323–30. https://doi.org/10.1016/j.bjae.2018.06.004. Epub 2018 Aug 28.
2. İyigün T, Kaya M, Gülbeyaz SÖ, Fıstıkçı N, Uyanık G, Yılmaz B, Onan B, Erkanlı K. Patient body image, self-esteem, and cosmetic results of minimally invasive robotic cardiac surgery. Int J Surg. 2017;39:88–94. https://doi.org/10.1016/j.ijsu.2017.01.105. Epub 2017 Jan 29.
3. Carpentier A, Loulmet D, Carpentier A, et al. First open heart operation (mitral valvuloplasty) under videosurgery through a minithoracotomy. C R Acad Sci III. 1996;319:221–5.
4. Gammie JS, Chikwe J, Badhwar V, et al. Isolated mitral valve surgery: the Society of Thoracic Surgeons Adult Cardiac Surgery Database analysis. Ann Thorac Surg. 2018;106(3):716–27. https://doi.org/10.1016/j.athoracsur.2018.03.086.
5. Cosgrove DM III, Sabik JF, Navia JL. Minimally invasive valve operations. Ann Thorac Surg. 1998;65(6):1535–8; discussion 1538–9. https://doi.org/10.1016/s0003-4975(98)00300-2.
6. Chitwood WR Jr, Wixon CL, Elbeery JR, Moran JF, Chapman WH, Lust RM. Video-assisted minimally invasive mitral valve surgery. J Thorac Cardiovasc Surg. 1997;114(5):773–80; discussion 780–2. https://doi.org/10.1016/S0022-5223(97)70081-3.
7. Svensson LG. Minimal-access "J" or "j" sternotomy for valvular, aortic, and coronary operations or reoperations. Ann Thorac Surg. 1997;64(5):1501–3. https://doi.org/10.1016/S0003-4975(97)00927-2.
8. Santana O, Xydas S, Williams RF, LaPietra A, Mawad M, Hasty F, Escolar E, Mihos CG. Outcomes of minimally invasive double valve surgery. J Thorac Dis. 2017;9(Suppl 7):S602–6. https://doi.org/10.21037/jtd.2017.05.62.
9. Giunta M, Recchia EG, Capuano P, Toscano A, Attisani M, Rinaldi M, Brazzi L. Management of harlequin syndrome under ECPELLA support: a report of two cases and a proposed approach. Ann Card Anaesth. 2023;26(1):97–101. https://doi.org/10.4103/aca.aca_176_21.
10. Aybek T, Doss M, Abdel-Rahman U, Simon A, Miskovic A, Risteski PS, Dogan S, Moritz A. Echocardiographic assessment in minimally invasive mitral valve surgery. Med Sci Monit. 2005;11(4):MT27–32. Epub 2005 Mar 24.
11. Santana O, Reyna J, Benjo AM, Lamas GA, Lamelas J. Outcomes of minimally invasive valve surgery in patients with chronic obstructive pulmonary disease. Eur J Cardiothorac Surg. 2012;42(4):648–52. https://doi.org/10.1093/ejcts/ezs098. Epub 2012 May 3
12. Ross AF, Ueda K. Pulmonary hypertension in thoracic surgical patients. Curr Opin Anaesthesiol. 2010;23(1):25–33. https://doi.org/10.1097/ACO.0b013e328334cb59.
13. Ashok V, Francis J. A practical approach to adult one-lung ventilation. BJA Educ. 2018;18(3):69–74. https://doi.org/10.1016/j.bjae.2017.11.007. Epub 2017 Dec 6.
14. Toscano A, Barbero C, Capuano P, Costamagna A, Pocar M, Trompeo A, Pasero D, Rinaldi M, Brazzi L. Chronic postsurgical pain and quality of life after right minithoracotomy mitral valve operations. J Card Surg. 2022;37(6):1585–90. https://doi.org/10.1111/jocs.16400. Epub 2022 Mar 11.
15. Mesbah A, Yeung J, Gao F. Pain after thoracotomy. BJA Educ. 2016;16:1–7. https://doi.org/10.1093/bjaceaccp/mkv005.
16. MacDougall P. Postthoracotomy shoulder pain: diagnosis and management. Curr Opin Anaesthesiol. 2008;21(1):12–5. https://doi.org/10.1097/ACO.0b013e3282f2bb67.
17. Guastella V, Mick G, Soriano C, Vallet L, Escande G, Dubray C, Eschalier A. A prospective study of neuropathic pain induced by thoracotomy: incidence, clinical description, and diagnosis. Pain. 2011;152(1):74–81. https://doi.org/10.1016/j.pain.2010.09.004. Epub 2010 Nov 13.
18. Svircevic V, Nierich AP, Moons KG, Diephuis JC, Ennema JJ, Brandon Bravo Bruinsma GJ, Kalkman CJ, van Dijk D. Thoracic epidural anesthesia for cardiac surgery: a randomized trial. Anesthesiology. 2011;114(2):262–70. https://doi.org/10.1097/ALN.0b013e318201d2de.
19. Svircevic V, Nierich AP, Moons KG, Diephuis JC, Ennema JJ, Brandon Bravo Bruinsma GJ, et al. Thoracic epidural anesthesia for cardiac surgery: a randomized trial. Anesthesiology. 2011;114:262–70.
20. Horlocker TT, Vandermeulen E, Kopp SL, Gogarten W, Leffert LR, Benzon HT. Regional anesthesia in the patient receiving antithrombotic or thrombolytic therapy: American Society of Regional Anesthesia and Pain Medicine evidence-based guidelines (fourth edition). Reg Anesth Pain Med. 2018;43:263–309.
21. Hoogma DF, Rex S, Tournoy J, Verbrugghe P, Fieuws S, Al Tmimi L. Erector spinae plane block for minimally invasive mitral valve surgery: a double-blind, prospective, randomised placebo-controlled trial—a study protocol. BMJ Open. 2021;11:e045833. https://doi.org/10.1136/bmjopen-2020-045833.
22. Toscano A, Capuano P, Costamagna A, Burzio C, Ellena M, Scala V, et al. The serratus anterior plane study: continuous deep serratus anterior plane block for mitral valve surgery performed in right minithoracotomy. J Cardiothorac Vasc Anesth. 2020;34:2975–82.

23. Toscano A, Capuano P, Galatà M, Tazzi I, Rinaldi M, Brazzi L. Safety of ultrasound-guided serratus anterior and erector spinae fascial plane blocks: a retrospective analysis in patients undergoing cardiac surgery while receiving anticoagulant and antiplatelet drugs. J Cardiothorac Vasc Anesth. 2022;36(2):483–8. https://doi.org/10.1053/j.jvca.2021.05.037. Epub 2021 May 24.
24. Horlocker TT, Neal JM, Kopp SL. Practice advisory on the bleeding risks for peripheral nerve and interfascial blockade: going out on a limb. Can J Anaesth. 2019;66(11):1281–5. https://doi.org/10.1007/s12630-019-01467-9. Epub 2019 Aug 21.
25. Toscano A, Capuano P, Costamagna A, Burzio C, Ellena M, Scala V, Pasero D, Rinaldi M, Brazzi L. The serratus anterior plane study: continuous deep serratus anterior plane block for mitral valve surgery performed in right minithoracotomy. J Cardiothorac Vasc Anesth. 2020;34(11):2975–82. https://doi.org/10.1053/j.jvca.2020.05.021. Epub 2020 May 27.
26. Hoogma DF, Van den Eynde R, Oosterlinck W, Al Tmimi L, Verbrugghe P, Tournoy J, Fieuws S, Coppens S, Rex S. Erector spinae plane block for postoperative analgesia in robotically-assisted coronary artery bypass surgery: results of a randomized placebo-controlled trial. J Clin Anesth. 2023;87:111088. https://doi.org/10.1016/j.jclinane.2023.111088. Epub 2023 Mar 1.
27. Toscano A, Capuano P, Costamagna A, Canavosio FG, Ferrero D, Alessandrini EM, Giunta M, Rinaldi M, Brazzi L. Is continuous erector spinae plane block (ESPB) better than continuous serratus anterior plane block (SAPB) for mitral valve surgery via mini-thoracotomy? Results from a prospective observational study. Ann Card Anaesth. 2022;25(3):286–92. https://doi.org/10.4103/aca.aca_69_21.
28. Sun Y, Luo X, Yang X, Zhu X, Yang C, Pan T, Du Y, Zhang R, Wang D. Benefits and risks of intermittent bolus erector spinae plane block through a catheter for patients after cardiac surgery through a lateral mini-thoracotomy: a propensity score matched retrospective cohort study. J Clin Anesth. 2021;75:110489. https://doi.org/10.1016/j.jclinane.2021.110489. Epub 2021 Sep 1.
29. Aston D, Zeloof D, Falter F. Anaesthesia for minimally invasive cardiac surgery. J Cardiovasc Dev Dis. 2023;10(11):462. https://doi.org/10.3390/jcdd10110462.

Ministernotomy

15

Paolo Capuano, Tarek Senussi, Giulio Carinci, Antonio De Bellis, and Francesco Santini

15.1 Introduction

During the past 50 years, median sternotomy has been the gold standard approach in cardiac surgery with excellent long-term outcomes.

However, since the 1990s, technological advancement, improved surgical techniques and anesthetic expertise, as well as patient expectations have led to an increased demand for minimally invasive cardiac surgery (MICS).

MICS refers to a constellation of surgical techniques that minimize surgical trauma through smaller incisions compared with a conventional sternotomy.

Although there is no universally agreed definition, the American Heart Association (AHA) defines MICS as any procedure performed via a "small chest wall incision that does not include the conventional full sternotomy" [1].

15.2 Ministernotomy: Definition and Technique

15.2.1 Overview

MICS is an attractive option for many patients; however, there are drawbacks including procedure-specific complications, considerable surgical training and skill required, and need for careful patient selection as minimally invasive procedures are not appropriate for all.

Owing to its similarity to a full midline sternotomy, ministernotomy (MS) has become one of the most popular MICS approaches besides mini-thoracotomy [2].

MS was described for the first time by Holman and Willet in 1949; they used a partial vertical sternotomy with transection of the sternum at the second intercostal space for pericardiotomy [3]. It consisted of a 6–10 cm midline vertical incision through the skin and sternum, completed by

P. Capuano (✉)
Department of Anesthesia and Intensive Care, Istituto Mediterraneo per i Trapianti e Terapie ad alta Specializzazione (IRCCS-ISMETT), UPMCI (University of Pittsburgh Medical Center Italy), Palermo, Italy

T. Senussi
Department of Cardiac Anesthesia and Intensive Care, Cardiovascular Network, IRCCS Ospedale Policlinico San Martino, Genoa, Italy

G. Carinci
Department of Medical Science, Surgery and Neurosciences, Anesthesia and Intensive Care Unit, University Hospital of Siena, Siena, Italy

A. De Bellis
Department of Cardiac Surgery, San Michele Hospital, Maddaloni-Caserta, Italy

F. Santini
Division of Cardiac Surgery, Ospedale Policlinico San Martino, Genoa, Italy

Department of Integrated Surgical and Diagnostic Sciences, University of Genova, Genoa, Italy
e-mail: francesco.santini@unige.it

G. Sepolvere, S. Silvetti (eds.), *Fast-Track in Cardiac Anesthesia*,
https://doi.org/10.1007/978-3-031-70899-2_15

a transverse sternal incision [4, 5], thus allowing access to the cardiac structures.

During the years, numerous types of MS incisions have been proposed, such as upper reversed T incision, right-side partial sternotomy, an upper J incision, S-shaped partial sternotomy, right parasternal incision, lower half MS, L-shaped incision, reversed Z-shaped sternotomy, I-shaped MS , and reversed C-shaped MS [6–8] these techniques have been performed in a variety of operations including aortic valve replacement, mitral valve replacement, coronary bypass grafting operation, ascending aorta aneurysm, aortic root replacement with composite graft, and combined cardiac operations [9, 10].

MS has also been used in redo procedures with the aim to avoid the dissection of ventricular adhesions, allowing the surgeon to expose only a limited required area [11].

MS has been associated with shorter ventilation time after surgery, less postoperative pain, shorter intensive care unit (ICU) stay and hospital stay, as well as less blood loss within 24 h of surgery compared to conventional full sternotomy, although patients undergoing MS had longer cross-clamp and cardio-pulmonary bypass (CPB) time [12].

Better ventilation parameters and shorter intubation time after MS procedures are explained by less pain related to the surgical wound, due to limited sternal split, smaller surgical wound, and preserved lower sternal integrity.

Moreover, the maintained integrity of the lower sternum is associated with a diminished risk of sternal dehiscence.

15.2.2 Cardiac Surgery Through MS

Laparoscopic surgery pushed the development of minimally invasive procedures in all surgical disciplines. MICS is widely spread around the world, and many surgeons have introduced and developed their own technique.

While on the one hand there is an increasing demand from patients for a small surgical incision, on the other, these incisions are foreign to traditional cardiac surgeons and require a long learning curve to be used safely and routinely [13].

A routinely used mini-access is represented by the MS, a term coined in 1994 to describe a series of sternal incisions for cardiac surgery other than the complete median sternotomy. Since the sternum in the adults is inflexible, the bone is divided in the midline from the jugulus to the second, third, or fourth intercostal space in an inverted “J” or “T” shape (Fig. 15.1).

Other definitions such as inverted “L,” “S,” and “C” or hemisternotomy, partial sternotomy, and limited sternotomy can also be found in the literature.

An upper MS can be used for all the operations on the aortic and mitral valves, as well as on the aortic root and the ascending aorta. As previously mentioned, the adult sternum is rigid; as such, the sternum must not only be divided in the midline, but also with “J” or “T” shape in an intercostal space. It is important to emphasize that the incision should only cut through the sternum; the surrounding tissues including the internal mammary arteries should be left intact. In case of “T” incision, once the sternal edge has been cut transversely, there is no need to further advance into the intercostal space. If the division is made only in the right or left intercostal space (“J” or “L” incisions), tension may be exerted on the internal mammary artery, and excessive sternal spreading should be avoided. The amount of sternal spreading to provide a good exposure to the base of the heart may vary with the size of the patient, the presence of emphysema, and whether

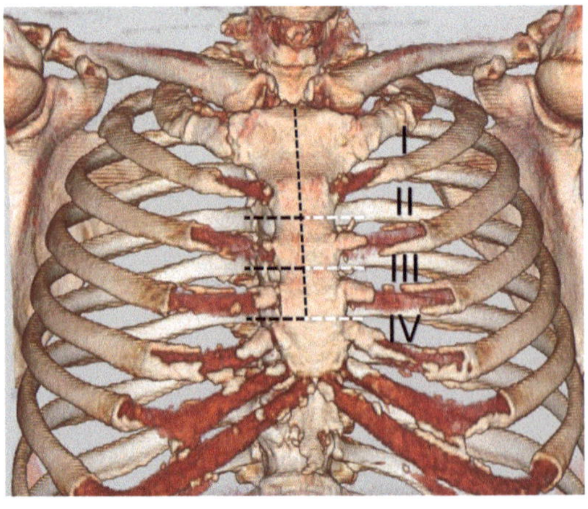

Fig. 15.1 Ministernotomy: different options based on individual anatomy (see text)

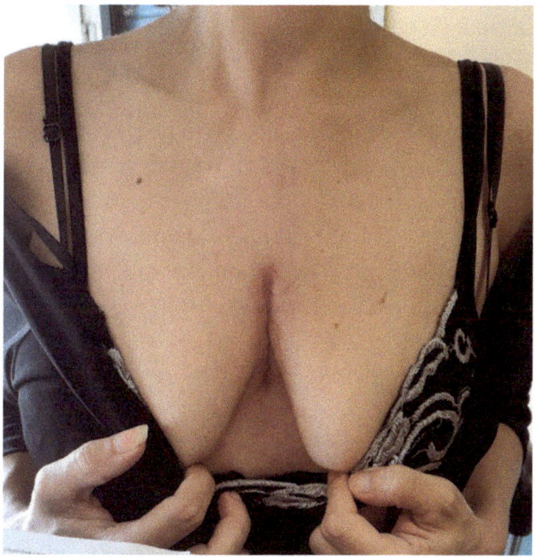

Fig. 15.2 Cosmetic result after minimally invasive aortic valve replacement via ministernotomy approach

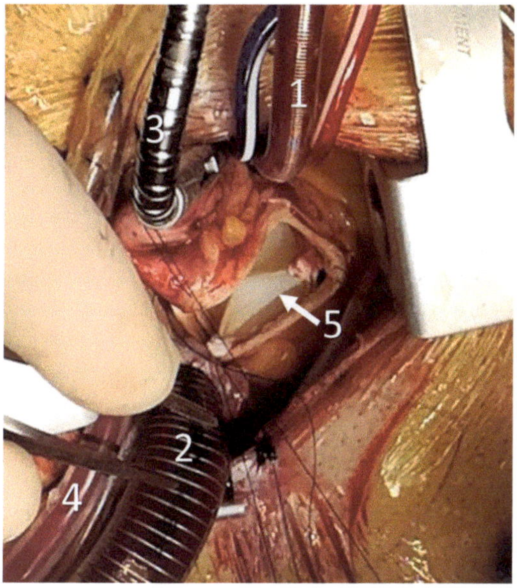

Fig. 15.3 Ministernotomy approach, intraoperative situs after cannulation: 1, aortic cannula; 2, venous cannula; 3, aortic clamp; 4, left ventricular vent; 5, biological aortic valve prosthesis

the heart is located transversely or longitudinally within the thorax. Usually, it is sufficient to incise the sternum at the third or the fourth intercostal space. In case of emphysema or when aortic root replacement is planned, the fourth space is preferential. As familiarity with the technique increases, a third or even second intercostal space MS may be increasingly employed. An angio-CT may be useful for surgical planning. The skin incision usually remains below 8 cm of the total length (Fig. 15.2).

An oscillating saw with a narrow blade is usually employed for osteotomy. Once the bone has been divided, a small retractor (e.g., Finochietto or Yan retractor) is positioned and the upper sternal edges are spread apart. The thymic tissue is divided and the pericardium opened in the midline using electrocautery. Once opened, the edges of the pericardium are pulled onto the skin using sutures, in order to improve exposure. Purse-string sutures for cannulation are placed on the ascending aorta in a standard position. Venous cannulation can be performed with the use of a standard double-stage cannula or using an oval double-stage venous cannula or a tri-stage venous return cannula positioned in the right atrial appendage. Alternatively, arterial, venous, or both cannulas can be inserted through the femoral vessels in the inguinal region percutaneously (echo-guided) or through surgical cut-down. Transesophageal echocardiography represents an essential guide to check the positioning of the metal guidewires before the advancements of the cannulas (Fig. 15.3).

Cardioplegia can be administered antegradely or, more rarely, retrogradely in a standard way in the aorta, right atrium, or coronary ostia, depending on preferences and needs.

Once CPB has started, the left heart can be vented, by means of a dedicated cannula, in several ways: through the superior right pulmonary vein, via the main pulmonary artery, through the aortic valve annulus, and through the roof of the left atrium.

The aortic valve is easily visualized by ministernotomy. A right-angle aortic cross-clamp is placed on the aorta. Aortotomy is performed based on the surgeon's preference. The rest of the aortic procedure proceeds in a standard fashion. If a central venous cannulation strategy has been chosen, a gentle traction on the cannula further makes the aortic annulus more accessible, improving surgical exposure. In the case of peripheral venous cannulation, assisted drainage helps to maintain right chambers collapsed, facilitating exposure of the aortic valve.

Aortic valve repair or replacement (AVR) is then completed in a standard fashion, usually by means of conventional surgical instruments. Sutures for traditional biological or mechanical prostheses can be tied directly or through the use of an automated suture fastener device (Cor-Knot, LSI Solutions) [13, 14].

Once the valve procedure is completed, closure of the aorta proceeds according to the surgeon's preference. The deairing maneuvers are guided by transesophageal echocardiography, which identifies potential air traps. A gentle shaking of the heart, combined with ventilation of the lungs and temporarily limiting venous return, is usually sufficient to remove air bubbles from cardiac chambers.

Atrial and/or ventricular wires are routinely placed for a temporary pacemaker and brought out through the intercostal space. It is important to place pacemaker wires on the right ventricle when the heart is decompressed and before weaning the patient from CPB.

AVR in ministernotomy can potentially improve postoperative recovery, shorten intensive care and hospital stay, and increase overall patient satisfaction due to less pain and superior cosmetic results than median sternotomy [15–23].

However, minimally invasive procedures are also associated with a higher grade of complexity and subsequently longer CPB and aortic cross-clamp times than conventional surgery with complete sternotomy. Given that prolonged CPB time and aortic cross-clamp time have been proven to be independent predictors of morbidity and mortality in both low- and high-risk cardiac patients, pros and cons of surgical approach must be evaluated on an individual base [24–26].

In this perspective, rapid deployment valves (RDVs) for AVR have been introduced into clinical practice to bypass these issues [27].

An RDV implant, associated with a reduction of CPB time in combination with MS, allows to improve postoperative outcomes with a particular significant benefits in frail population [27–30].

Through MS, it is possible to perform reoperations on the aortic valve, after accurate evaluation of preliminary CT scan. Partial upper hemiresternotomy approach for reoperative AVR takes less time and less postoperative bleeding than complete resternotomy. These beneficial effects can be achieved without compromising the surgical exposure. The reduced blood loss depends on the limited dissection required. With the reoperative MS, only those structures absolutely necessary for surgery are dissected free. The cannulation sites can be accomplished according to needs. Cannulation sites in redo procedures may also include axillary artery, innominate vein, and percutaneous femoral vein.

The use of innominate vein or femoral vein percutaneous cannulation is very helpful in minimizing the dissection of the right atrium, which may be of limited access due to surgical adhesions and restricted surgical exposure [31, 32].

Nowadays, minimally invasive mitral valve surgery (MIMVS) through a right minithoracotomy has become well established and widely practiced all around the world. In the 1990s, MS was pioneered as an access for MIMVS [33].

MS represented an alternative approach to the mitral valve usually through an extended transseptal incision. This access provides a familiar surgical field for traditional or young surgeons. Direct cannulation of the aorta and venae cavae is possible in almost all cases, and the use of a vacuum-assisted drainage allows the use of small-caliber cannulas. The extended transseptal incision provides an excellent exposure to the mitral valve for repair or replacement. Almost all patients with isolated mitral valve disease can be candidates for this approach. Contraindications include the need for coronary artery bypass grafting requiring extensive exposure of the heart and reoperations [34, 35].

With the spreading of minimally invasive techniques in cardiac surgery and off-pump coronary artery bypass grafting (OPCABG), alternatives to full sternotomy have been proposed in coronary artery bypass surgery as well.

A left inferior L-reversed hemisternotomy has been proposed as an alternative technique to perform coronary revascularization of the left anterior descending artery (LAD) by means of left internal mammary artery (LIMA) [36].

This approach is supposed to allow standard off-pump surgery, with its relative benefits, without particular patient selection and conventional instruments for OPCABG.

This technique is performed through a low surgical skin incision, median lower division of the sternum, and left transection in the third intercostal space. Through this access, it is possible to harvest the LIMA in a standard fashion, up to the second-third intercostal space. Exposure of the LAD is obtained through a C-shaped cut of the pericardium and properly placed stay sutures, while off-pump surgery is performed in a standard fashion with the aid of suction devices, proximal looping suture, and intracoronary shunt device [37].

Partial sternotomy represents a safe alternative for the repair of congenital heart defects in pediatric and adult patients. While pediatric population is beyond the aim of this chapter, the most common congenital heart defects in the adult being corrected through this access are represented by atrial septal defect and atrioventricular canal. Lower sternotomy up to the second-third intercostal space allows a standard surgical technique for the correction of these defects [38].

Patients with advanced heart failure symptoms (New York Heart Association functional class IIIB–IV) refractory to maximal medical management, who are inotrope dependent, or who are on temporary circulatory support are candidates for durable mechanical circulatory support. Left ventricular assist device (LVAD) surgery through a full median sternotomy still remains the gold standard for device implantation. Nevertheless, evolving clinical indications together with recent advances in device miniaturization have fueled the development of minimally invasive implantation approaches by means of different techniques, promoting less bleeding and infectious.

One of these approaches is represented by the combination of partial sternotomy and left thoracotomy. The "Hannover technique" is performed through a partial J-sternotomy for aortic access and cannulation. Venous cannulation is performed through right atrial or femoral vein cannulation, and the apex is exposed via a left minithoracotomy, in order to secure the VAD sewing ring. After positioning the inflow cannula, the outflow vascular graft is tunneled towards the ascending aorta, where it is anastomosed in standard fashion [39, 40].

Furthermore, upper sternotomy has also been used to achieve access to the ascending aorta for transcatheter aortic valve implantation procedures, when other peripheral vascular routes resulted unfeasible.

An increasing number of patients in need for a percutaneous treatment of aortic valve pathology is treated every year.

While transfemoral route is the most spread approach, challenging anatomy or peripheral arterial pathology may lead to choosing alternative access, and transaortic route by partial J-sternotomy is indeed an option. After adequate exposure of ascending aorta, purse strings are placed at the selected cannulation site, from where the delivery system can be advanced through the aortic valve and the prosthesis deployed under fluoroscopy [41].

15.3 Anesthesiological Management for MS

15.3.1 Preoperative Assessment

The main principles of anesthesia for routine full sternotomy apply to an MS approach, but the limited nature of the incision presents some specific challenges of which the anesthesiologist must be aware.

Preoperative assessment is similar to other cardiac operations, and a multidisciplinary approach and detailed preoperative planning are essential to achieve better outcomes for patients.

Routine examinations must include electrocardiogram, chest X-ray, blood test including coagulation tests, and preoperative echocardiogram.

15.3.2 Cardiovascular Evaluation

Alongside the primary cardiac pathology, it is imperative to assess for any concurrent cardiac or vascular abnormalities. A comprehensive examination of patients' peripheral vasculature is essential when considering peripheral bypass cannulation [42]. The existence of plaques, aneurysms, dissections, tortuosity, or foreign vascular materials (such as grafts or stents) may contraindicate peripheral cannulation. If endoballoon clamping is being considered, a higher degree of aortic valve insufficiency and aortic vascular diseases, such as an aneurysmal ascending aorta or effacement of the sinotubular junction, should be ruled out [43]. Computed Tomography (CT) angiography could be incorporated into the evaluation process for MS. In fact, CT allows to better understand vascular anatomy and, at the same time, provides information about lung's morphology and airways. Moreover, for MS approach, CT also provides information about the aorta and its relationship with the sternum.

15.3.3 Gastrointestinal

The feasibility to conduct intraoperative transesophageal echocardiography (TEE) is crucial, and if TEE is contraindicated, it essentially rules out the surgical procedure itself.

Absolute contraindications to TEE include the presence of esophageal webs or strictures, tumors, lacerations, diverticula, or active upper gastrointestinal (GI) bleeding. Common relative contraindications to TEE comprise a history of radiation to the head, neck, or mediastinum; prior surgery of the upper GI tract; esophageal varices; active peptic ulcer disease; and hiatal hernia. If any of these conditions are present, the risks and benefits of TEE must be carefully evaluated.

15.3.4 General Issues

Surgical challenges may arise in cases of morbid obesity, which can hinder surgical access and make the patient unsuitable for MS, especially when coupled with very large breasts [44]. Furthermore, extremely obese patients may necessitate additional drainage cannulas for increased CPB flow.

On the contrary, in smaller patients with a limited thoracic cavity, achieving adequate surgical exposure may prove difficult. Additionally, the size of their femoral vessels may prevent direct cannulation [45].

15.3.5 Intraoperative Management

Anesthesia induction and maintenance, as for any cardiac surgery, are commonly achieved using intravenous agents. Likewise, hemodynamic management follows the same principles as conventional cardiac surgery.

There are few differences from a standard cardiac surgery setup:

- Placement of external defibrillation pads is mandatory, as the use of internal defibrillation paddles is not always feasible during MS.
- Transesophageal echocardiography is also essential during MS.
  A TEE comprehensive study of the heart function should be performed at the beginning of the case and during cannulation, since incorrect positioning of CPB cannulas can lead to severe consequences, including unintentional cannulation of the hepatic veins or perforation of the right atrium, right ventricle, or interatrial septum.
  TEE can play a crucial role in evaluating left ventricle distension. During the administration of cardioplegic solution, aortic regurgitation may lead to left ventricle distension and insufficient myocardial protection. Furthermore, TEE is crucial in evaluating the effective arrest of the heart following the administration of cardioplegia, especially considering the limited visibility in the operative field during surgery.
  Also, the MS incision, that is usually about one-third of the normal sternotomy length, limits not only surgical access but also the view of the myocardium, especially to the right ventricle. Hence, TEE is the key tool for assessing the size and function of the right

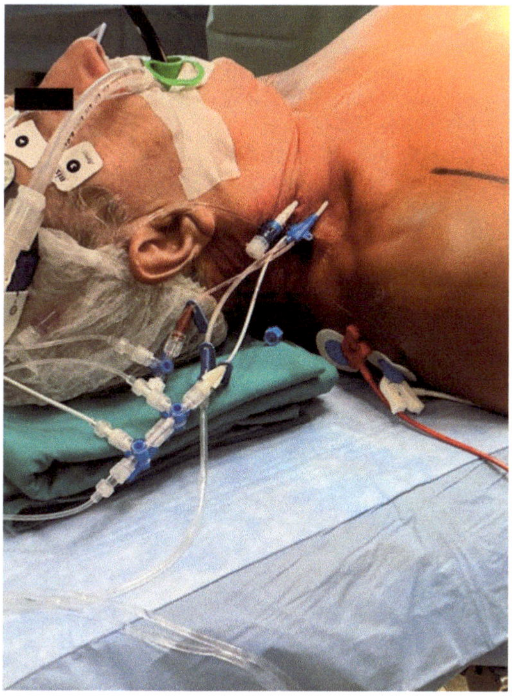

Fig. 15.4 Placement of central venous multi-lumen catheter and 8 French sheath introducer in the jugular vein for possible temporary pacing

ventricle particularly during the process of separation from CPB.

- To achieve the goal of a fast-track extubation, short-acting drugs should be preferred for anesthesia induction and maintenance.
- Routinely, a central venous multi-lumen must be used, and a 6–8 French sheath introducer must be placed in the jugular vein for possible temporary pacing (Fig. 15.4).

15.4 Postoperative Care and Analgesia

Patients undergoing MS require admission to a cardiothoracic intensive care unit. Peripheral CPB cannulation sites must be monitored for hematoma, thrombus, and pseudoaneurysm formation, and the integrity of limb perfusion distal to the cannulation sites needs to be regularly assessed.

In the absence of major complications, MS patients are typically placed on a "fast-track" protocol, where they are gradually weaned from sedation and extubated as soon as it is deemed appropriate. Some institutions prefer an "ultra-fast tracking" approach, aiming for extubation in the operating theatre.

15.4.1 Opioid-Sparing Analgesia

Over the years, opioids have been a fundamental component of a "balanced cardiac anesthetic technique," offering pain relief while preventing a sympathetic response during cardiac surgery. Despite their effectiveness as analgesics, opioids are associated with various side effects including respiratory depression, delirium, hyperalgesia, constipation, or urinary retention, all of which can hinder patient recovery and increase morbidity [45]. Enhanced Recovery After Surgery (ERAS) protocols in noncardiac surgery have led to a gradual shift away from high doses of opioids in the perioperative period, with opioid-free anesthesia OFA gaining popularity in general surgical specialties [46].

In recent years, cardiac anesthesiologists have also begun to reduce the use of high opioid doses in favor of multimodal analgesia [47]. The innervation of the chest wall allows for peripheral nerve blockade, providing stable cardiovascular conditions as well as effective pain relief. This, along with a combination of adjunct drugs, can offer effective and safe perioperative conditions for cardiac surgery. Understanding the pharmacokinetics of these drugs allows for their discontinuation to be appropriately timed, facilitating early or even on-table extubation when clinically suitable.

Actually, ERAS recommends an opioid-sparing approach, in order to achieve an enhanced and faster recovery from surgery.

Actually, ERAS protocols aim to limit unnecessary opioids, MV, and inotropic support; avoid nonessential invasive monitoring; and improve mobility and expedite discharge. Implementation of ERAS measures in the routine clinical practice also requires a considerable effort to standardize care, which may vary across different institutions. On the other hand, care standardization should result in better outcomes via decreasing variations and improving efficiency [48].

In this scenario, new locoregional anesthesia techniques, the so-called fascial plane block, are emerging as a valid tool to promote fast-track extubation, especially in minimally invasive cardiac surgery [49].

Therefore, analgesia for MS may be achieved via parasternal intercostal plane block (PIP), a pectoralis nerve block (PECS I and II), or an erector spinae plane (ESP) block. Thoracic epidural catheterization is feasible but not recommended due to the requirement for systemic heparinization.

For patients undergoing MS approach, PIP block can indeed be particularly effective for pain management.

PIP block, in fact, targets the anterior cutaneous branches from T2 to T6 intercostal nerves, covering the anterior and medial chest wall.

PIP block can be divided into superficial PIP block, targeting the fascial plane between the pectoralis major muscle and the external intercostal muscle, and deep PIP block, in which the local anesthetic is deposited in the fascial plane between the internal intercostal muscle and the transversus thoracic muscle.

Evidence about the analgesic efficacy of PIP block for sternotomy pain has been derived from several RCTs and meta-analyses.

Although the superiority of one technique over the other has not been defined, considering the increased risk of pneumothorax and IMA injury associated with deep PIP, the superficial PIP is actually considered safer to perform in the context of a fast-track program [50].

References

1. Di Bacco L, Miceli A, Glauber M. Minimally invasive aortic valve surgery. J Thorac Dis. 2021;13(3):1945–59. https://doi.org/10.21037/jtd-20-1968.
2. Phan K, Xie A, Tsai YC, Black D, Di Eusanio M, Yan TD. Ministernotomy or minithoracotomy for minimally invasive aortic valve replacement: a Bayesian network meta-analysis. Ann Cardiothorac Surg. 2015;4(1):3–14. https://doi.org/10.3978/j.issn.2225-319X.2014.08.01.
3. Julian OC, Lopez-Belio M, Dye WS, Javid H, Grove WJ. The median sternal incision in intracardiac surgery with extracorporeal circulation; a general evaluation of its use in heart surgery. Surgery. 1957;42(4):753–61.
4. Schmitto JD, Mokashi SA, Cohn LH. Minimally-invasive valve surgery. J Am Coll Cardiol. 2010;56:455–62.
5. Karimov JH, Santarelli F, Murzi M, et al. A technique of an upper V-type ministernotomy in the second intercostal space. Interact Cardiovasc Thorac Surg. 2009;9:1021–2.
6. De Amicis V, Ascione R, Iannelli G, Di Tommaso L, Monaco M, Spampinato N. Aortic valve replacement through a minimally invasive approach. Tex Heart Inst J. 1997;24(4):353–5.
7. Kasegawa H, Shimokawa T, Matsushita Y, Kamata S, Ida T, Kawase M. Right-sided partial sternotomy for minimally invasive valve operation: "open door method". Ann Thorac Surg. 1998;65(2):569–70. https://doi.org/10.1016/s0003-4975(97)01332-5.
8. Svensson LG, D'Agostino RS. "J" incision minimal-access valve operations. Ann Thorac Surg. 1998;66(3):1110–2. https://doi.org/10.1016/s0003-4975(98)00655-9.
9. Vigano M, Rinaldi M, D'Armini AM, Boffini M, Zattera GF, Alloni A, Dore R. Ascending aortic aneurysms treated by cuneiform resection and end-to-end anastomosis through a ministernotomy. Ann Thorac Surg. 2002;74:S1789–S1791; discussion S1792–9.
10. Sun L, Zheng J, Chang Q, Tang Y, Feng J, Sun X, Zhu X. Aortic root replacement by ministernotomy: technique and potential benefit. Ann Thorac Surg. 2000;70(6):1958–61. https://doi.org/10.1016/s0003-4975(00)02147-0.
11. Svensson LG, Nadolny EM, Kimmel WA. Minimal access aortic surgery including re-operations. Eur J Cardiothorac Surg. 2001;19(1):30–3. https://doi.org/10.1016/s1010-7940(00)00597-2.
12. Brown ML, McKellar SH, Sundt TM, Schaff HV. Ministernotomy versus conventional sternotomy for aortic valve replacement: a systematic review and meta-analysis. J Thorac Cardiovasc Surg. 2009;137(3):670–679.e5. https://doi.org/10.1016/j.jtcvs.2008.08.010. Epub 2008 Oct 23.
13. Gundry SR. Aortic valve replacement by ministernotomy. Oper Tech Cardiac Thorac Surg. 1998;3:47–53.
14. Morgant MC, Malapert G, Petrosyan A, Pujos C, Jazayeri S, Bouchot O. Comparison of automated fastener device Cor-Knot versus manually-tied knot in minimally-invasive isolated aortic valve replacement surgery. J Cardiovasc Surg. 2020;61(1):123–8. https://doi.org/10.23736/S0021-9509.19.10792-6.
15. Rosengart TK, Feldman T, Borger MA, et al. Percutaneous and minimally invasive valve procedures: a scientific statement from the American Heart Association Council on Cardiovascular Surgery and Anesthesia, Council on Clinical Cardiology, Functional Genomics and Translational Biology

Interdisciplinary Working Group, and Quality of Care and Outcomes Research Interdisciplinary Working Group. Circulation. 2008;117:1750–67.
16. Merk DR, Lehmann S, Holzhey DM, et al. Minimal invasive aortic valve replacement surgery is associated with improved survival: a propensity-matched comparison. Eur J Cardiothorac Surg. 2015;47:11–7.
17. Furukawa N, Kuss O, Aboud A, et al. Ministernotomy versus conventional sternotomy for aortic valve replacement: matched propensity score analysis of 808 patients. Eur J Cardiothorac Surg. 2014;46(2):221–6.
18. Bonacchi M, Prifti E, Giunti G, Frati G, Sani G. Does ministernotomy improve postoperative outcome in aortic valve operation? A prospective randomized study. Ann Thorac Surg. 2002;73:460–5.
19. Moustafa MA, Abdelsamad AA, Zakaria G, Omarah MM. Minimal vs median sternotomy for aortic valve replacement. Asian Cardiovasc Thorac Ann. 2007;15:472–5.
20. Sharony R, Grossi EA, Saunders PC, et al. Minimally invasive aortic valve surgery in the elderly: a case-control study. Circulation. 2003;108(Suppl 1):II43–7.
21. Bakir I, Casselman FP, Wellens F, et al. Minimally invasive versus standard approach aortic valve replacement: a study in 506 patients. Ann Thorac Surg. 2006;81:1599–604.
22. Aris A, Cámara ML, Montiel J, Delgado LJ, Galán J, Litvan H. Ministernotomy versus median sternotomy for aortic valve replacement: a prospective, randomized study. Ann Thorac Surg. 1999;67:1583–7.
23. Dogan S, Dzemali O, Wimmer-Greinecker G, et al. Minimally invasive versus conventional aortic valve replacement: a prospective randomized trial. J Heart Valve Dis. 2003;12:76–80.
24. Salis S, Mazzanti VV, Merli G, et al. Cardiopulmonary bypass duration is an independent predictor of morbidity and mortality after cardiac surgery. J Cardiothorac Vasc Anesth. 2008;22(6):814–22.
25. Al-Sarraf N, Thalib L, Hughes A, et al. Cross-clamp time is an independent predictor of mortality and morbidity in low- and high-risk cardiac patients. Int J Surg. 2011;9(1):104–9.
26. Salsano A, Giacobbe DR, Sportelli E, et al. Aortic cross-clamp time and cardiopulmonary bypass time: prognostic implications in patients operated on for infective endocarditis. Interact Cardiovasc Thorac Surg. 2018;27(3):328–35.
27. Chien S, Clark C, Maheshwari S, et al. Benefits of rapid deployment aortic valve replacement with a mini upper sternotomy. J Cardiothorac Surg. 2020;15(1):226.
28. Ramsaransing K, Hindori V, Kougioumtzoglou A, Kaya A, Verbeek E. Minimally invasive sutureless aortic valve replacement with the Perceval S bioprosthesis through ministernotomy: a single-center experience. Cureus. 2020;12(10):e11212.
29. Pollari F, Mamdooh H, Hitzl W, Grossmann I, Vogt F, Fischlein T. Ten years' experience with the sutureless aortic valve replacement: incidence and predictors for survival and valve durability at follow-up. Eur J Cardiothorac Surg. 2023;63(2):ezac572.
30. Barnhart GR, Accola KD, Grossi EA, et al., TRANSFORM Trial Investigators. TRANSFORM (Multicenter Experience With Rapid Deployment Edwards INTUITY Valve System for Aortic Valve Replacement) US clinical trial: performance of a rapid deployment aortic valve. J Thorac Cardiovasc Surg. 2017;153(2):241–51.e2.
31. Bichell DP, Balaguer JM, Aranki SF, et al. Axilloaxillary cardiopulmonary bypass: a practical alternative to femorofemoral bypass. Ann Thorac Surg. 1997;64:702–5.
32. Zlotnick AY, Gilfeather M, Adams DH, Cohn LH, Couper GS. Innominate vein cannulation for venous drainage in minimally invasive aortic valve surgery. Ann Thorac Surg. 1999;67:864–5.
33. Abu-Omar Y, Fazmin IT, Ali JM, Pelletier MP. Minimally invasive mitral valve surgery. J Thorac Dis. 2021;13(3):1960–70.
34. Gillinov AM, Cosgrove DM. Minimally invasive mitral valve surgery: mini-sternotomy with extended transseptal approach. Semin Thorac Cardiovasc Surg. 1999;11(3):206–11.
35. Radwan M, Salewski C, Hecker F, et al. Mitral valve surgery via upper ministernotomy: single-centre experience in more than 400 patients. Medicina (Kaunas). 2021;57(11):1179.
36. Riess FC, Schofer J, Kremer P, et al. Beating heart operations including hybrid revascularization: initial experiences. Ann Thorac Surg. 1998;66(3):1076–81.
37. Modrau IS, Nielsen PH, Bøtker HE, et al. Feasibility and early safety of hybrid coronary revascularisation combining off-pump coronary surgery through J-hemisternotomy with percutaneous coronary intervention. EuroIntervention. 2015;10(10):e1–6.
38. Garcia Vieites M, Cardenas I, Loyola H, et al. Lower mini-sternotomy in congenital heart disease: just a cosmetic improvement? Interact Cardiovasc Thorac Surg. 2015;21(3):374–8.
39. Hanke JS, Rojas SV, Avsar M, Haverich A, Schmitto JD. Minimally-invasive LVAD implantation: state of the art. Curr Cardiol Rev. 2015;11(3):246–51.
40. Hanke JS, Dogan G, Shrestha M, Haverich A, Schmitto JD. Innovations in implantation techniques of ventricular assist devices. JTCVS Open. 2021;8:28–32.
41. Bapat V, Attia R. Transaortic transcatheter aortic valve implantation: step-by-step guide. Semin Thorac Cardiovasc Surg. 2012;24(3):206–11.
42. Malik V, Jha AK, Kapoor PM. Anesthetic challenges in minimally invasive cardiac surgery: are we moving in a right direction? Ann Card Anaesth. 2016;19(3):489–97. https://doi.org/10.4103/0971-9784.185539.
43. Klein P, Klop IDG, Kloppenburg GLT, van Putte BP. Planning for minimally invasive aortic valve replacement: key steps for patient assessment. Eur J Cardiothorac Surg. 2018;53(Suppl_2):ii3–8. https://doi.org/10.1093/ejcts/ezy086.

44. Müller L, Höfer D, Holfeld J, et al. Indications and contra-indications for minimally invasive mitral valve surgery. J Vis Surg. 2018;4:255.
45. Lavand'homme P, Steyaert A. Opioid-free anesthesia opioid side effects: tolerance and hyperalgesia. Best Pract Res Clin Anaesthesiol. 2017;31:487–98.
46. Forget P. Opioid-free anaesthesia. Why and how? A contextual analysis. Anaesth Crit Care Pain Med. 2019;38(2):169–72. https://doi.org/10.1016/j.accpm.2018.05.002. Epub 2018 Sep 13.
47. Noss C, Prusinkiewicz C, Nelson G, Patel PA, Augoustides JG, Gregory AJ. Enhanced recovery for cardiac surgery. J Cardiothorac Vasc Anesth. 2018;32(6):2760–70. https://doi.org/10.1053/j.jvca.2018.01.045.
48. Spadaccio C, Salsano A, Pisani A, Nenna A, Nappi F, Osho A, D'Alessandro D, Sundt TM, Crestanello J, Engelman D, Rose D. Enhanced recovery protocols after surgery: a systematic review and meta-analysis of randomized trials in cardiac surgery. World J Surg. 2024;48(4):779–90. https://doi.org/10.1002/wjs.12122. Epub 2024 Feb 29.
49. Capuano P, Sepolvere G, Toscano A, Scimia P, Silvetti S, Tedesco M, Gentili L, Martucci G, Burgio G. Fascial plane blocks for cardiothoracic surgery: a narrative review. J Anesth Analg Crit Care. 2024;4(1):20. https://doi.org/10.1186/s44158-024-00155-5.
50. Toscano A, Capuano P, Perrucci C, Giunta M, Orsello A, Pierani T, Costamagna A, Tedesco M, Arcadipane A, Sepolvere G, Buono G, Brazzi L. Which ultrasound-guided parasternal intercostal nerve block for post-sternotomy pain? Results from a prospective observational study. J Anesth Analg Crit Care. 2023;3(1):48. https://doi.org/10.1186/s44158-023-00134-2.

16 TAVI

Denti Paolo, Azzola Nicolò Guicciardi, Rapetti Francesca, and Maisano Francesco

16.1 Introduction

Aortic valve disease (AVD) is the most common disease in elderly patients in Europe [1] and North America. Every patient who needs therapy should be evaluated by the Heart Team, a team composed of interventional cardiologists, cardiothoracic surgeons, cardio-anesthesiologist, radiologists, echocardiographers that consider risks and benefits of each individual patient for surgical aortic valve replacement (SAVR) or transcatheter aortic valve implantation (TAVI).

Since its introduction in 2002 TAVI was considered a valid option only for those patients who had prohibitive surgical risk [2] but in the last decades has been validated within high- and intermediate-risk patients and has increasingly replaced SAVR with good outcomes [3].

The trials about surgical risk scores demonstrate that TAVI is superior to medical therapy in extreme-risk patients [4], and non-inferior to SAVR in high [5–7] and intermediate-risk patients at 5-year follow-up [3, 4, 8, 9].

TAVI is also non-inferior to SAVR in low-risk patient at a 2-year follow-up, as the PARTNER 3 and Evolut Low Risk trials recently demonstrate [7, 10, 11].

This chapter aims to provide a comprehensive overview of the management of patients undergoing TAVI from procedure planning to follow-up in an ERAS perspective and present our fast-track TAVI protocol.

16.2 Procedure Planning

16.2.1 Long-Life Management of Aortic Valve Disease

Firstly considered as an alternative to SAVR in old and high-risk patients, in the last decade TAVI became a widely chosen option in patients with AVD. The number of TAVI performed in the United States has increasingly grown until overcoming SAVR [12], and these estimates are predicted to rise.

Although both ACC/AHA [13] and ESC/EACTS [14] guidelines recommend surgery in young patients without relevant comorbidities, they reported different age cut-off and considered of pivotal importance in decision-making process exclusively age and surgical risk.

D. Paolo (✉) · A. N. Guicciardi · M. Francesco
Valve Center, Cardiac Surgery Department, San Raffaele University Hospital, Milan, Italy
e-mail: denti.paolo@hsr.it; azzola.nicolo@hsr.it; maisano.francesco@hsr.it

R. Francesca
Department of Cardiac Anesthesia and Intensive Care, Cardiovascular Network, IRCCS Ospedale Policlinico San Martino, Genoa, Italy
e-mail: francesca.rapetti@hsanmartino.it

G. Sepolvere, S. Silvetti (eds.), *Fast-Track in Cardiac Anesthesia*,
https://doi.org/10.1007/978-3-031-70899-2_16

However in the last few years, concomitantly with the spreading and improved outcomes of TAVI, greater attention has raised on long-life management of patients with AVD [15]. New issues and concerns have been developed such as bioprosthetic valve durability, reintervention strategies, and coronary access availability.

Indeed, since more and more patients chose TAVI at younger age, within the next years the number of a second procedure after TAVI is destined to raise consistently [16]. Although TAVI in TAVI represent a valid solution as second procedure, it may result challenging since not always suitable, and it often requires technical expertise including leaflet modification techniques to prevent coronary obstruction [17–19]. Furthermore, TAVI explant has been demonstrated until now to be at higher risk of death and morbidity if compared to SAVR reintervention [20].

Last, despite TAVI was initially developed and employed to address aortic stenosis (AS) treatment, recently new devices have been designed and approved to target specifically aortic insufficiency [21].

Given this background, the first intervention on the aortic valve is crucial and irreversibly sign the patient's history. Hence, a comprehensive evaluation of the patient should take place in the context of the Heart Team, accordingly to current guidelines [13, 14]. Still, Heart Team should deliberate on patients in hospital stay, assessing eventual warning issues (clinically, anatomically, or electrocardiographically relevant) that may undermine the feasibility of a fast-track protocol.

In a patient-centered view, TAVI rule-out decision-making process should be based on three pillars: clinical assessment, anatomical evaluation, and patient will. Plus, in order to improve TAVI outcomes in terms of safety and procedural success we endorse the transcatheter treatment of AVD in high-volume centers with a cardiac surgery ward in situ to eventually manage procedure-related complications [22].

16.2.2 Anatomy Assessment and Imaging Evaluation

Although the first diagnosis of severe AS is mainly done with transthoracic echocardiogram [14], computer tomography angiography (CTA) is nowadays the gold standard to assess if TAVI is suitable and to determine procedural strategy [23].

CTA should be performed ideally before index hospitalization both to avoid kidneys injury due to cumulative contrast liquid exposition, especially in patients with impaired renal function, and to reduce in-hospital length of stay [23]. However, CTA during index hospitalization may be considered in the two following settings. First, if patients present reduced glomerular filtration rate, peri-examination hydration and bloods level of creatinine monitoring are recommended. Further, in those with known allergy to contrast liquid, a pre-medication with steroidal anti-inflammatory drugs, according to local protocols, is mandatory [23].

For TAVR planning, the CTA protocol involves an ECG-synchronized scan of the aortic root [24]. Additionally, a non-ECG-synchronized CTA of the aorta and iliofemoral vessels is conducted to assess vascular access. Typically, the contrast is injected at a flow rate of 4.0–6.0 mL/s, with an estimated total volume of 50–100 cc [24]. The CTA scan can be initiated using bolus tracking, with the region of interest set in the descending aorta.

The CTA analysis purpose is to assess aortic valve-related elements such as virtual basal ring dimension (measured at 10–30% of the cardiac cycle) [23], leaflets morphology, calcium burden, coronary ostial height, sinus of Valsalva diameter, sinotubular junction diameter, and ascending aorta diameter. Furthermore, for a complete and safety procedural planning aortic route and access viability study is mandatory. To assess aortoiliofemoral vascularization, CTA scans should cover the aorta, iliac arteries, and common femoral arteries. Additionally, starting the scan at the head can help evaluate the carotid and subclavian arteries for alternative vascular access points [25].

Here we highlight anatomical findings that should raise the attention of the interventionalist and may require further caution and observation in patient's index hospitalization because more prone to critical complication:

- Large annulus.
- Poorly or heavily calcified annulus.
- Bicuspid aortic valves with calcified raphe.
- Calcified left ventricular outflow tract.
- Low coronary ostia.
- Ascending aorta enlargement.
- Tortuous and calcific aortic route.
- Calcified and narrow peripheral access.

Still, an early CTA evaluation allows to point out all the critical issues that make treatment strategy decision of the Heart Team aware and safe.

16.2.2.1 Index Hospitalization and Medication

If diagnostic and therapeutic rule-out is already defined, patients are admitted to hospital on the same date of the index procedure. Patient must be in the fasted state and must be in wash-out from drugs that interfere with heart rhythm increasing the risk of postoperative conduction blocks [26]. Antiplatelets or anticoagulant drugs are not contraindicated preoperatively [27]. Detailed indications for anticoagulant drugs management in patients undergoing TAVI are reported in the 2021 consensus document of the ESC Working Group on Thrombosis and the European Association of Percutaneous Cardiovascular Interventions [27].

ECG evaluation is mandatory and essential to detect preexisting conduction disturbances (right bundle branch block (RBBB) and atrio-ventricular I grade block (AVI)) that increase the risk of new pacemaker permanent implantation (PPI).

16.3 Procedure-Related Highlights

16.3.1 Access Sites: Transfemoral Approach

The most common approach for TAVI is transfemoral. It can be performed both surgically (Fig. 16.1) or percutaneous. Although data derived from randomized controlled trials are lacking on this topic, it has been demonstrated that the percutaneous transfemoral TAVI approach is associated with shorter procedural times, lower rates of major vascular complications, bleeding, transfusion requirements, access-site bleeding, and shorter length of hospital stay than a surgical cut-down approach. However, femoral stenosis and dissections seem to be more frequent using the percutaneous approach [28]. Currently, we recommend the use of a surgical approach when facing hostile calcific access,

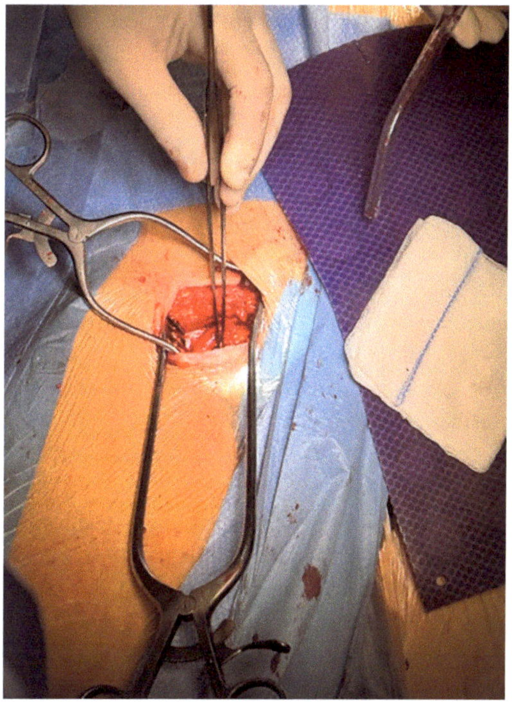

Fig. 16.1 Surgical femoral vascular access

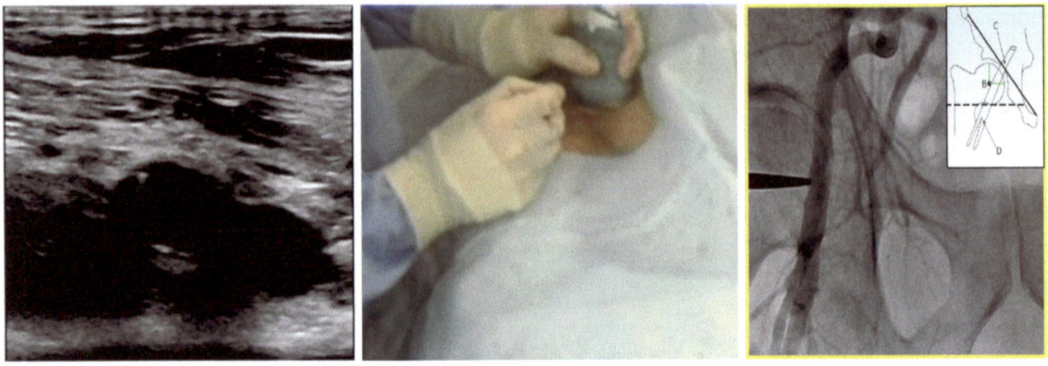

Fig. 16.2 Echo-guided and fluoroscopic puncture

with an increased risk of access complications. Percutaneous echo-guided femoral puncture is preferable, rather than fluoroscopic guided. (Fig. 16.2).

Percutaneous transfemoral approach requires both therapeutic and diagnostic access sites. Valve deployment is performed through the first access (14–20 Fr), while the second is typically used to advance diagnostic pigtail and manage any access complication (6–8 Fr). Main access side should be determined accordingly to route diameter, calcification, and tortuosity. Diagnostic access location is mainly operator dependent and could be both radial and transfemoral (same-site or opposite-site). Many retrospective experiences report a beneficial role of radial access in terms of bleeding and vascular adverse events [29, 30]. However, currently available literature may be influenced by selection bias and does not consider the impact of dedicated vascular closure devices. Further, femoral diagnostic access enhances the possibility to face main access complications.

After confirming the correct valve positioning via fluoroscopy, the femoral access site is generally closed with a vascular closure device or sutures, depending on the medical team's practices [31]. A fluoroscopic control of the main access is recommended before removing the diagnostic access.

16.3.2 Access Sites: Trans-axillary Approach

The subclavian approach for TAVI is safe and feasible, demonstrating procedural outcomes comparable to the femoral approach over the medium term [32]. It should be considered a viable alternative not only in cases where femoral access is impossible, but also in vasculopathic patients with at least challenging femoral artery accessibility [33]. A subclavian access is obtained through the subclavian artery, typically with a surgical incision (Fig. 16.3). Through the axillary artery, a guide catheter is advanced into the ascending aorta under fluoroscopic guidance. This step may require a greater curve in the catheter due to the angle of the subclavian artery compared to the aorta. Subsequently, the closed aortic valve is inserted into the correct position. The new valve is expanded using a balloon, compressing the native valve against the aortic wall and securing the new valve in place. Then the subclavian access site is surgically closed.

16.3.3 Access Sites: Transapical Approach

During the TAVI transapical procedure, a left anterolateral mini thoracotomy is performed at the fifth or sixth intercostal space to access the

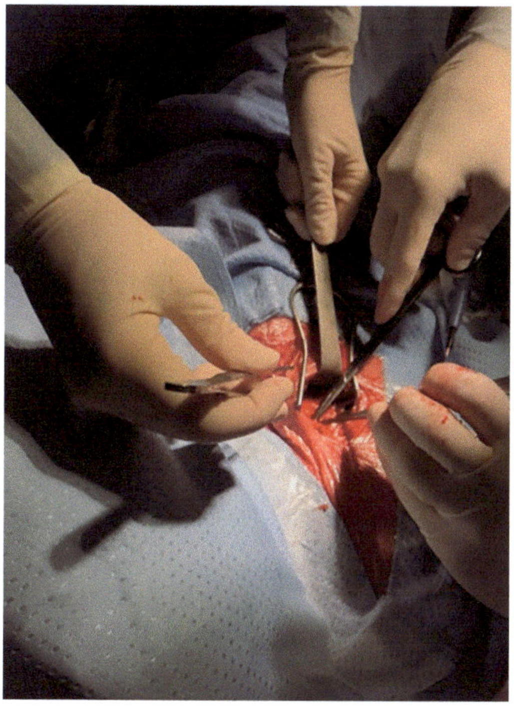

Fig. 16.3 Subclavian approach for trans-axillary TAVI

heart apex directly. The procedure is performed under general anesthesia to better manage the patient in case of complications that may occur due to heart damage, coronary ischemia, embolism, or bleeding. To ensure good postoperative analgesia, it is recommended to perform serratus anterior block to minimize surgical site pain and ensure optimal respiratory weaning, ideally already in the operating room when possible.

In these patients, it is crucial to stabilize hemodynamic, especially before proceeding with valve implantation, potentially using volume expansion and low-dose inotropic agents to maintain a mean blood pressure above 80 mmHg. The procedure is guided by fluoroscopy and supplemented with transesophageal echocardiography for precise monitoring. The aortic valve is crossed antegrade after puncturing the apex with a needle; balloon valvuloplasty occurs during rapid ventricular pacing (RVP), carefully maintaining mean arterial pressure above 60 mmHg, typically set between 170/min and 220/min to aid valve deployment, with angiographic guidance ensuring proper positioning of the valve in the annulus, supported by echocardiographic confirmation [34, 35].

16.3.4 Temporary PM Management

TAVI procedure requires pacemaker (PM)-induced rapid pacing at 180–200 heart rate and subsequent drop of pressure during valve deployment or balloon-assisted pre- and post-dilatation if required. Furthermore, PM plays a pivotal role in the management of post-procedural heart rhythm disturbances management. Namely, although TAVI outcomes surprisingly improved in the last years, PPI remains one of the most frequent procedure-related adverse events.

Temporary PM's location can be both trans-jugular and transfemoral (Fig. 16.4.) The first approach is suggested when patient has risk factors for PPI, including anatomical, ECG, and procedure-related issues. Namely, it allows early mobilization also in those who experienced heart rhythm abnormalities. However, trans-jugular venous route may result more challenging to be allocated in the right ventricular apex and is related with longer in-hospital length of stay. On the other hand, transfemoral venous access is to be considered in patients with low risk for rhythm-related adverse events to reduce procedure-related times and removed at the end of the procedure in the operating room. The latter strategy may result more feasible for the operator, but if temporary PM should be kept in place as protection, early mobilization could be compromised.

Last, rapid pacing can be performed also electrifying the stiff wire, with a technique named "pacing through the wire." Although fast and safe, this strategy is feasible accordingly to the operator experience and may seem reasonable in high-volume centers for low-risk patients.

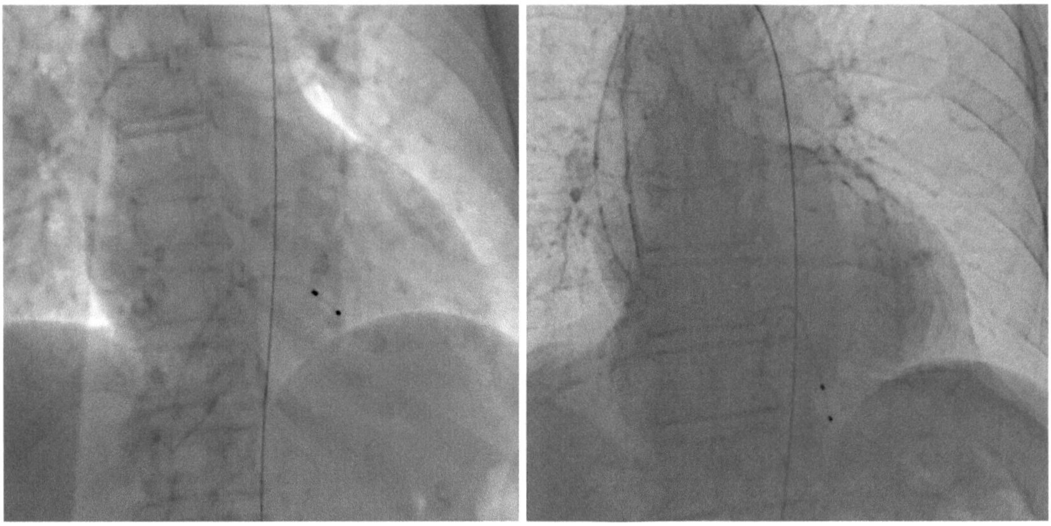

Fig. 16.4 Fluoroscopic view of transfemoral and trans-jugular temporary PM

16.3.5 Cerebral Embolic Protection

Debris embolization from the valve or blood vessels can lead to peri-procedural strokes, raising morbidity and mortality rates [36]. Despite a lack of clinical symptoms, diffusion-weighted perfusion imaging reveals defects in 68–93% of patients following TAVI [36]. Although the stroke risk associated with TAVI is decreasing with newer-generation devices and is comparable to that of surgical aortic valve replacement, it continues to be a significant and concerning complication [37]. Hence, cerebral embolic protection (CEP) devices have been developed. They consist in filters allocated in the arteriosus anonymous trunk and left common carotid artery generally via radial access. Although randomized clinical trials didn't show a significant impact of CEP on cerebral adverse event among the general population [38], CEP should be considered in patients undergoing TAVI with an increased risk of embolic consequence, including those with heavily calcified valve or requiring leaflet modification techniques.

16.3.6 After Valve Delivery

Once, the prosthesis is delivered, before the sheath removal, transthoracic echocardiogram (TTE) should be promptly performed both to assess the presence of pericardial effusion and to assess valves gradients and paravalvular leaks. This allows to safely evaluate procedural success and identify early complications. Alternatively, hemodynamic assessment of the gradients may be performed, and contrast-enhanced fluoroscopy could be used. Of note, during the whole procedure the exposure to X-rays and liquid of contrast is warranted to guarantee procedure safety and control but should be limited to that is strictly necessary.

After sheaths removal and adequate hemostasis, patient can be led to recovery room or ICU for monitoring.

16.4 Anesthesiologic Management for TAVI

16.4.1 Preoperative Assessment

The TAVI procedure is a minimally invasive treatment for AS. During this procedure, anesthesia plays a crucial role in ensuring the patient's comfort and the success of the intervention. Considering how the indications of TAVI became wider than before, extended both to very critical patients or very low risks patients, the anesthesiologist approach can sometimes make the difference in management after surgery and in duration of hospital length of stay therefore in the outcome. According to the ERAS [11]and cardiac ERAS guidelines [39, 40], patients must be approached with multimodal and interdisciplinary model in order to stratify preoperative risks and optimize perioperative condition (Table 16.1) [39, 41].

High-surgical risk is typically defined by a logistic EuroScore predicting mortality risk over 15%, Society of Thoracic Surgeons' score over 10%, or challenging factors like a porcelain aorta, prior cardiac surgery with grafts, severe adhesions, radiation therapy history, liver cirrhosis, immobile patients avoiding sternotomy, or pronounced frailty. Each patient requires personalized risk assessment, acknowledging that scoring systems aid but do not fully encompass all considerations.

Table 16.1 Cardiac ERAS guidelines [39] on multimodal and interdisciplinary model to stratify preoperative patients' risks and optimize perioperative condition

Preoperative examination	Preoperative counseling and information preferably in the presence of relatives Medical optimization including cardiac, renal, endocrine, and pulmonary evaluation Nutritional status assessment and promotion of a protein-rich diet before procedure Smoking and alcohol cessation before procedure
Perioperative treatment	8 h fasting, anxiolytic medication, gabapentin 300 mg, and acetaminophen 1000 mg given orally
Intraoperative strategy	Opioid spare—Opioid-free multimodal analgesia, loco-regional anesthesia first choice when feasible
Postoperative phase	Early extubation, early mobilization out of bed to chair or ambulating as much as tolerated Acetaminophen 1000 mg every 6 h Gabapentin 300 mg twice daily, if necessary, medication preferable orally PONV prophylaxis and bowel motility evaluation, glycemic control, and early alimentation Early removal of central venous access, pacing wires, urinary catheter

16.4.1.1 Cardiac Evaluation

The initial assessment of patients with aortic stenosis focuses on evaluating their overall medical condition, the severity of the valve abnormality, and its impact on daily life. A comprehensive history and physical examination are essential, particularly in assessing exercise tolerance and the rate of symptom progression as the valve area narrows. Key symptoms of aortic stenosis include exertional or resting dyspnea, chest pain or discomfort, and syncope.

Echocardiography is crucial for assessing the severity of aortic stenosis and for cardiac risk stratification prior to intervention, typically based on estimated valve area and mean pressure gradient. In cases of reduced cardiac function, special attention should be given to "low flow - low gradient" scenarios [44], where velocity and gradient measurements may not accurately reflect the true severity of aortic valve stenosis.

Other parameters that require careful evaluation include left and right ventricular ejection fractions, chamber dimensions, estimated pulmonary artery pressure, regional wall motion abnormalities, concomitant coronary artery disease, and other valve abnormalities (e.g., mitral valve). These factors are critical in guiding anesthetic management during the procedure, particularly in deciding whether the placement of a central venous catheter or an invasive arterial pressure monitoring is necessary at the outset.

16.4.1.2 Major Comorbidities Evaluation

Other medical comorbidities are crucial in determining the potential prognostic benefits of an intervention and the patient's likelihood of recovery. Respiratory conditions, such as chronic obstructive pulmonary disease, pulmonary fibrosis, and other chronic pulmonary pathologies, are particularly concerning, especially if the patient requires domiciliary oxygen therapy or has significantly reduced lung function (e.g., FEV1 <50% predicted). Neurological conditions, including cognitive and physical impairments, prior strokes, or movement disorders such as Parkinson's disease, and renal impairment with an eGFR <30 mL/min, with or without dialysis dependence, further complicate the risk assessment. Gastrointestinal comorbidities, such as hepatic cirrhosis (Child-Pugh B or C), esophageal varices, and active gastrointestinal bleeding, pose additional risks, particularly when antiplatelet therapy is contraindicated.

16.4.2 Intraoperative Assessment

16.4.2.1 Anesthetic Strategies

With growing experience, further development of the devices, and the expansion to intermediate-risk or even in some cases high-risk patients, there is increasing interest in performing this procedure under loco-regional anesthesia rather than the previously favored approach of general anesthesia or sedation. The proposed benefits of loco-regional anesthesia include: reduced procedure time, shorter stay in the cardiac intensive care unit or even postoperative discharge to a cardiology ward with telemetric monitoring, less hemodynamic instability in reaction to sedative drugs, and consequently reduced need for intraprocedural vasopressor support. The presence of a cardiac anesthetist ensures the safe management of any complications that may arise during the various stages of the procedure. Additionally, during the delicate phase of aortic valve implantation, the anesthetist provides temporary sedation to the patient so that they do not perceive the sensation of palpitations caused by rapid pacing. However, this approach lacks airway protection, increasing the risk of obstruction, and may cause patient distress due to mandatory positioning on the surgical table. Conversely, general anesthesia provides definitive airway control and allows for the use of transesophageal echocardiography, which aids in precise hemodynamic monitoring and valve placement. However, it is linked to a higher risk of hemodynamic instability, increased need for inotropic support, longer recovery times, and extended hospital stays.

Despite the expansion towards intermediate-risk or even low-risk patients, TAVI remains a procedure predominantly performed in elderly patients with numerous comorbidities. Therefore, the pathophysiological changes in elderly patients require careful consideration during procedures with the potential risk of serious hemodynamic disturbances, including low or high blood pressure that is sometimes difficult to manage, decreased respiratory capacity and decreased metabolic compensation, and the risk of onset or worsening of renal insufficiency, regardless of the type of anesthesia used.

The standard management of severe aortic stenosis focuses on preserving myocardial perfusion using vasopressors and maintaining cardiac output with positive inotropes, despite the limitations of a fixed left ventricular outflow tract obstruction. Maintaining sinus rhythm is crucial, as loss of atrial contraction, especially with ventricular hypertrophy, can be disastrous. Many inotropic agents can induce atrial dysrhythmias, making it challenging to balance cardiac output support while preserving sinus rhythm. In these kind of procedures, an anesthesiologist with specific sub-specialty training in cardiac anesthesia is highly recommended.

16.4.2.2 Monitoring

ECG: A 5-lead electrocardiogram should be used.

Pressure Monitoring: Invasive arterial pressure monitoring is essential. The radial or brachial artery, managed by the anesthesiologist, is the most convenient access point for continuous monitoring during all stages of the procedure and allows for blood sampling without interrupting the procedure. Alternatively, a side port of an arterial sheath placed by the proceduralist can be used. Both devices can be removed upon discharge from the recovery room if no complications arise.

Venous Access: Large-bore venous access (at least 16G) is mandatory to reduce the risk of severe hemorrhage from femoral vessels or cardiac wall perforation. In high-risk patients, an invasive central venous line may be necessary for the administration of vasoactive and inotropic agents. The anesthesiologist may opt for a femoral venous sheath from the surgical field or a dedicated line in the internal jugular or subclavian vein, which also allows for central venous pressure monitoring.

Pulmonary Artery Pressure Monitoring: Invasive pulmonary artery pressure monitoring is considered risky in TAVI patients, who often have poor left ventricular systolic function and bundle branch block; the introduction of a pulmonary artery catheter may precipitate complete heart block and hemodynamic shock.

Cerebral Monitoring: Cerebral oximetry can be useful for assessing the adequacy of cerebral perfusion, while bispectral index (BIS) or entropy monitoring can aid in the titration of anesthetic drugs.

16.4.2.3 Loco-Regional Anesthesia

During the transfemoral approach, we always recommend using loco-regional anesthesia in the crural region not only for the percutaneous puncture but also to manage potential complications due to the arterial puncture, like stenosis or vessels ruptures, especially in those patients with severe or moderate vessel calcification and peripheral vascular disease or when the minimal artery diameter is smaller than the sheath.

The iliohypogastric and ilioinguinal nerve block is used, with 10 mL of long active local anesthetic (e.g., Ropivacaine 0.2%), spread between the transversus abdominis and internal oblique muscle planes, in the proximity of the two nerves (Fig. 16.5). Additionally, a medial-lateral spread of 20–40 mL of local anesthetic (e.g., Ropivacaine 0.2%) underneath the fascia iliaca ensures anesthesia of the hypogastric region, the inguinal crease, and the upper medial thigh in case of surgery. When sedation is needed to increase patient cooperation, the best choice is dexmedetomidine (0.2–1.4 mcg/kg/h).

To provide effective anesthesia at the subclavicular access site during the procedure, we use the Pecs I nerve block, devised to anesthetize the medial and lateral pectoral nerves, which innervate the pectoralis muscles. This is achieved by injecting a long active local anesthetic (e.g., Ropivacaine 0.375% 10–15 mL) into the fascial plane between the pectoralis major and minor muscles. This provides effective anesthesia, but it is often necessary to infiltrate the skin and subcutaneous tissue with 2% lidocaine, 10 mL, before surgical incision due to potential uneven distribution of the anesthetic in superficial planes.

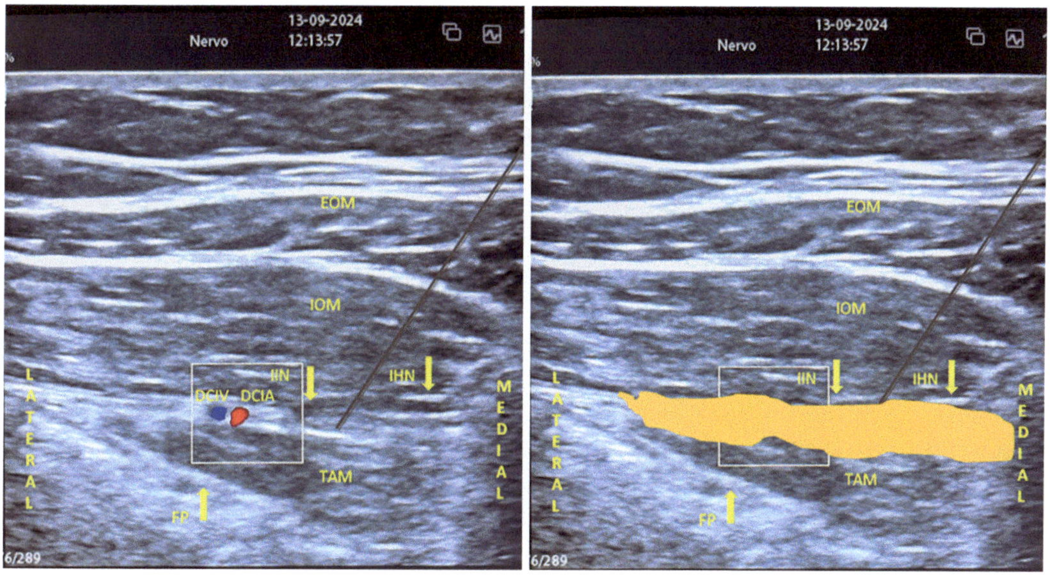

Fig. 16.5 Ultrasound anatomy of the iliohypogastric and ilioinguinal nerve (*TAM* transverse abdominal muscle, *IOM* internal oblique muscle, *EOM* external oblique, *IIN* ilioinguinal nerve, *IHN* iliohypogastric nerve, *FP* fascia peritoneum, *DCIA* deep circumflex iliac artery, *DCIV* deep circumflex iliac vein). The iliohypogastric and ilioinguinal nerves lie in the plane between the TAM and the IOM. They are often seen side by side or up to 1 cm apart, typically hypoechoic ovals

In both approaches, the patient's position in this type of procedure is often uncomfortable, so sedation is typically required to keep the patient still on the operating table. In such cases, dexmedetomidine (0.2–1.4 mcg/kg/h) is the preferred medication.

During the rapid pacing, a deeper sedation is needed to avoid discomfort and possible involuntary movements dangerous for the valve deployment. Depending on patient condition, valuable options are midazolam (bolus 1–5 mg) or propofol (bolus 0.5–1 mg/kg). Sometimes remifentanil may be added for a light analgesia (0.02–0.1 mcg/kg/min).

For the transapical approach, general anesthesia is mandatory. In this case, we recommend to perform a serratus anterior block before the surgical incision in order to spare opioids during surgery and to ensure adequate postoperative analgesia that allows a fast recovery and an early discharge from hospital. In this case, long active local anesthetic must spread between the latissimus dorsi and serratus anterior muscles or underneath the serratus anterior muscle (e.g., Ropivacaine 0.25–0.375% 30–40 mL).

16.4.3 Postoperative Care and Analgesia

16.4.3.1 Post-Procedural Monitoring

After the procedure, patients were transferred to the ICU for close monitoring. A fast-track protocol is implemented to facilitate early extubation of mechanically ventilated patients and gradual weaning from vasoactive medications. Postoperative pain management includes paracetamol at a dose of 1 g every 6 h to effectively control pain and minimize opioid usage. Most patients who undergo regional anesthesia typically do not require additional pain medication. Antiplatelet therapy is restarted promptly once the bleeding risk is assessed to be minimal.

Patients are transferred from the ICU or recovery room to an intermediate care unit when the following conditions are met: oxygen saturation (SpO_2) is 94% or higher on a face mask with FIO2 of 0.5 or less, stable cardiac status without significant arrhythmias, urine output exceeding 0.5 mL/kg/h, no need for intravenous inotropes or vasopressors, and absence of seizures. Early mobilization in the intermediate care unit is encouraged within 6–24 h post-procedure, depending on the patient's clinical status. The recommended length of stay after the implant is 3–4 days. Common postoperative complications include arrhythmias, renal function impairment, and access-site complications, warranting daily ECG monitoring, blood tests, and physical exams. Prior to discharge, chest X-rays and transthoracic echocardiography (TTE) are required. Early removal of the bladder and central venous catheters is advised to reduce the risk of hospital-acquired infections and shorten hospitalization.

Discharge criteria are designed to ensure patient safety and readiness for home care, requiring hemodynamic stability, normal cardiac rhythm, a clean and dry surgical site, absence of fever, normal bowel function, and the ability to walk and self-feed independently.

16.5 FAST-TRACK Protocol in Patients Undergoing TAVI

Although many fast-track protocols have been proposed and studied [42, 43], here we want to report our standard of care employed in daily practice. This structured perioperative care protocol aimed to optimize recovery, reduce hospital stay length, and minimize the risk of postoperative complications, thereby promoting a smoother transition from hospital to home (Fig. 16.6).

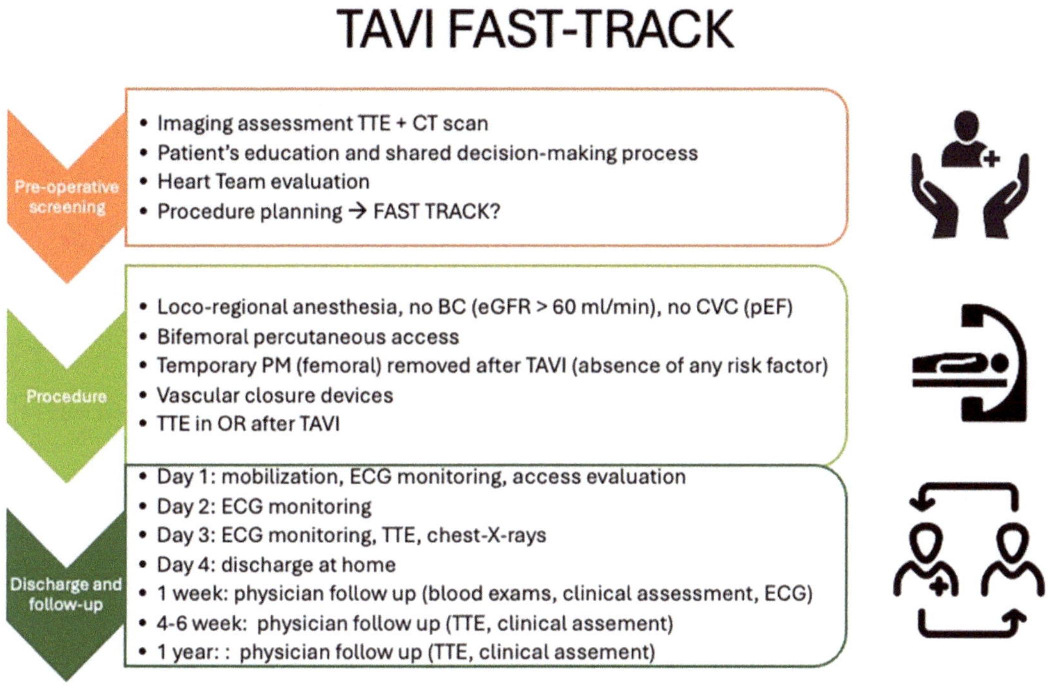

Fig. 16.6 Fast-track TAVI. Main issues of fast-track protocol in patients undergoing TAVI. *TTE* transthoracic echocardiogram, *CT* computerized tomography, *BC* bladder catheter, *eGFR* estimated glomerular filtration rate, *CVC* central venous catheter, *pEF* preserved ejection fraction, PM pacemaker, *TAVI* transcatheter aortic valve implant, *OR* operating room

16.5.1 Procedure Planning

Patient selection occurs out-hospital through imaging screening and risk assessment evaluation.

- CT scan should be performed early to prevent damage from liquid of contrast.
- Patient-centered approach with shear decision-making process is crucial.
- Heart team evaluation aim to establish early if a patient is eligible for fast-track protocol.

16.5.2 Index Hospitalization

- At day 0, patient is admitted to hospital and procedure is performed. Fast-track or setting is depicted in Fig. 16.7.
- Neither BC nor CVC are employed unless eGFR is <60 mL/min or left ventricular ejection fraction is EF >50%.
- Local-regional anesthesia is preferable.
- If feasible, transfemoral percutaneous access is preferable, secondary access on the opposite femoral side.
- Temporary PM is led through femoral venous access and removed at the end of the procedure in patients without any preoperative risk factors (presence of I grade AV block, RBBB, bicuspid aortic valve, calcium in the LVOT) or any adverse event occurred during the implant.
- Percutaneous vascular closure devices are mandatory both for the main and the secondary access.
- TTE in OR or cath-lab is necessary to exclude adverse events and evaluate procedure success.

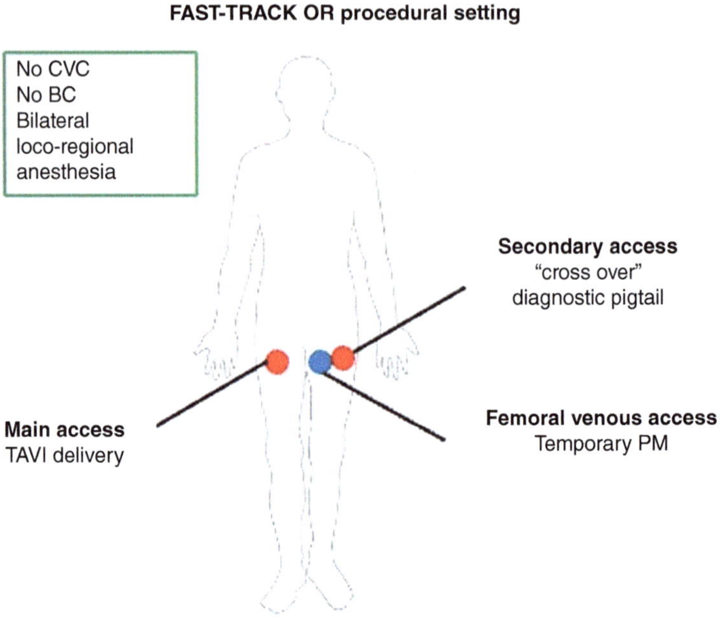

Fig. 16.7 Procedural setting in the operating room

- After short period monitoring (1–2 h) in ICU or dedicated recovery room, patient is transferred to intermediate care unit.
- At day 1, early mobilization is recommended and ECG monitoring and blood test (renal function, hemoglobin level, cardiac enzymes) as well.
- Patients underwent to valve in valve procedure or with a pre-procedural permanent PM could be discharge at home at day one.
- At day 3–4, discharge at home is feasible after TTE and chest X-rays. ECG must remain stable after the implant.

16.5.3 Follow-Up

- At 1 week, a visit with general practitioner or referral physician is scheduled to assess blood test, ECG, and access.
- At 4–6 weeks, patient undergoes TTE and cardiologist evaluation.
- Yearly follow-up.

16.6 Conclusion

In the treatment of AVD TAVI is nowadays of paramount importance. The number of procedures, technological development, and operators' expertise are growing consistently. Although considered minimally invasive and with lower risk compared to surgical approach, TAVI procedure requires careful patient selection and adequate in-hospital management. Safe and effective fast-track protocols are desirable and aim to improve TAVI outcomes, reducing in-hospital length of stay and adverse events.

References

1. Iung B, Delgado V, Rosenhek R, et al. Contemporary presentation and management of valvular heart disease: the EURObservational research Programme Valvular Heart Disease II Survey. Circulation. 2019;140(14):1156–69. https://doi.org/10.1161/CIRCULATIONAHA.119.041080.

2. Arora S, Misenheimer JA, Ramaraj R. Transcatheter aortic valve replacement: comprehensive review and present status. Tex Heart Inst J. 2017;44(1):29–38. https://doi.org/10.14503/THIJ-16-5852.
3. Reardon MJ, Van Mieghem NM, Popma JJ, et al. Surgical or transcatheter aortic-valve replacement in intermediate-risk patients. N Engl J Med. 2017;376(14):1321–31. https://doi.org/10.1056/NEJMoa1700456.
4. Leon MB, Smith CR, Mack MJ, et al. Transcatheter or surgical aortic-valve replacement in intermediate-risk patients. N Engl J Med. 2016;374(17):1609–20. https://doi.org/10.1056/NEJMoa1514616.
5. Deeb GM, Reardon MJ, Chetcuti S, et al. 3-Year outcomes in high-risk patients who underwent surgical or transcatheter aortic valve replacement. J Am Coll Cardiol. 2016;67(22):2565–74. https://doi.org/10.1016/j.jacc.2016.03.506.
6. Smith CR, Leon MB, Mack MJ, et al. Transcatheter versus surgical aortic-valve replacement in high-risk patients. N Engl J Med. 2011;364(23):2187–98. https://doi.org/10.1056/NEJMoa1103510.
7. Mack MJ, Leon MB, Thourani VH, et al. Transcatheter aortic-valve replacement with a balloon-expandable valve in low-risk patients. N Engl J Med. 2019;380(18):1695–705. https://doi.org/10.1056/NEJMoa1814052.
8. Thourani VH, Kodali S, Makkar RR, et al. Transcatheter aortic valve replacement versus surgical valve replacement in intermediate-risk patients: a propensity score analysis. Lancet. 2016;387(10034):2218–25. https://doi.org/10.1016/S0140-6736(16)30073-3.
9. Makkar RR, Thourani VH, Mack MJ, et al. Five-year outcomes of transcatheter or surgical aortic-valve replacement. N Engl J Med. 2020;382(9):799–809. https://doi.org/10.1056/NEJMoa1910555.
10. Popma JJ, Deeb GM, Yakubov SJ, et al. Transcatheter aortic-valve replacement with a self-expanding valve in low-risk patients. N Engl J Med. 2019;380(18):1706–15. https://doi.org/10.1056/NEJMoa1816885.
11. Ljungqvist O, Scott M, Fearon KC. Enhanced recovery after surgery: a review. JAMA Surg. 2017;152(3):292. https://doi.org/10.1001/jamasurg.2016.4952.
12. Carroll JD, Mack MJ, Vemulapalli S, et al. STS-ACC TVT registry of transcatheter aortic valve replacement. J Am Coll Cardiol. 2020;76(21):2492–516. https://doi.org/10.1016/j.jacc.2020.09.595.
13. Otto CM, Nishimura RA, Bonow RO, et al. 2020 ACC/AHA guideline for the management of patients with valvular heart disease: a report of the American College of Cardiology/American Heart Association joint committee on clinical practice guidelines. Circulation. 2021;143(5):923. https://doi.org/10.1161/CIR.0000000000000923.
14. Vahanian A, Beyersdorf F, Praz F, et al. 2021 ESC/EACTS guidelines for the management of valvular heart disease. Eur Heart J. 2022;43(7):561–632. https://doi.org/10.1093/eurheartj/ehab395.
15. Tarantini G, Nai FL. Lifetime strategy of patients with aortic stenosis. JACC Cardiovasc Interv. 2021;14(15):1727–30. https://doi.org/10.1016/j.jcin.2021.06.029.
16. Dvir D, Khan J, Kornowski R, et al. Novel strategies in aortic valve-in-valve therapy including bioprosthetic valve fracture and BASILICA. EuroIntervention. 2018;14(AB):AB74–82. https://doi.org/10.4244/EIJ-D-18-00667.
17. Bruce CG, Greenbaum AB, Babaliaros VC, Rogers T, Lederman RJ, Khan JM. Safeguards and pitfalls for bioprosthetic or native aortic scallop intentional laceration to prevent iatrogenic coronary artery obstruction during transcatheter aortic valve replacement—the BASILICA technique. Ann Cardiothorac Surg. 2021;10(5):700–7. https://doi.org/10.21037/acs-2021-tviv-26.
18. Chan KYE, Tai-Leung Chan D, Lam CCS, et al. First-in-human undermining iatrogenic coronary obstruction with radiofrequency needle (UNICORN) procedure during valve-in-valve transcatheter aortic valve replacement. Circ Cardiovasc Interv. 2022;15(11):928–31. https://doi.org/10.1161/CIRCINTERVENTIONS.122.012399.
19. Azzola Guicciardi N, Buzzatti N, Saccocci M, Maisano F. Simplified balloon-BASILICA: a different perspective. Catheter Cardiovasc Interv. 2024;104:419. https://doi.org/10.1002/ccd.31121.
20. Hirji SA, Percy ED, McGurk S, et al. Incidence, characteristics, predictors, and outcomes of surgical explantation after transcatheter aortic valve replacement. J Am Coll Cardiol. 2020;76(16):1848–59. https://doi.org/10.1016/j.jacc.2020.08.048.
21. Vahl TP, Thourani VH, Makkar RR, et al. Transcatheter aortic valve implantation in patients with high-risk symptomatic native aortic regurgitation (ALIGN-AR): a prospective, multicentre, single-arm study. Lancet. 2024;403(10435):1451–9. https://doi.org/10.1016/S0140-6736(23)02806-4.
22. Marin-Cuartas M, De Waha S, Naumann S, et al. Incidence and outcomes of emergency intraprocedural surgical conversion during transcatheter aortic valve implantation: insights from a large tertiary care centre. Eur J Cardiothorac Surg. 2023;63(6):ezad142. https://doi.org/10.1093/ejcts/ezad142.
23. Blanke P, Weir-McCall JR, Achenbach S, et al. Computed tomography imaging in the context of transcatheter aortic valve implantation (TAVI)/transcatheter aortic valve replacement (TAVR). JACC Cardiovasc Imaging. 2019;12(1):1–24. https://doi.org/10.1016/j.jcmg.2018.12.003.

24. Litmanovich DE, Ghersin E, Burke DA, Popma J, Shahrzad M, Bankier AA. Imaging in transcatheter aortic valve replacement (TAVR): role of the radiologist. Insights Imaging. 2014;5(1):123–45. https://doi.org/10.1007/s13244-013-0301-5.
25. Blanke P, Schoepf UJ, Leipsic JA. CT in transcatheter aortic valve replacement. Radiology. 2013;269(3):650–69. https://doi.org/10.1148/radiol.13120696.
26. Saito T, Yoshijima N, Hase H, et al. Impact of beta blockers on patients undergoing transcatheter aortic valve replacement: the OCEAN-TAVI registry. Open Heart. 2020;7(2):e001269. https://doi.org/10.1136/openhrt-2020-001269.
27. Ten Berg J, Sibbing D, Rocca B, et al. Management of antithrombotic therapy in patients undergoing transcatheter aortic valve implantation: a consensus document of the ESC working group on thrombosis and the European Association of Percutaneous Cardiovascular Interventions (EAPCI), in collaboration with the ESC Council on Valvular Heart Disease. Eur Heart J. 2021;42(23):2265–9. https://doi.org/10.1093/eurheartj/ehab196.
28. Nakamura M, Chakravarty T, Jilaihawi H, et al. Complete percutaneous approach for arterial access in transfemoral transcatheter aortic valve replacement: a comparison with surgical cut-down and closure. Catheter Cardiovasc Interv. 2014;84(2):293–300. https://doi.org/10.1002/ccd.25130.
29. Das TM, Shin J, Czarny MJ, Nanavati J, Resar JR, Hasan RK. Radial versus femoral secondary access for transcatheter aortic valve replacement: a systematic review and meta-analysis. Catheter Cardiovasc Interv. 2022;99(4):1225–33. https://doi.org/10.1002/ccd.30009.
30. Junquera L, Urena M, Latib A, et al. Comparison of transfemoral versus transradial secondary access in transcatheter aortic valve replacement. Circ Cardiovasc Interv. 2020;13(3):e008609. https://doi.org/10.1161/CIRCINTERVENTIONS.119.008609.
31. Toggweiler S, Gurvitch R, Leipsic J, et al. Percutaneous aortic valve replacement. J Am Coll Cardiol. 2012;59(2):113–8. https://doi.org/10.1016/j.jacc.2011.08.069.
32. Schofer N, Deuschl F, Conradi L, et al. Preferential short cut or alternative route: the transaxillary access for transcatheter aortic valve implantation. J Thorac Dis. 2015;7(9):1543–7. https://doi.org/10.3978/j.issn.2072-1439.2015.07.27.
33. Petronio AS, De Carlo M, Bedogni F, et al. 2-year results of CoreValve implantation through the subclavian access. J Am Coll Cardiol. 2012;60(6):502–7. https://doi.org/10.1016/j.jacc.2012.04.014.
34. Useini D, Beluli B, Christ H, et al. Transapical transcatheter aortic valve implantation in patients with aortic diseases. Eur J Cardiothorac Surg. 2021;59(6):1174–81. https://doi.org/10.1093/ejcts/ezab050.
35. Walther T, Dewey T, Borger MA, et al. Transapical aortic valve implantation: step by step. Ann Thorac Surg. 2009;87(1):276–83. https://doi.org/10.1016/j.athoracsur.2008.08.017.
36. Fanning JP, Walters DL, Platts DG, Eeles E, Bellapart J, Fraser JF. Characterization of neurological injury in transcatheter aortic valve implantation: how clear is the picture? Circulation. 2014;129(4):504–15. https://doi.org/10.1161/CIRCULATIONAHA.113.004103.
37. Everett EA, Everett W, Brier MR, White P. Appraisal of health states worse than death in patients with acute stroke. Neurol Clin Pract. 2021;11(1):43–8. https://doi.org/10.1212/CPJ.0000000000000856.
38. Kapadia SR, Makkar R, Leon M, et al. Cerebral embolic protection during transcatheter aortic-valve replacement. N Engl J Med. 2022;387(14):1253–63. https://doi.org/10.1056/NEJMoa2204961.
39. Williams JB, McConnell G, Allender JE, et al. One-year results from the first US-based enhanced recovery after cardiac surgery (ERAS Cardiac) program. J Thorac Cardiovasc Surg. 2019;157(5):1881–8. https://doi.org/10.1016/j.jtcvs.2018.10.164.
40. Engelman DT, Ben Ali W, Williams JB, et al. Guidelines for perioperative care in cardiac surgery: enhanced recovery after surgery society recommendations. JAMA Surg. 2019;154(8):755. https://doi.org/10.1001/jamasurg.2019.1153.
41. Chen S, Dizon JM, Hahn RT, et al. Predictors and 5-year clinical outcomes of pacemaker after TAVR. JACC Cardiovasc Interv. 2024;17(11):1325–36. https://doi.org/10.1016/j.jcin.2024.03.034.
42. Barbanti M, Van Mourik MS, Spence MS, et al. Optimising patient discharge management after transfemoral transcatheter aortic valve implantation: the multicentre European FAST-TAVI trial. EuroIntervention. 2019;15(2):147–54. https://doi.org/10.4244/EIJ-D-18-01197.
43. Chopra M, Luk NHV, De Backer O, Søndergaard L. Simplification and optimization of transcatheter aortic valve implantation—fast-track course without compromising safety and efficacy. BMC Cardiovasc Disord. 2018;18(1):231. https://doi.org/10.1186/s12872-018-0976-0.
44. Ludwig S, Goßling A, Waldschmidt L, Linder M, Bhadra OD, Voigtländer L, Schäfer A, Deuschl F, Schirmer J, Reichenspurner H, Blankenberg S, Schäfer U, Westermann D, Seiffert M, Conradi L, Schofer N. TAVR for low-flow, low-gradient aortic stenosis: prognostic impact of aortic valve calcification. Am Heart J. 2020;225:138–48. https://doi.org/10.1016/j.ahj.2020.03.013. Epub 2020 Apr 8. PMID: 32502877.

17 ERAS in Robotic Cardiac Surgery

Matteo Parrinello, Giovanni Albano, and Alfonso Agnino

17.1 Introduction

Since the first robotic totally endoscopic CABG (TECAB) by Loulmet and colleagues in 1998, the safety and efficacy of robotic cardiac surgery have long been proven.

Robotic minimally invasive cardiac surgery (MICS) has the potential to boost patient outcomes further when combined with Enhanced Recovery After Surgery (ERAS): robotic arms allow otherwise impossible angles of approach to organs and tissues, require even smaller incision ports compared to conventional laparoscopic/thoracoscopic surgery, and enhance field clarity and surgical tool maneuverability for their operators.

Robotic cardiac surgery case numbers in Europe are growing fast, including a large spectrum of procedures. Conversion rates are low, and clinical outcomes are favorable, showing a safe conduct of these high-tech minimally invasive procedures [1, 2].

Robotic cardiac surgery, together with other MICS in general, can be expected to set a new benchmark and compete with the results of transcatheter mitral valve (MV) procedures [2]. Intermediate and long-term results of robotic mitral valve reapair (MVR) demonstrate at least equal efficacy and durability compared with their non-robotic MICS counterparts [3].

Robotic approaches are limited to a restricted group among all cardiac surgery patients. The typical candidate is younger and fitter than average, presents electively for surgery, and is at his first thoracic procedure. Therefore, although not being completely representative of the cardiac surgery patient population, candidates to robotic procedures present key features that make them ideal for ERAS protocols.

The benefits of robotic cardiac surgery include reduced need for transfusions, shorter intensive care unit (ICU) and hospital length of stay, lower incidence of atrial fibrillation, acute kidney injury, stroke, permanent pacemaker (PM) implantation, shorter mechanical ventilation hours, lower readmission rates, lower conversion to open MVR, improved postoperative quality of life, and faster return to work. These may justify the higher procedural costs and even make it overall more cost-effective [1, 2, 4].

Furthermore, implementing ERAS protocols in MICS was associated with saving up to 2000€/patient compared to traditional approaches. This can be crucial in healthcare systems with ever-increasing expenditures and a fast-growing number of surgical candidates.

M. Parrinello (✉) · G. Albano
Anesthesiology Department, Humanitas Gavazzeni, Bergamo, Italy
e-mail: matteo.parrinello@gavazzeni.it; giovanni.albano@gavazzeni.it

A. Agnino
Heart-Surgery Department, Humanitas Gavazzeni, Bergamo, Italy
e-mail: alfonso.agnino@gavazzeni.it

G. Sepolvere, S. Silvetti (eds.), *Fast-Track in Cardiac Anesthesia*,
https://doi.org/10.1007/978-3-031-70899-2_17

17.2 Surgical Considerations

17.2.1 Preoperative Diagnostic Workup

In robotic cardiac surgery, preoperative evaluation plays a key role in the success of the procedure, which needs to be individualized on each patient.

Radiological imaging including chest X-ray, computed tomography (CT), and magnetic resonance imaging (MRI) is commonly performed to delineate cardiac anatomy and its relationships with surrounding thoracic structures.

This is of utmost importance to guide thoracic port positioning (Fig. 17.1) and avoid competition between the instruments and the anatomical structures during surgery.

In robotic coronary surgery, preoperative CT or CT-ANGIO scans are also crucial to gather information on the size, position, and quality of the left internal mammary artery (LIMA) and left anterior descending artery (LAD). Indeed, the degree and site of coronary calcifications as well as the potential intramyocardial course of LAD should be assessed.

For robotic epicardial atrial fibrillation (AF) ablation, MRI provides 3D anatomical reconstruction of left atrium (LA), pulmonary vein (PV), and left atrial appendage (LAA) while also evaluating LA fibrosis via assessment of late enhancement [5].

Last, in robotic mitral valve repair (MVRCT), angio scan is extended to iliac/femoral vessels, to evaluate their status and size in the event of peripheral cannulation for cardiopulmonary bypass (CPB).

Preoperative assessment is completed with transthoracic (TTE) or transesophageal echocardiography (TEE) as routine clinical practice, along with electrocardiography (ECG), and routine biochemical exams. Coronary angiography is routinely performed on patients undergoing robotic MVR, but it is not mandatory prior to robotic AF ablation, provided that the patient has no risk factors for ischemic heart disease (IHD).

17.2.2 Surgical Technique

17.2.2.1 Robotic Epicardial Atrial Fibrillation Ablation (REAFA)

To perform REAFA, the patient is positioned supine, with a square pad located behind the left scapula to moderately bump up the left hemithorax.

The surgeon marks the third, fifth, sixth, seventh, and eighth left intercostal spaces to guide port positioning. After left-lung deflation, the ports are placed in the intercostal spaces.

In this phase, TEE is routinely repeated to confirm the absence of LAA thrombosis.

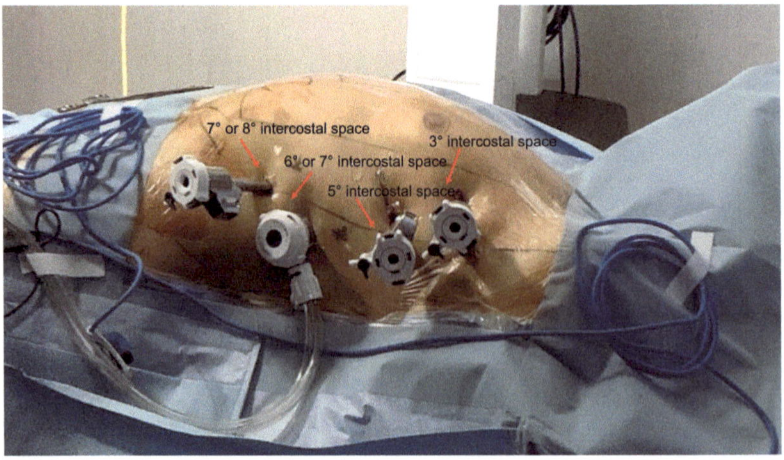

Fig. 17.1 Port positioning for AF ablation. The red arrows indicate alternative positions for the third port depending on the patient's anatomy

Carbon dioxide (CO_2) insufflation is started with a target intrathoracic pressure of 8–10 mmHg. The robot platform is placed at the patient's right side, and robotic arms are anchored to the designated working ports. A 30° endoscopic camera (Intuitive) is inserted to navigate the thorax, pericardium, and heart structures with enhanced views (10× magnification).

An S-shaped esophageal temperature probe (S-Cath Esophageal Temperature Probe, Circa Scientific) (Fig. 17.2a, b), equipped with a series of 12 sensors and its proprietary CIRCA monitoring system, is inserted into the esophagus to monitor temperature during ablation and avoid thermal damage, with a threshold set at 37.2 °C [5].

The surgeon identifies and carefully opens the pericardium under the phrenic nerve. The left atrial appendage (LAA) is identified and gently moved to visualize and subsequently dissect Marshall's ligament.

Unipolar, suction-assisted, radiofrequency (RF) ablation is executed using a 3 cm, self-irrigated, EPi-Sense Coagulation Device (AtriCure Inc., Mason, OH, USA; Fig. 17.2c). This device integrates RF energy, direct visualization, and impedance monitoring to deliver continuous RF coagulation of cardiac tissue.

The probe is introduced into the pericardial space; RF energy is delivered at a preset level of 30 W for 90 seconds, to engrave transmural coagulative lesions, while a vacuum seal ensures stable contact between the EPi-sense lead and LA walls. The system exploits continuous saline irrigation to prevent overheating of the probe.

The EPi-sense probe is also equipped with sensing electrodes, and it is connected to the CardioTek recording system. LA electrograms are monitored in real time by an electrophysiologist.

The first coagulation line is impressed on the LA roof, between left and right superior pulmonary veins. The desired outcome is a steady and continuous drop of impedance. If local atrial electrograms persist, or if the impedance drop does not reach the desired level (<10 Ohm), a second ablation is performed.

The surgeon then impresses a second ablation line connecting the superior and inferior left pulmonary veins. He then lifts the LA and, after identifying superior vena cava, burns a third line on the LA floor. The ablation proceeds medially at the opening of the right pulmonary veins and on the entire LA posterior wall.

Finally, the surgeon completes the ablation with two coagulation lines at the base of the LAA and between the base and the apex of the LAA (Figs. 17.3 and 17.4).

The procedure ends with LAA closure by means of an epicardial clip (AtriClip Device, AtriCure Inc., Mason, OH, USA; Fig. 17.2d), which prevents LAA thrombosis and cerebral embolization. The anesthesiologist provides real-time TEE guidance for LAA clip positioning and confirms the correct closure of LAA.

17.2.2.2 Robotic Assisted Minimally Invasive Coronary Artery Bypass Graft (RA-MICABG)

Patient positioning is the same as for robotic AF ablation. The second, fourth, and seventh left intercostal spaces are then marked for port positioning. Based on preoperative radiological studies, the surgeon also marks the fourth/fifth intercostal space for mini-thoracotomy.

Left capnothorax is then achieved with a mean CO_2 pressure of 4–10 mmHg, to collapse the left lung and displace the heart to the right to gain maneuvering space. The patient's anatomy dictates the ideal CO_2 pressure, as a small heart-to-thorax size ratio requires lower CO_2 pressures for the creation of a comparable working space.

The endoscopic camera takes the 8 mm port in the fourth intercostal space. Robotic instruments enter via the second and third ports, located in the second and seventh intercostal spaces, respectively (Fig. 17.5). When LIMA harvesting is completed, we either use the incision in the seventh intercostal space, or a distinct subxiphoid access, to place the arm of the coronary stabilizer (Octopus Nuvo Tissue Stabilizer, Medtronic, Minneapolis, MN, USA).

CO_2 insufflation is continued through the third port with a target intrathoracic pressure of 6–10 mmHg. The Da Vinci X robot system (Intuitive Surgical, Inc., Sunnyvale, CA, USA) is

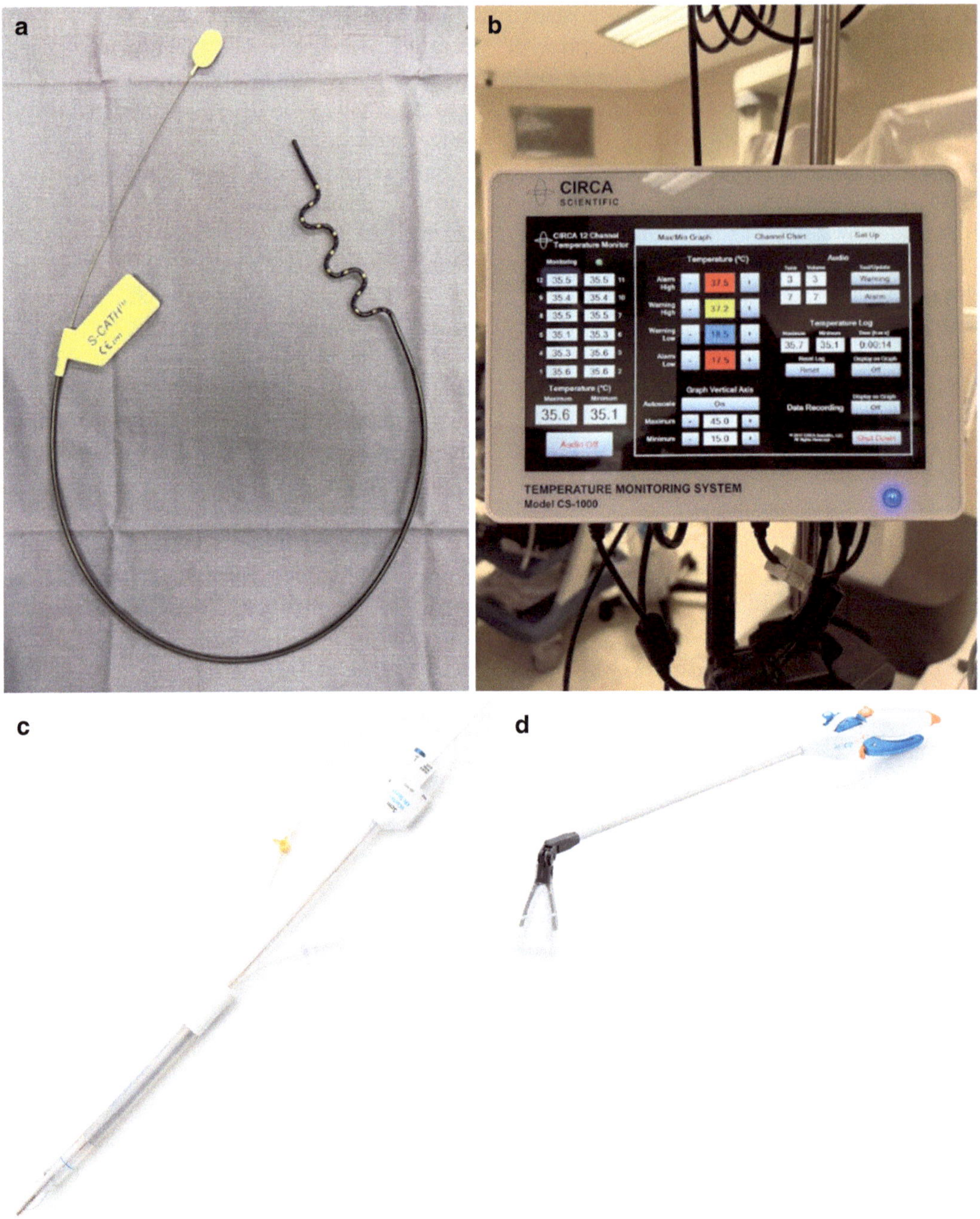

Fig. 17.2 (**a**): S-Cath Esophageal Temperature Probe (CIRCA Scientific, Englewood, CO, USA). The 10-F, 65 cm probe deploys an array of 12 fully insulated, fast-response temperature sensors on a uniquely designed soft, flexible, "S" shape providing edge-to-edge coverage. A soft-tipped, rigid metallic guidewire straightens the catheter during deployment and is then retrieved to let the probe recover its operational shape. Combined with the proprietary CIRCA monitoring system (**b**), it provides a 20 Hz refresh rate and detects esophageal temperature changes. (**c**) EPi-Sense Coagulation Device and (**d**) AtriClip Device (both by AtriCure Inc., Mason, OH, USA)

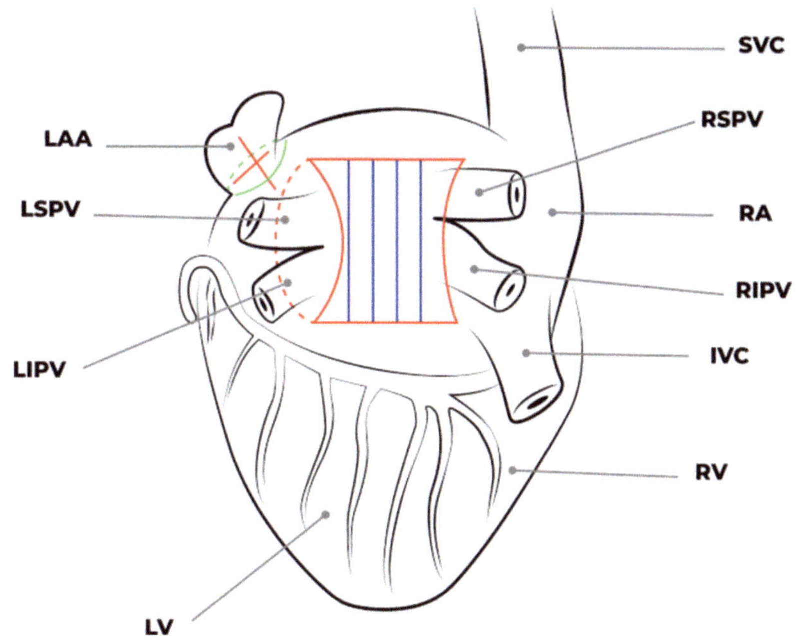

Fig. 17.3 Ablation line scheme

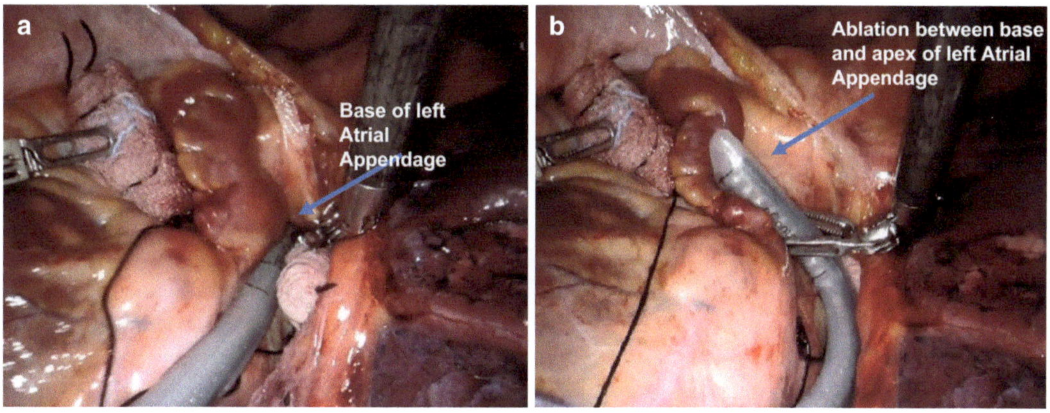

Fig. 17.4 Ablation line at the base of the left atrial appendage and between the base and apex of the LAA

placed at the patient's right side, and robotic arms are anchored to the designated working ports.

The surgeon carefully opens the pericardium above the phrenic nerve; pericardial fat is removed if necessary. The pericardium is opened a second time under the phrenic nerve; in case of bleeding or pericardial effusion, this hole will drain fluids into the left pleura.

The LAD and the possible site for LIMA-LAD anastomosis are identified, and a clip is placed nearby as reference point.

The LIMA graft is harvested using a low-energy monopolar electrocautery spatula and high-energy bipolar cautery forceps via skeletonized technique: bipolar cautery forceps are used to seal and divide small collateral branches, while metal clips are used for larger branches.

When the harvest is completed, LIMA is heparinized, then clamped distally with a bulldog, and cut free, while the thoracic stump is sealed with metal clips.

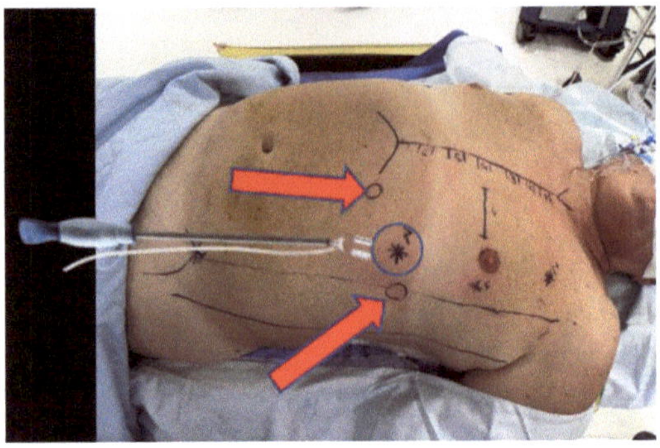

Fig. 17.5 Port positioning for RA-MICABG. Red arrows indicate alternative port positioning for the third port according to the patient's anatomy

The appropriate intercostal space is determined based on the LAD site identified previously, and a mini-thoracotomy (4–5 cm) is generally performed at the fourth/fifth intercostal space.

A vacuum, flexible Octopus Nuvo Tissue Stabilizer (Medtronic, Minneapolis, MN, USA) is placed at the site of anastomosis.

The off-pump LIMA-LAD anastomosis is performed under direct vision with the surgeon's standard technique. Finally, intraoperative graft quality control is performed using a Transit Time Flowmeter (Mira-Q, Medistim, Oslo, Norway) that provides accurate estimations of graft hemodynamics by the pulsatility index, diastolic filling (%), and mean flow.

17.2.2.3 Robotic Assisted Mitral Valve Surgery (RA-MVS)

Pre- and intraoperative TEE is routinely performed to study mitral valve morphology and determine the mechanisms underlying MV pathology.

The patient is positioned supine with a square pad behind the right scapula, to moderately bump up the right hemithorax.

According to pre-procedural radiological planning, a working port (assisting port) of 1.5–2 cm is created at the third/fourth right intercostal space anterior to the midaxillary line; four 8 mm instrument ports are created, respectively, at the third/fourth intercostal (camera arm), second intercostal midclavicular line (left arm), fourth intercostal (dynamic left atrial retractor), and sixth intercostal (right arm). Care is taken to prevent instrument conflict (Fig. 17.6).

Surgeons cannulate both the femoral artery and vein peripherally for cardiopulmonary bypass (CPB), using Seldinger technique, and advance the guidewires and cannulas under continuous TEE surveillance. An additional superior vena cava drainage cannula is placed percutaneously by the anesthesiologist via the right internal jugular vein (RIJV).

The robotic platform is placed at the patient's left side, and robotic arms are anchored to the designated working ports.

When ready, CPB is started according to institutional standards. The pericardium is opened above the phrenic nerve, and heart structures are exposed. A dedicated cannula is introduced in the ascending aorta through the working port, serving both to deliver cold crystalloid HTK (histidine–tryptophan–ketoglutarate) cardioplegia, and as an aortic vent for de-airing once the procedure has been completed.

The aorta is cross-clamped using either a transthoracic Chitwood clamp or alternatively an endoaortic balloon, according to the patient's anatomical characteristics. The left atrium is opened along Sondergaard's groove, and a dynamic LA retractor is employed to obtain adaptive exposure of the mitral leaflet and annulus portions throughout the procedure.

Mitral repair or replacement is performed using surgeon's standard technique. After suture of the left atriotomy, particular care is given to de-airing before weaning from CPB and robotic arm removal from the patient.

17.3 Anesthetic Considerations in Robotic Cardiac Surgery

Integrating ERAS with robotic MICS means adopting ERAS evidence-based core principles, which in 2018 guidelines consisted of 22 recommendations, in a fast-growing field that includes by definition the newest technologies and the most refined surgical techniques. The resulting approach embraces preoperative, intraoperative,

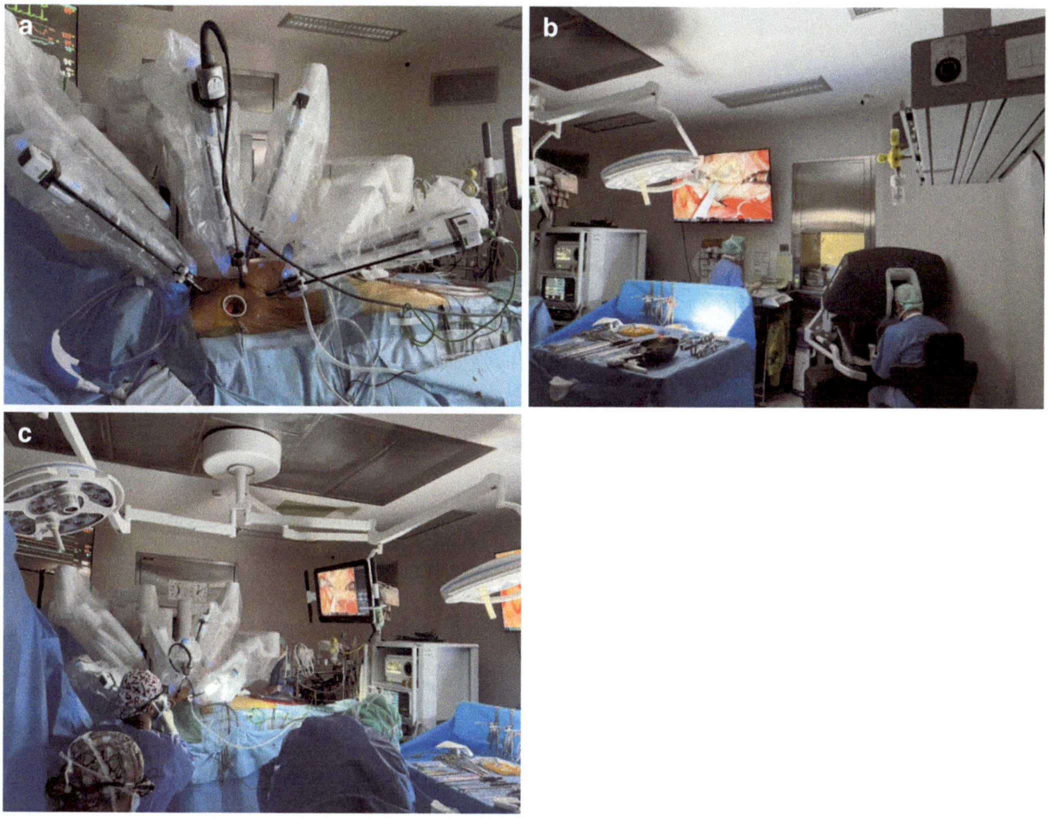

Fig. 17.6 OR layout during RA-MVS with Da Vinci X robot system (Intuitive Surgical, Inc., Sunnyvale, CA, USA). (**a**) Port positioning for RA-MVS. (**b**) Robotic console placed at the patient's right outside the sterile field. (**c**) OR display

and postoperative care and can be summarized as follows.

17.3.1 Preoperative Evaluation

- Appropriate patient selection for RA-MICS is essential in reducing the risk of perioperative complications, and formulation of a preliminary plan for immediate postoperative care is mandatory. Studies have demonstrated that TECAB grafting is beneficial in morbidly obese patients who have a greater risk of deep sternal wound infection [6].
- Cardiac prehabilitation includes several initiatives such as aerobic exercise, respiratory muscle training, smoking cessation, decreasing alcohol consumption, improving sleep patterns, weight control, and optimization of medical comorbidities [7].
- Preoperative physiotherapeutic exercises decrease sympathetic overreactivity and improve insulin sensitivity.
- Anemia is a recognized risk factor of surgical mortality. Preoperative use of iron has been shown to reduce postoperative anemia and the need for red blood cells.
- Robot techniques require one-lung ventilation (OLV) and carbon dioxide insufflation. Patients with chronic obstructive pulmonary disease (COPD), restrictive or infiltrative diseases of the lung, or pulmonary hypertension should be considered for additional pulmonary testing.
- Optimizing perioperative nutrition can improve a wide range of patient outcomes.

Supplemental nutritional support is recommended for the last 2 weeks before the scheduled surgery by means of a high-energy high-carbohydrate diet.
- Minimize fasting.
- Preoperative oral carbohydrate loading of 25–50 g reduces insulin resistance and perioperative hyperglycemia. In the absence of clinical trials on this topic, institutions are likely to assess the individual risk/benefit profile [7].
- Cardiac ERAS programs should strive to achieve optimal preoperative glycemic control, defined as hemoglobin A1C levels <6.5, because this has been associated with a decrease in deep sternal wound infection and ischemic events and improved long-term survival [8].

17.3.2 Intraoperative Management

17.3.2.1 Airway Management

During robotic procedures, OLV is recommended. This can be achieved through a double-lumen endotracheal tube (DLET) or with a standard single-lumen endotracheal tube (SLET) along with a bronchial blocker (BB).

It was thought that placing a double-lumen tube, despite the better collapse of the non-ventilated lung, was more insidious because it required a tube exchange to a single-lumen tube if the patient was not a candidate for extubation at the end of the procedure [6].

However, in common practice, this is almost never necessary for two reasons. First, nearly every patient is extubated in the operating room at the conclusion of surgery, a process that is aided tremendously by the use of regional anesthesia with minimization of systemic opioid administration. Second, the duration of mechanical ventilation in the ICU following robotic cardiac surgery is seldom more than an hour or two, and the availability of smaller suction catheters eases pulmonary toilet [8].

With most patients getting extubated shortly after the procedures and with increased familiarity of the ICU staff with DLET, the need to exchange the tube at the end of the surgical procedure, for the most part, has been eliminated [9].

The DLET provides several advantages. It has a lower probability of moving after positioning and allows the application of continuous positive airway pressure and suction to the deflated lung.

The anatomic variability of the right upper lobe may complicate bronchial blocker positioning on the right and render these procedure unfeasible; moreover, the difficult positioning and easy displacement of bronchial blocker during surgery are key reasons to use a double-lumen tube for robotic surgery.

Near-supine positioning results in unfavorable areas of ventilation versus perfusion when one-lung ventilation begins. If the patient cannot tolerate one-lung ventilation, intermittent apnea in coordination with the surgeon and ultimately initiating CPB may be required.

17.3.2.2 Capnothorax

The insufflation of CO_2 into the right chest is commonly performed following deflation of the right lung. Insufflation of CO_2 into the chest reduces the amount of intracardiac air present at the conclusion of CPB and diminishes the likelihood of a surgical site fire. Hemodynamic compromise resulting from a tension capnothorax is possible though really rare.

If pressure in the right hemithorax does not exceed 10 mmHg and rates of insufflation are held below 2–3 L/min, the risk of a tension capnothorax is reduced [6].

17.3.2.3 Aortic Clamping

Transthoracic aortic cross-clamping and endoaortic balloon occlusion through an endoclamp aortic catheter are the two main strategies used for aortic clamping and myocardial protection. Both have proven their efficacy. The endoaortic balloon avoids using the additional incision required for the external clamp and aortic manipulation for root cannula insertion and provides a less crowded surgical field. However, its positioning requires specific training. It is specifically indicated in redo procedures and in all cases in which pleural adhesions are suspected.

The balloon occluder also has a central lumen through which antegrade cardioplegia may be delivered into the aortic root. The delivery of antegrade cardioplegia in this way is dependent on a competent aortic valve. In the event the patient has more than trivial aortic insufficiency, protection of the heart is heavily dependent on the retrograde cardioplegia given through a catheter placed by the anesthesiologist in the coronary sinus passing through a right internal jugular vein (RIJV) sheath. The anesthesiologist then controls the correct catheter positioning with TEE.

17.3.2.4 TEE

Proficiency and confidence with TEE imaging by the anesthesiologist are essential for success.

TEE is used to confirm surgical indication, for cannulation, and to monitor for complications, including but not limited to balloon occluder migration, aortic dissection, pericardial tamponade, and potentially liver laceration.

The need for real-time guidance during placement of guidewires and cannulae represents a unique role for TEE during robotic cardiac surgery.

The addition of color Doppler can verify the flow of cardioplegia into the coronary sinus during CPB and correct positioning of the aortic clamp. The delivery of antegrade cardioplegia is also routinely imaged. Although an electrically silent ECG is reassuring, it is safer to visualize the flow of cardioplegia into the left main and right coronary arteries. The use of TEE during the initial administration of cardioplegia also excludes the presence of significant aortic regurgitation and left ventricular distension [8].

17.3.2.5 Defibrillation

If external defibrillation is required, all instruments must be removed from the chest, and reinflation of the lung occurs before shock delivery. Reinflation of the lung is mandatory as the capnothorax significantly impedes conduction of the electrical discharge via defibrillation.

17.3.2.6 Separation from CBP

- Rewarming: Intraoperative hypothermia can delay emergence and cause increased oxygen consumption.
- Vasoactive and inotropic support, if necessary.
- FiO_2 can be increased in support of maintaining an adequate partial pressure of oxygen after CBP, but the minimum necessary FiO_2 is recommended. Concomitant restauration of volume status will start the weaning process.
- Unilateral pulmonary edema: Unilateral pulmonary edema is a phenomenon associated with minimally invasive cardiac surgeries, specifically those requiring CPB. Manifestations include profound hypoxia, hypercapnia, pulmonary hypertension, and hemodynamic instability. It is associated independently with chronic obstructive pulmonary disease, preexisting pulmonary hypertension, moderate or severe right ventricular dysfunction, and increased time on CPB. The lung on the operative side suffers an ischemia-reperfusion injury. It is first identified typically by the presence of copious frothy yellow/pink fluid originating from the lung on the operative side.
- Acquired coagulopathy: Obtain TEG/ROTEM, and send blood for platelet count when the rewarming begins; treat the bleeding, not the TEG/ROTEM or lab values. If there is no bleeding, no products are administered.

17.3.2.7 Fast-Track Extubation Candidacy

One of the major advantages of the robotic approach is the potential to put these patients on a fast-track or ultrafast-track extubation; the ideal patients have limited to no significant comorbidities, and the minimally invasive nature makes adequate pain management a reasonable goal.

Operating room extubation (ORE) for suitable patients avoids discomfort from prolonged intubation and ventilation, avoids administration of unnecessary sedation medications, and may help to maintain better hemodynamics in an awake, spontaneously breathing patient. Data suggest that ORE is associated with reduction in duration of ICU and hospital lenght of stay [9].

Regional anesthesia (i.e., thoracic epidural and paravertebral blocks, erector spinae plane, serratus anterior plane), total intravenous anesthesia, and short-acting inhalation anesthetics have been used to facilitate recovery and ORE.

Furthermore, multiple studies demonstrated that there was no delay in subsequent procedures as a result of ORE [9, 10].

Studies conducted on patients undergoing a fast-track cardiac surgery suggest that extubation guidelines must include:

1. Left ventricular ejection fraction >40% with minimal inotropic support.
2. Normal right ventricular function.
3. Stable rhythm or reliable pacing wires.
4. Patient awake and able to follow simple commands.
5. Adequate muscle strength and respiratory effort.
6. Vital capacity greater than 25 ml/kg.
7. Tidal volume greater than 5 ml/kg.
8. Respiratory rate < 18/min.
9. $EtCO_2$ less than 50 mmHg.
10. No significant metabolic acidosis.
11. Normothermia.
12. Absence of significant mediastinal bleeding or coagulopathy: chest tube output <100 ml in 30 min.

Patients not fulfilling ORE criteria should be transferred to the ICU and extubated within 4 h. More detail about ultra fast track and ORE are explain in assigned chapter.

17.3.2.8 Pain Management

Multimodal pain management must aim at complete analgesic coverage while minimizing opioid consumption, favoring locoregional techniques, and combining various drugs to avoid toxic doses of single molecules.

In robotic cardiac surgery, pain is reduced owing to the absence of a median sternal incision. Pain management is very important because of the interest in fast-tracking these patients. Narcotics should be used sparingly at the end of the procedure to prevent delay in extubation, stabilization, and discharge from the hospital. Multimodal analgesia, including neuraxial and regional anesthetic techniques, should be considered strongly. Neuraxial anesthesia may be contraindicated in patients undergoing procedures with drug-eluting stents necessitating the use of antiplatelet medication, and many anesthesiologists are reluctant to utilize neuraxial techniques prior to administration of a large dose of heparin [8]. Because the surgery involves several small incisions, a number of regional anesthesia and analgesic techniques may be employed. New advancements in ultrasound-guided chest wall nerve and plane blocks may prove to be most beneficial. Paravertebral and erector spinae plane blocks have been studied extensively in cardiac surgery and have been shown to be effective in providing postoperative analgesia while reducing the effects of sympathetic blockade in minimally invasive robotic cardiac surgery. Intraoperative intercostal blocks are also used commonly. Serratus anterior plane blocks have been shown to provide significant benefit for robotic cardiac surgery. Pectoralis I and II blocks have been demonstrated in minimally invasive mitral valve surgery and may provide analgesic benefits alone or in conjunction with the serratus anterior plane block, depending on port placement. Intercostal nerve cryoablation has been described as an effective method for the relief of thoracotomy incisions during minimally invasive direct CABG procedures [11].

17.3.3 Postoperative Management

- Early mobilization after cardiac surgery is crucial to the success of ERAS.
- Mobilization has been shown to reduce postoperative pulmonary complications and thromboembolic events. It has several benefits, including improved lung and tissue oxy-

genation, as well as increased muscle mass and strength.

- Inadequate pain and nausea control can disempower patients and limit their ability to mobilize.
- Postoperative systematic delirium screening tool use at least once per nursing shift [7].
- Early detection of kidney stress and interventions to avoid acute kidney injury (AKI) after surgery [7].
- Core bundle of practices to reduce surgical site infections.
- Perioperative glycemic control is essential to avoid both hypo- and hyperglycemic states. Continuous insulin infusions should be considered over bolus doses in the early perioperative period.

17.4 A Practical Guide

In this subsection we will provide a protocol used in some centers that perform robotic MICS daily.

17.4.1 Preoperative Evaluation

Patient selection represents the first step in preoperative assessment. As with conventional surgery, all patients evaluated for robotic surgery should undergo a comprehensive preoperative assessment, including clinical history, physical examination, 12-lead electrocardiogram, and appropriate imaging studies. All patients should receive computed tomography angiography of the chest, abdomen, and pelvis before surgery for the assessment of the thoracic and abdomen aorta to rule out significant atherosclerotic disease that may result in serious perioperative vascular complications.

Robotic surgery is facilitated by single-lung ventilation at different moments during the operation. Patients with severe chronic pulmonary disease or pulmonary hypertension should be evaluated carefully to determine if they can tolerate this safely. In some patients, OLV can be reduced or even avoided at the expense of longer duration of CPB.

17.4.1.1 Patient Blood Management (PBM)

The activities included in the PBM program aim to optimize the preoperative hematopoietic structure of anemic patients undergoing elective surgery and at high risk of perioperative transfusion in order to plan an adequate transfusion strategy.

In the preoperative period, the three pillars of PBM include the following:

- Optimize erythropoiesis: detect anemia.
- Identify and treat the underlying diseases causing the anemia.
- Reassess the patient if necessary.
- Treat martial deficiency and iron-deficiency anemia, anemia of chronic diseases, and functional iron deficiencies.

This evaluation is multiparametric and is essentially based on the in-depth analysis of the following indices, at an optimal distance of at least 14–28 days before surgery:

- Basal hemoglobin with simultaneous evaluation of erythrocyte indices.
- Evaluation of martial balance: serum iron, ferritin, transferrin, and transferrin saturation percentage.
- Evaluation of creatinine and creatinine clearance.

All patients are evaluated at the pre-admission by the anesthetist, and if considered eligible for treatment, they will be contacted by telephone for an appointment in which they will be subjected to martial therapy with ferric carboxymaltose. 3–4 weeks after the therapy, the patient will repeat a blood count, and if the anemia is corrected, he will undergo surgery (Fig. 17.7).

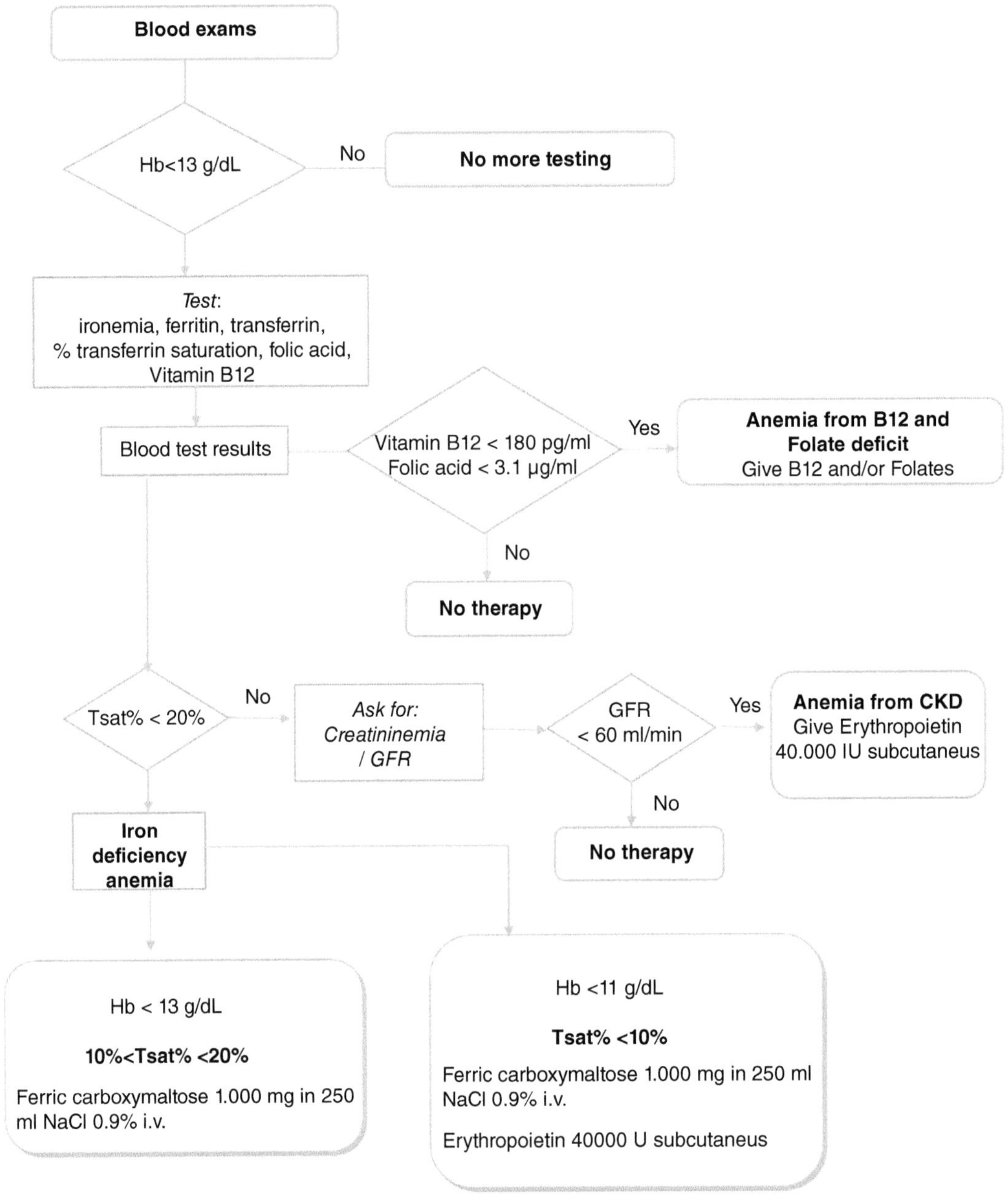

Fig. 17.7 An example of an anemia diagnostic and therapeutic protocol

17.4.2 Intraoperative Management

17.4.2.1 Induction of GA

- Anxiolysis with midazolam, 2–3 mg bolus.
- Arterial line placement: If endoaortic balloon occlusion of the ascending aorta with antegrade cardioplegia is planned, then bilateral radial arterial catheters are placed. Under these circumstances, damping of the right radial arterial pressure waveform is presumed to represent migration of the endoaortic balloon with innominate artery occlusion. Intraoperative cerebral oximetry has also been suggested to detect endoaortic balloon migration. A decline in right-sided cerebral oxime-

ter readings should prompt TEE confirmation of aortic balloon position.

- Locoregional anesthesia as part of a multimodal analgesia strategy to minimize intraoperative opioid use together with the need for high-dose postoperative rescue analgesia with opiates/NSAIDs: We mainly perform the ESP block, strictly under ultrasound (US) guidance, for its simplicity and effectiveness, combined with its very low risk of complications (pneumothorax, bleeding). This block is performed twice at two different levels (usually T3–T5), with the patient sitting on the OR bed, either in the preoperative room or in the OR itself. Care should be taken to avoid vascular structures along the needle's path, and pleura should as well be identified and avoided. Advantages of ESP block include spread of local anesthetic over multiple dermatomes covering all of the surgical incisions. Compared with a thoracic epidural catheter, ESP blocks are associated with a reduced risk of neuraxial hematoma in a heparinized patient and a lower risk of hypotension from sympathetic blockade. The inclusion of ESP block into our anesthetic management plan along with the associated decrease in the use of the systemic opioid medication has allowed us to extubate almost all the patients in the operating room at the conclusion of surgery.
- Bair hugger with underbody blanket is positioned and activated.
- General anesthesia induction with short-acting opioids (fentanyl 1.5 mcg/kg) and gradual propofol injection (1.5–2.5 mg/kg) under continuous EEG monitoring (SedLine vs. BIS technologies at our institution).
- Muscle relaxation is obtained with rocuronium 0.6–1 mg/kg.
- 1 g of tranexamic acid is administered as a bolus at induction and 1 g at CPB weaning.
- To perform a multimodal analgesia, a bolus of 1–1.5 mg/kg of lidocaine and 1 g of $MgSO_4$ are administered at induction.
- Shortly before awakening the patient, a bolus of 8 mg ondansetron is administered in order to prevent postoperative nausea and vomiting (PONV).

17.4.2.2 Airway Management

A dual-lumen left endotracheal tube (DLETT) is positioned. Correct tube positioning is evaluated with a fiberscope. Orotracheal intubation can be performed alternatively with a single-lumen tube and a bronchial occluder.

Although initial placement of DLETT is more challenging, if no concerns about the difficulty of the airway are present, experts prefer it since it permits to suction the excluded lung, to apply external positive end expiratory pressure (PEEP) or jet ventilation if OLV is not tolerated, and it's easier to deflate the right lung when compared to an SLETT with the bronchial blocker.

In robotic assisted cardiac surgery, the lung exclusion is of utmost importance: it must be perfectly achieved to have a perfect surgical view of the field, and the OLV is more challenging because the capnothorax is at higher pressure, and it lasts more, if compared with minimally invasive cardiac surgery.

The need to apply continuous positive airways pressure (CPAP) or reinflate the non-ventilated lung is not so rare.

Effective lung exclusion and tolerance to one-lung ventilation are then tested, while the surgical sterile field is prepared.

17.4.2.3 CBP Preparation, Patient Positioning, and TEE

- Once DLETT is securely in place, a 15 Fr cannula for superior vena cava drainage is positioned just proximal to the site of CVC insertion. This is performed by the anesthesiologist under continuous ultrasound (US) guidance, with the help of the scrub nurse. The perfusionist will then hand the afferent circuit of the CPB machine for de-airing and connection to the SVC cannula.
- In the few centers that perform robotic atrial fibrillation (AF) surgery, an S-shaped esophageal temperature probe equipped with a series of 12 sensors is inserted into the esophagus to monitor temperature during ablation and avoid thermal damage, with a threshold set at 37.2 °C. The probe has an inner stylet; only when this is removed after positioning will the probe assume the S-shape designed to increase

the surface in contact with the esophagus. In other centers, where epicardic AF ablation is performed in the cath-lab without robotic assistance, the correct positioning of the probe is monitored through X-ray; the tip of the probe must be seen 2 cm under tracheal carina.

- In the OR setting, the DLT is used as a marker; the DLT bronchial tip stands 4 cm after the carina. Therefore, the probe must be fixed 2 cm less deep than the tube (Fig. 17.8). Only in case of impossibility of DLT placement the traditional X-ray control is performed.
- During patient positioning, care should be taken to avoid neural injuries due to compression.
- TEE is performed in order to confirm surgical indication and the correct positioning of all the devices. TEE is of utmost importance throughout all the surgery, and especially during mitral valve repair and left appendage closure, which is TEE guided. During AF ablation, it is mandatory to exclude the presence of clots in the atrial appendage, to control the correct site of closure and the correct distance from circumflex artery.
- CPB times, if the surgeon has developed the correct expertise, are similar as surgery through a median sternotomy. Anyways, adequate cardioprotection is crucial, and specific differences related to the procedure, including the fact that rewarming of the heart occurs faster in a closed chest, need to be considered.

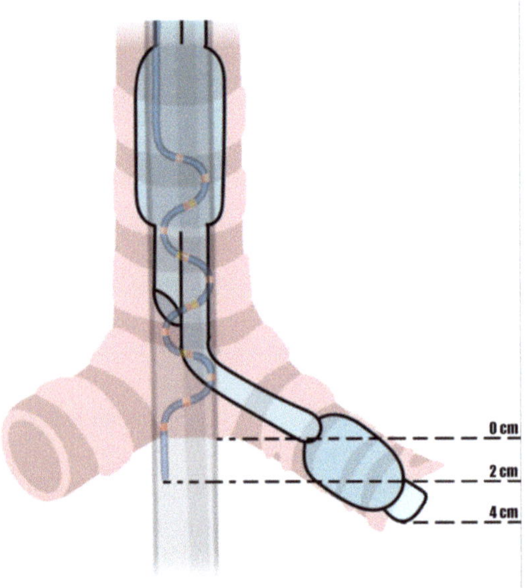

Fig. 17.8 Correct temperature probe positioning using the DLT as a marker

- In the case of surgical bleeding that cannot be resolved promptly, an urgent sternotomy should be performed. The need for sternotomy is really rare.

17.4.2.4 Pain Management

- Acetaminophen 1 g ev + ibuprofen 600 mg or ketorolac 30 mg ev + dexamethasone 8 mg 60 min before the end of surgery.
- Surgeons irrigate the pleura with local anesthetics.

17.4.3 Postoperative Management

- Early extubation improves the quality of patient recovery.
- Fast-track extubation after cardiac surgery remains globally poorly defined, with protocols for early extubation ranging from 6 or less hours to 24 h postoperatively.
- In high-quality centers, patients undergoing robotic cardiac surgery are awakened and extubated in the OR, unless clinical conditions (i.e., insufficient rewarming, insufficient pain control, suspicion of glottis edema, or other airway malprotection) prevent it. In this case, patients are transferred to the ICU, where these conditions are treated and resolved, and the patient is promptly extubated.
- In those centers, average OR extubation rate is 70% for MVR and >80% for FA ablation and CABG.
- Regardless of extubation status, all patients are transported directly to the ICU on a monitored ICU bed.
- Pain is managed with acetaminophen 1 g i.v. every 6 h (18–24–6) + ibuprofen 600 mg or ketorolac 30 mg i.v. every 12 h (18–6) + $MgSO_4$ 2 g ev (added in the maintenance fluids). Rescue dose if NRS >3 with morphine 3 mg i.v. every 6 h.

- FKT starts 3 h after the arrival of the patient in the ICU.
- The patient is moved to an armchair, and motor and respiratory physiotherapy are started. He is than taught some exercises he must then execute autonomy during the day. He is then put in a standing position, with the aid of physiotherapists. The patient is invited to use as soon as possible his own devices, i.e., glasses, hearing aids, and cellphone.
- At supper, the patient will eat a light diet supplemented with protein integrators (i.e., Fortimel).
- On day 1 post-op, chest tubes are clamped early in the morning and removed after a chest X-ray for control is performed.
- The patient is free to eat a normal diet from day 1 post-surgery, and he is invited to drink 1500 ml of water daily.
- Physiotherapy continues with armchair, standing position, and aided walk.
- Usually, at 11 of the same day, the patient is discharged to cardiosurgery ward; arterial line and bladder catheter are removed, fluid infusion is stopped, and analgesic therapy is switched to oral medications.

References

1. Cerny S, Oosterlinck W, Onan B, Singh S, Segers P, Bolcal C, et al. Robotic cardiac surgery in Europe: status 2020. Front Cardiovasc Med. 2022;8:8.
2. Mori M, Parsons N, Krane M, Guy TS, Grossi EA, Dearani JA, et al. Robotic mitral valve repair for degenerative mitral regurgitation. Ann Thorac Surg. 2024;117:96–104. Elsevier Inc
3. Palmen M, Navarra E, Bonatti J, Franke U, Cerny S, Musumeci F, et al. Current state of the art and recommendations in robotic mitral valve surgery. Interact Cardiovasc Thorac Surg. 2022;35. Oxford University Press
4. Akowuah EF, Maier RH, Hancock HC, Kharatikoopaei E, Vale L, Fernandez-Garcia C, et al. Minithoracotomy vs conventional sternotomy for mitral valve repair: a randomized clinical trial. JAMA. 2023;329(22):1957–66.
5. Agnino A, Giroletti L, Graniero A, Gerometta P, Parrinello M, Albano G, et al. Robotic-assisted Epicardial hybrid ablation and left appendage closure in persistent atrial fibrillation: first European experience. J Clin Med. 2024;13(6)
6. Bernstein W, Walker A. Anesthetic issues for robotic cardiac surgery. Ann Card Anaesth. 2015;18(1):58–68.
7. Gregory AJ, Grant MC, Manning MW, Cheung AT, Ender J, Sander M, et al. Enhanced recovery after cardiac surgery (ERAS cardiac) recommendations: an important first step—but there is much work to be done. J Cardiothorac Vasc Anesth. 2020;34:39–47.
8. Rehfeldt KH, Andre JV, Ritter MJ. Anesthetic considerations in robotic mitral valve surgery. Ann Cardiothorac Surg. 2017;6(1):47–53.
9. Rodrigues ES, Lynch JJ, Suri RM, Burkhart HM, Li Z, Mauermann WJ, et al. Robotic mitral valve repair: a review of anesthetic management of the first 200 patients. J Cardiothorac Vasc Anesth. 2014;28(1):64–8.
10. Subramaniam K, DeAndrade DS, Mandell DR, Althouse AD, Manmohan R, Esper SA, et al. Predictors of operating room extubation in adult cardiac surgery. J Thorac Cardiovasc Surg. 2017;154(5):1656–65.
11. Fitzgerald MM, Bhatt HV, Schuessler ME, Guy TS, Ivascu NS, Evans AS, et al. Robotic cardiac surgery. Part I: Anesthetic considerations in totally endoscopic robotic cardiac surgery (TERCS). J Cardiothorac Vasc Anesth. 2020;34:267–77. W.B. Saunders

Part IV

Early Extubation After Cardiac Procedures

Risks and Benefits 18

Simona Silvetti, Giuseppe Sepolvere, Antonio Salsano, and Andrea De Martino

18.1 Introduction

Early extubation after cardiac surgery is an aim of ERAS program; despite that, it is not well defined who is the best patient to receive this practice or if there are some patients that should be excluded.

The cardiac surgery patients' outcomes are often affected by many preoperative and various intraoperative factors that affect organ function. Although cardiac impairment is a given, lot of conditions related to cardiac surgery also induce pulmonary dysfunction. Cardiac surgery causes damage to tissues, organs, and peripheral nerves; smooth and striated muscle spasm compression of visceral structures; costal cartilage tissue trauma; ribs and sternum fractures; and inflammatory conditions determining impaired respiratory mechanics, and this will be accompanied by reduced mobility, leading to pulmonary complications or muscle atrophy. Furthermore, feeling pain induces breath more rapidly and less deeply, with cough inhibition and mucus expectoration [1, 2].

For these conditions and also because all cardiac surgery is a high-risk invasive procedure, usually after cardiac surgery, the patients require a more or less longer ICU recovery, receive an intensive monitoring, and continue mechanical ventilation. The extubation after cardiac surgery is a tricky maneuver, and anesthesiologists usually perform it in ICU after adequate evaluations.

In the recent past, all patients undergoing cardiac surgery (without complications) were weaned from the ventilator 12–24 h after surgery; today, this time is considered a prolonged ventilation. In fact, it is well known that mechanical ventilation leads to a high incidence of postoperative complications, which affects the prognosis of patients.

In early 2017, a group of cardiac surgeons, anesthesiologists, and intensivists first met to establish the Enhanced Recovery After Cardiac Surgery (ERACS) Society to achieve some goals for patients undergoing heart surgery. One

The original version of the chapter has been revised. A correction to this chapter can be found at https://doi.org/10.1007/978-3-031-70899-2_26

S. Silvetti (✉)
Department of Cardiac Anesthesia and Intensive Care, Cardiovascular Network, IRCCS Ospedale Policlinico San Martino, Genoa, Italy

G. Sepolvere
Department of Anesthesia and Cardiac Surgery Intensive Care Unit, San Michele Hospital, Maddaloni, Caserta, Italy

A. Salsano
Cardiac Surgery Division, Ospedale Policlinico San Martino, Genoa, Italy

Disc Department, University of Genoa, Genoa, Italy

A. De Martino
Cardiac Surgery Division, Ospedale Policlinico San Martino, Genoa, Italy

G. Sepolvere, S. Silvetti (eds.), *Fast-Track in Cardiac Anesthesia*,
https://doi.org/10.1007/978-3-031-70899-2_18

of the most important ERAS targets is the "early extubation." Nowadays, we define early extubation as ERACS definition until 6 h after surgery [3], but in the past, many studies have established a fast-track criterion for endotracheal tube removal within 12 h [4] to 2 h after surgery [5]. Over the years, not only the definition has changed but also the objective of early extubation maneuver. In 1980, the goal was to reduce opioid administration and obtain lower risk of pulmonary complications [6]. In the 1990, the fast-track movement in cardiac surgery was initiated by Dr. Engelman with the aim to limit the ICU stay [7]. Finally, today, according to the 2016 Cochrane review [8], fast-track cardiac care has the objective of reducing ICU and hospital stay.

In 1995, Cheng et al. [8] asked in their manuscript, "Is early tracheal extubation (<8 h) appropriate for the cardiac surgical population in the 1990s?" Also, is early extubation really cost saving to healthcare budgets? And they concluded, "All patients who underwent cardiac surgery should be valued for an early tracheal extubation. Early extubation does reduce ICU and hospital stay and costs." They also underlined the importance of a prompt program of care to obtain the maximum benefits from this clinical practice [9].

Over the time, many manuscripts about fast-track cardiac anesthesia have consistently confirmed as said and demonstrated that this methodology is safe and associated with reduced complications and length of stay [10, 11]. On the contrary, less well known are the risks that come from early extubation in this kind of patients. In this chapter, we analyzed benefits and risks for early extubation after cardiac procedures in adult patients (Fig. 18.1).

18.2 Benefits

The rationale behind early extubation is grounded in its multiple physiological and psychological benefits. Physiologically, early removal of the endotracheal tube reduces the risks associated with prolonged mechanical ventilation, such as ventilator-associated pneumonia and other pulmonary complications. It also favors hemodynamic stability and reduces the need for sedatives, thereby decreasing the incidence of delirium and other cognitive dysfunctions, a common complication in the elderly post-cardiac surgery population.

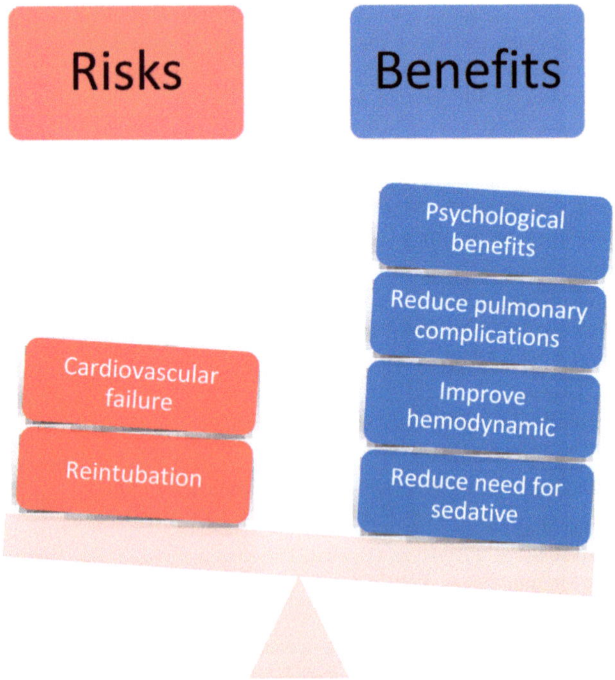

Fig. 18.1 Benefit and risks from early extubation

From a psychological perspective, patients benefit from an enhanced sense of control and comfort, experiencing less distress and disorientation often associated with mechanical ventilation.

In this section, we will analyze all beneficial effect from early extubation.

First, early extubation reduces pulmonary complications including laryngeal-trachea trauma and ventilator-associated pneumonia. This may result from improved clearance of pulmonary secretion and earlier return of ciliary function [6], earlier mobilization, and improved cardiac performance [12]; furthermore, prolonged mechanical ventilation has been previously related with higher rates of bacterial colonization [13]. A 2014 meta-analysis [14] showed that the prevalence of ventilator-associated pneumonia in all cardiac surgery patients was 6.37%, increasing to 35.2% in patients with greater than 48 h of mechanical ventilation.

Second, a favorable hemodynamic effect is an expected consequence: removal of tracheal tube induces a decrease in positive-pressure ventilation with consequent decrease in venous return and right ventricular afterload; no less relevant, the tracheal intubation in awake patients is poorly tolerated, and the patient discomfort often pressurizes the anesthesiologist to increase sedative drug administration, but this mechanism may produce cardiovascular instability with both vasodilation and myocardial depression. Intubated patients commonly require increased fluid infusion or vasoconstrictor agents to manage vasodilation and hypotension, avoiding sedative drug, and the hemodynamic management could be easier (Fig. 18.2).

Third, higher doses of sedation required in intubated patients, particularly in elderly patients, may contribute to delirium, confusion, and delayed return of cognitive function. Delirium after cardiac surgery has an estimated incidence of 26–52% and has been associated with a longer period of mechanical ventilation in the elderly [15].

Among others, prolonged intubation time is also linked to a longer time to restart normal feeding with consequent problems and gastrointestinal complications.

Patients free from hemodynamic, pulmonary complications and delirium could be early mobilized, and it leads to improved muscle strength and a lower risk of postoperative complications such as deep vein thrombosis and pressure ulcers. Early mobilization in cardiac surgery patients represents one of the most important items of ERAS protocols.

As explained, the benefits of early extubation are a lot and lead to reduced hospital cost (Fig. 18.3). In fact, early extubation was associated with an abbreviated ICU and hospital length [16, 17] of stay, and readmission to the ICU also declined by 50% [18]. The broader impact on hospital resources extends to reducing the overall burden on the healthcare system. By shortening ICU stays and hospitalizations, early extubation protocols free up valuable resources that can be redirected to other patients, thereby increasing the overall efficiency and capacity of the health-

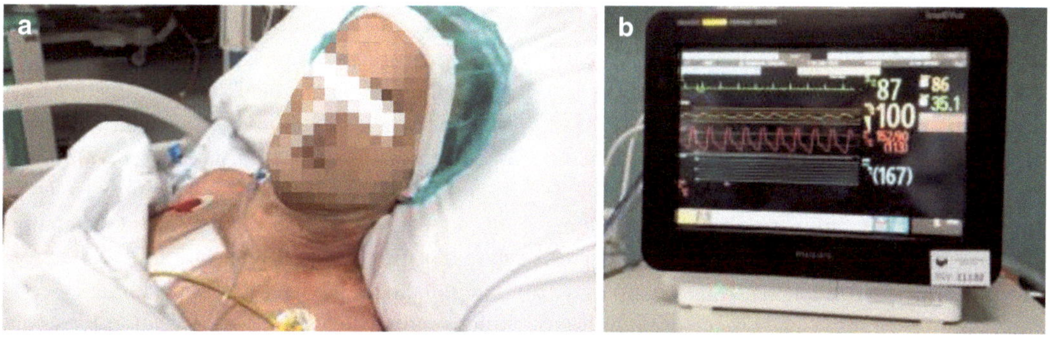

Fig. 18.2 Early extubation. (**a**) Patient underwent multiple coronary artery bypass grafting. (**b**) Good hemodynamic and respiratory stability. In this figure, the patient who underwent multiple coronary artery bypass grafting was early extubated after receiving both parasternal and rectus sheath blocks at the end of the surgery

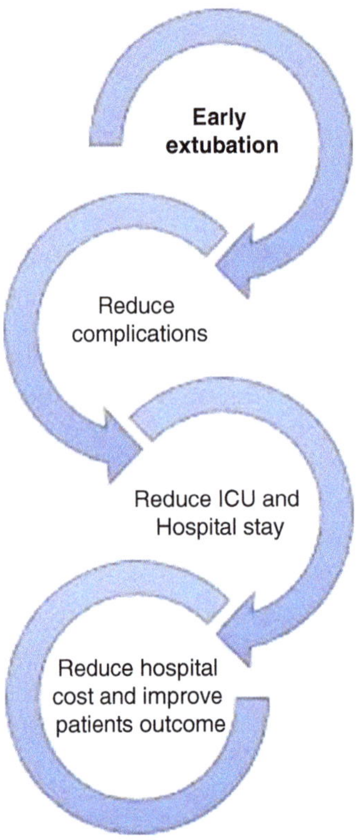

Fig. 18.3 Benefit from early extubation leads to reduced hospital cost

care system. This optimization of resources can lead to reduced wait times for ICU beds and improved access to critical care services for patients who need them most [19].

Given the countless advantages related to the early extubation, cardiac surgery anesthesiologists are encouraged to implement the ERAS pathways and strategies significantly reducing extubation times and postoperative complications [20, 21]. It is noteworthy to point out that early extubation represents a feasible procedure if performed in the correct way: by a skilled team sharing the same goals, for a selected population patients. Implementing early extubation protocols requires a multidisciplinary approach involving surgeons, anesthesiologists, intensivists, nurses, and respiratory therapists. This collaborative effort ensures the safety and effectiveness of early extubation and fosters a culture of teamwork and continuous improvement within the healthcare setting. Continuous evaluation and adjustment of these protocols based on patient outcomes and feedback are essential to maintain their effectiveness and adapt to evolving clinical practices.

18.3 Risks

Although the early extubation benchmark is 6 h, the actual ventilation time that leads to increased complications is not known. And unfortunately, extubation within 6 h after some kinds of cardiac surgery may not be feasible because of postoperative respiratory and ventricular dysfunctions following prolonged cardiopulmonary bypass, hemodynamic instability, abnormal hemostasis, hypothermia, bleeding, and postoperative complications. Postoperative mechanical ventilation is routinely used after cardiac surgery to minimize myocardial oxygen consumption and work of breathing from spontaneous ventilation. In fact, weaning from positive-pressure ventilation has been compared to an exercise stress test for the cardiovascular system [17], and in post-cardiac surgery patients, this phenomenon is magnified. Extubation is associated with an abrupt increase of both the venous return to the heart and left ventricular afterload secondary to the inspiratory fall of intrathoracic pressure. These hemodynamic changes and an increase in work of breathing may result in increased pulmonary venous pressure with associated risk of pulmonary edema [18]. In addition, the conjunction of sudden increase in both the work of breathing and adrenergic tone may also raise myocardial oxygen consumption and induce ischemia in this susceptible heart. Accordingly, inadequate cardiovascular response to spontaneous breathing is one of the leading mechanisms of extubation failure. Nevertheless, cardiovascular insufficiency, a frequent condition after cardiac surgery, may also be a primary cause of weaning failure. To avoid this adverse event, an accurate patient evaluation should be performed before this clinical practice. Caution should be taken for the emergency conditions, for patients receiving ventricular assist device placement and cardiac transplantation due to the unstudied conditions in the context of early extubation.

The risks of early extubation have not been sufficiently studied. They are often related to both potential failure of extubation with subsequent reintubation and lack of protocols aimed at identifying appropriate criteria for adequate patient type of surgery stratification eligible for fast-track extubation.

18.4 Conclusion

Fast-track protocol in cardiac surgery was introduced as a system by which patients could be early extubated and early transferred out of the ICU. By reducing ICU and hospital length of stay, it was anticipated that fast-tracking would reduce hospital costs and improve hospital efficiency.

Despite the beneficial effects of early extubation, the application of this clinical practice must be meticulously managed, balancing the benefits with potential risks. A thorough assessment is crucial and required to identify suitable candidates while considering individual patient risk factors and the complexity of the surgical procedure. This selective approach ensures that the advantages of early extubation can be harnessed effectively without compromising patient safety. In fact, not all patients are suitable candidates for early extubation. Tailoring the approach to each patient's specific needs and risk factors ensures that the benefits of early extubation can be maximized without compromising patient safety [21].

Despite these premises, the uptake of fast track has been variable. Obviously, many factors influence the timing of extubation after cardiac surgery, including patient comorbidities and intraoperative and postoperative complications. With this variability, it is challenging to make a single standard for time to extubation. Furthermore, there are many differences in practice patterns, in availability resources, and in levels of monitoring in the ICU.

In conclusion, the successful implementation of protocols within the ERACS framework for cardiac surgery patients marks a significant advancement in postoperative care. This multidisciplinary approach, involving careful preoperative planning, intraoperative management, and a postoperative care, leads to improved patient outcomes, increased patient satisfaction, reduced ICU stays, and enhanced resource utilization. To disseminate this pathway as best as possible, not only a knowledge of benefits and risk of this maneuver should be clear for any anesthesiologist and surgeon, but also an institutional research and planning are required.

References

1. Kaplan JA. Kaplan's Essentials of cardiac anesthesia for cardiac surgery. 2nd ed. Elsevier; 2017.
2. Sasseron AB, Figueiredo LC, Trova K, Cardoso AL, Vieira Lima NMF, Olmos SC, et al. Does the pain disturb respiratory function after heart surgeries? Rev Bras Cir Cardiovasc. 2009;24(4):490–6.
3. Engelman DT, Ben Ali W, Williams JB, Perrault LP, Reddy VS, Arora RC, et al. Guidelines for perioperative care in cardiac surgery: enhanced recovery after surgery society recommendations. JAMA Surg. 2019;154(8):755–66.
4. Arom KV, Emery RW, Petersen RJ, Schwartz M. Cost-effectiveness and predictors of early extubation. Ann Thorac Surg. 1995;60(1):127–32.
5. Pettersson PH, Settergren G, Owall A. Similar pain scores after early and late extubation in heart surgery with cardiopulmonary bypass. J Cardiothorac Vasc Anesth. 2004;18(1):64–7.
6. Quasha AL, Loeber N, Feeley TW, Ullyot DJ, Roizen MF. Postoperative respiratory care: a controlled trial of early and late extubation following coronary-artery bypass grafting. Anesthesiology. 1980;52(2):135–41.
7. Engelman RM, Rousou JA, Flack JE 3rd, Deaton DW, Humphrey CB, Ellison LH, et al. Fast track recovery. Ann Thorac Surg. 1994;58(6):1742–6.
8. Wong WT, Lai VK, Chee YE, Lee A. Fast-track cardiac care for adult cardiac surgical patients. Cochrane Database Syst Rev. 2016;9:CD003587.
9. Cheng DC. Pro: early extubation after cardiac surgery decreases intensive care unit stay and cost. J Cardiothorac Vasc Anesth. 1995;9:460–4.
10. Zhu F, Lee A, Chee YE. Fast-track cardiac care for adult cardiac surgical patients. Cochrane Database Syst Rev. 2012;10:CD003587.
11. MacLeod JB, D'Souza K, Aguiar C, Brown CD, Pozeg Z, White C, et al. Fast track after cardiac surgery: it is safe? J Cardiothorac Surg. 2022;17:69.
12. Vieillard-Baron A, Naeije R, Haddad F, Bogaard HJ, Bull TM, Fletcher N, et al. Diagnostic workup, etiologies and management of acute right ventricle failure : a state-of-the-art paper. Intensive Care Med. 2018;44(6):774–90.
13. Cheng DCH, Wall C, Djaiani G, Peragallo RA, Carroll J, Li C, et al. Randomized assessment of resource use

in fast-track cardiac surgery 1-year after hospital discharge. Anesthesiology. 2003;98:651–7.
14. He S, Chen B, Li W, Yan J, Chen L, Wang X, et al. Ventilator-associated pneumonia after cardiac surgery: a meta-analysis and systematic review. J Thorac Cardiovasc Surg. 2014;148(6):3148–55.
15. Brown CH. Delirium in the cardiac surgical ICU. Curr Opin Anaesthesiol. 2014;27(2):117–22.
16. Hawkes CA, Dhileepan S, Foxcroft D. Early extubation for adult cardiac surgery patients. Cochrane Database Syst Rev. 2007:CD003587.
17. Guller U, Anstrom KJ, Holman WL, Allman RM, Samson M, Peterson ED, et al. Outcomes of early extubation after cardiac surgery in the elderly. Ann Thorac Surg. 2004;77:781–8.
18. Myles PS, Daly DJ, Djaiani G, Lee A, Cheng DCH. A systematic review of the safety and effectiveness of fast-track cardiac anesthesia. Anesthesiology. 2003;99:982–7.
19. Reich DL, Bodian CA, Krol M, Kuroda M, Osinski T, Thys DM. Intraoperative hemodynamic predictors of mortality, stroke, and myocardial infarction after coronary artery bypass surgery. Anesth Analg. 1999;89:814–22.
20. Grant MC, Crisafi C, Alvarez A, Arora RC, Brindle ME, Chatterjee S, et al. Perioperative care in cardiac surgery: a joint consensus statement by the enhanced recovery after surgery (ERAS) cardiac society, ERAS international society, and the Society of Thoracic Surgeons (STS). Ann Thorac Surg. 2024;117(4):669–89. https://doi.org/10.1016/j.athoracsur.2023.12.006.
21. Probst S, Cech C, Haentschel D, Scholz M, Ender J. A specialized post anaesthetic care unit improves fast-track management in cardiac surgery: a prospective randomized trial. Crit Care. 2014;18(4):468.

Patients' Selection 19

Simona Silvetti, Filippo Sanfilippo,
and Valentina Ajello

19.1 Introduction

In the Enhanced Recovery After Cardiac Surgery (ERACS) guidelines on perioperative care for patients undergoing cardiac surgery [1], the panel introduced the importance of early extubation and recommended that strategies to ensure extubation within 6 h of surgery should be pursued with a class of evidence IIa (level B-NR: moderate-quality evidence from at least one well-designed, well-executed nonrandomized or observational study).

Several reasons suggest the implementation of fast-track extubation protocols in patients undergoing cardiac surgery in order to promote an early recovery according to the ERACS principles and fast track extubation is now a well-accepted and widely utilized approach to post-operative cardiac surgical care. Therefore, whilst acknowledging the advantages and the value of ERACS, in order to avoid possible adverse effects and complications, it is imperative to properly select the patients that may have greatest benefits and lowest risks of failure and complications.

This chapter focuses mostly on the proper selection of those patients that may benefit the most from early extubation, and similarly to identify those at higher risk that may require a longer period of mechanical ventilation before the weaning takes place.

19.2 Which Patient?

In order to achieve early extubation, it would be necessary to implement a series of interventions that should be part of a time-directed protocol. The first and more important point should be considered a careful patients' selection. The appropriate identification of patients that may benefit from early extubation, whilst correctly separating from those who may need longer intubation and ventilation periods, is a key factor for a successful implementation of an ERACS program to benefit from such strategy whilst reducing the risks for patients. This represents a daily clinical challenge for the cardiac anesthesiologists facing a different demographic population as compared to the previous decades. Indeed, patients with multiple comorbidities and octa- and nonagenarians with increased frailty are daily encountered

S. Silvetti
Department of Cardiac Anesthesia and Intensive Care, Cardiovascular Network, IRCCS Ospedale Policlinico San Martino, Genoa, Italy

F. Sanfilippo
University Hospital Policlinico G. Rodolico-San Marco, Catania, Italy

Department of Surgery and Medical-Surgical Specialties, University of Catania, Catania, Italy

V. Ajello (✉)
Department of Cardiac Anesthesia, Tor Vergata University Hospital, Rome, Italy

G. Sepolvere, S. Silvetti (eds.), *Fast-Track in Cardiac Anesthesia*,
https://doi.org/10.1007/978-3-031-70899-2_19

during cardiac surgery procedures; moreover, also the surgical complexity has increased for these patients.

In this scenario, there are no currently standardized criteria for fast-track extubation, and each institution has eventually developed its own internal procedure in this regard. Indeed, the feasibility of fast-track extubation has to strongly consider local factors in terms of staffing, teaching programs, skills of the surgical and anesthetic teams, and many others. Consequently, the matter of understanding the most appropriate clinical criteria and the best approach for patient's selection, relies on a low quality of evidence. A standardized selection cannot be based solely on research conducted by individual centers, as it is influenced by local factors. Indeed, most of the evidence and literature available remain related to single-center experience reported with retrospective analyses. Further, in order to increase the sample size, authors usually pool together data from long periods, where several local factors such as change of policies, staffing, and processes are likely to influence the results. Nonetheless, the selection of the patient's candidate for a fast-track extubation remains complex and multifactorial, hence not truly appropriate for a randomized controlled trial or for an approach with blind design.

Therefore, in the following sections, we summarize the factors that could be considered in the patients' selection for early extubation in cardiac surgery. For a better understanding, we describe the patients' characteristics that seem to be associated with greater benefit and lowest risk of harm from this fast-track strategy and divide these characteristics in relation to the different phases of each cardiac surgery procedure, separating factors into

- Preoperative.
- Intraoperative or surgical.
- Postoperative.

These factors are gathered mainly from expert consensus and pathophysiological judgment. Until now, the evidence that we found in order to summarize these factors and gauge their impact derives mainly from retrospective studies investigating factors associated with early extubation without incurring in postoperative complications and/or reintubation. A list of the pre-, intra-, and postoperative factors is provided in Fig. 19.1, which can be used and adapted to promote fast-track extubation according to local policies.

19.2.1 Preoperative Factors

Preoperative factors are probably the most important ones in the consideration of undertaking an early extubation strategy. Indeed, it is unlikely that early extubation strategy is implemented for any patients if not preventively planned. In fact, when targeting early extubation, the cardiac anesthesiologist will adapt his clinical practice, for example reducing the amount of opioids administered and favoring locoregional anesthesia techniques to improve the management of acute postoperative pain.

Preoperative factors that are likely to influence the success of early extubation and can be divided into demographic factors on the one side, preexisting comorbidities and their severity on the other. Such conditions should be pooled together and weighted, deserving special attention from the cardiac anesthesiologist willing to implement early extubation.

Several studies in literature, particularly of retrospective design, have attempted to evaluate which clinical characteristics of cardiac surgery patients may be positively associated with early extubation.

Among the demographic factors described as potentially influencing the success of early extubation, age and gender play a role. Indeed, a recent large retrospective study conducted on approximately 8000 patients found that younger age and male gender are associated with early extubation [2]. Indeed, Arom et al. examined predictors of early extubation after CABG surgery and reported that female gender was associated with delayed extubation (defined as extubation beyond 12 h of surgery) [3]. Another study designed to assess the safety and efficacy of early extubation in patients undergoing

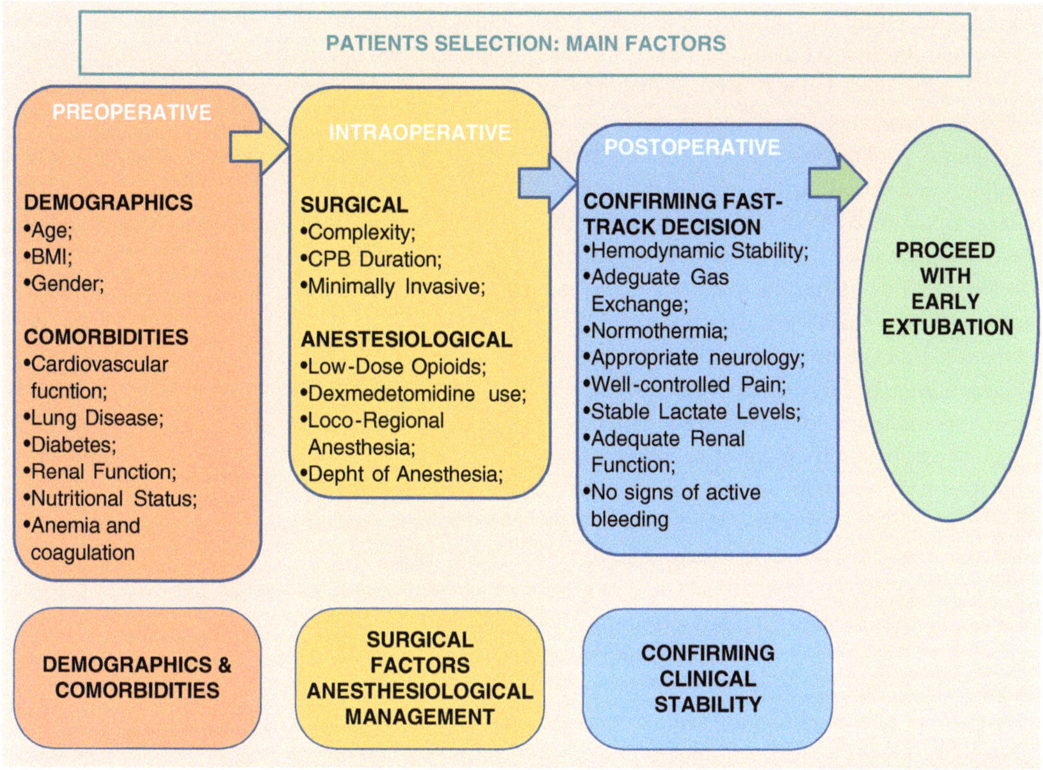

Fig. 19.1 Pre-intra and apost operative factors associated with early extubation in cardiac surgery

CABG surgery found that males were more likely to be extubated in a shorter period of time as compared to females. Using the same criteria for early extubation, Bezanson et al. investigated a population of 919 patients (age 65 years old or older). Over half of the patients ($n = 464$) were extubated within 6 h, and the authors performed a statistical analysis with stepwise logistic regression, which identified age (odds ratio 1.05) and female gender (odds ratio 1.48) as significant predictors of late extubation in this population of older patients undergoing CABG surgery [4]. Moreover, the authors created a model regarding the patient's comorbidities influencing early extubation, and in this pathophysiological model, the authors reported several factors significantly associated with failure of extubation within 6 h (with moderate discrimination). These factors were renal insufficiency (odds ratio 3.3), previous peripheral vascular surgery (odds ratio 2.9), nonelective preoperative clinical status (odds ratio 2.8), congestive heart failure (odds ratio 2.6), and reoperation (odds ratio 2.3).

Apart from age and gender, among the most studied demographic factors, obesity is increasingly recognized as a comorbidity influencing the success of early extubation. Hence, the body mass index (BMI) value is closely correlated with the possibility of including or not a patient in a fast-track process. Obesity is an independent risk factor for coronary artery disease and is a common comorbid condition in CABG surgery patients it has also been associated with an increased risk of complications in cardiac surgery, such as sternal wound infection and dehiscence, arrhythmias, and perioperative myocardial infarction. There is definitely an association between an increase in the duration of mechanical ventilation in obese patients compared to non-obese population. Obese patients are at increased risk of atelectasis due to the negative effects of weight and fat tissue on the thoracic wall and pulmonary compliance [5]. However, this belief has been questioned by one retrospective study that did not find differences in survival and potential complications (perioperative myocardial infarction, sternal wound or leg wound infection, acute renal failure, stroke, pneumonia, redo surgery for bleeding, and atrial arrhythmias) in patients undergoing cardiac surgery when comparing the obese population with nonobese patients. However, in this study, the population did not undergo a "fast-track" recovery protocol, and extubation times were similar between groups [6]. Extending the bibliographic research to retrospective studies on obese patients applying a fast-track extubation protocol, it becomes apparent that even if obese patients may safely undergo a fast-track recovery practice after cardiac surgery, the rate of failure of early extubation remains significantly higher than in nonobese patients. Moreover, the increased difficulties in managing airways in obese patients and their reduced functional capacity and reserve may cause harm in case of extubation failure. It seems reasonable that obese patients undergoing fast-track extubation should be closely monitored in the following operatory hours, especially if a difficult airway and/or ventilation is reported by the attending cardiac anesthesiologist during the induction of anesthesia. In theory, there is not a single BMI cutoff that precludes early extubation. However, it seems likely that obesity, particularly in severe cases, should be adequately accounted for when considering an early extubation, weighing risks and benefits of early extubation.

Furthermore, other than demographic factors, it is crucial to assess the patient's comorbidities when determining the suitability of early extubation protocols in cardiac surgery. In truth, from a research perspective, it is difficult to gauge the impact of these conditions, as usually the patients with moderate or severe organ dysfunction (heart, lung, kidney, liver, coagulation, central nervous system) are not undergoing fast-track extubation. Consequently, it is difficult to establish the weight of each comorbidity. Moreover, these conditions are not evaluated as a dichotomous but rather as a continuous variable with different degrees of dysfunction. For instance, a left ventricular ejection fraction (EF) of 45–50%, despite showing a slight reduction from normal values, can be well compensated and in the absence of other comorbidities should not work as a factor refraining from early extubation. On the other hand, a left ventricular EF below 35–40% probably would refrain most of the cardiac anesthesiologists from accelerating the weaning process. Indeed, among the comorbidities usually considered in the patient's selection for early extubation, the systolic function of the left ventricle, even if it remains a parameter with several limitations, is one of the most commonly considered. A study on almost 9000 adults [2] identified several factors associated with successful early extubation, and among others, the higher left ventricular EF was associated with earlier extubation. Similarly, a mild increase in creatinine does not refrain from undertaking the fast track, whilst the need for hemodialysis 2–3 times a week itself may open the space to a series of considerations on the most appropriate timing for extubation. Hence, such considerations are valid for the other comorbidities, such as lung or liver disease, and it would be ideal to use models with weights on each of the most common and impactful comorbidities. The Euroscore or the Society of Thoracic Surgeons (STS) score is used for weighting the risk of perioperative complications and mortality and could be useful to point out the patients at increased risk, which would generally coincide with the ones at greater risk of early extubation. It is also true that a simpler evaluation conducted with the American Society of Anesthesiologists (ASA) score may be used to evaluate its impact on fast-track extubation. In one study, high-risk patients with preoperative ASA score >3 and New York Heart Association (NYHA) class greater than III (together with intraoperative time >267 min) required significantly longer time to extubation than low-risk patients when the same fast-track cardiac anesthesia technique was used [7].

From this brief summary, it appears evident that several preoperative factors influence the likelihood of a successful early extubation, and each factor may have a different weight. Moreover, the analysis of these factors is rather complex as some variables are dichotomous (i.e., gender, presence of a certain disease, elective or nonelective surgery), but most of the parameters that should be considered are continuous (age and BMI, serum values of albumin and creatinine, diastolic and systolic function, etc.). We envisage that in the near future, the introduction and implementation of artificial intelligence based on data sharing from large databases may produce models wrestling in scoring systems that could help clinicians in balancing the risks of early extubation estimating the chances of success.

19.2.2 Intraoperative Factors

The study by Kiessling et al previous presented, highlights that an early extubation strategy is not suitable for every patient and that longer intraoperative courses will affect the preoperative plan. The preoperative conditions are only the first evaluation, many others intraoperative factors, explain in this part, could compromise the success of early extubation. Among the intraoperative factors that affect postoperative extubation times, we could summarize these three points

1. Surgical Duration and Complexity: Shorter, less complex surgeries are more amenable to early extubation strategies. Operations that do not involve prolonged bypass times or extensive hemodynamic instability lend themselves to quicker recovery and thus, earlier removal of the endotracheal tube.
2. Fluid Management: Optimal intra-operative fluid management ensures that the patient does not emerge from surgery overly fluid overloaded, which can affect pulmonary function and delay extubation.
3. Anesthetic Management: Use of short-acting anesthetic agents and minimal opioid usage during surgery can facilitate quicker return of consciousness and respiratory drive, which are essential for early extubation.

The type of surgical procedure undoubtedly plays an important role. The literature offers several information in this regard, with many studies that have investigated the presence of links between the type of surgery and the extubation time. For instance, the results of the retrospective study by Nguyen et al. [2] already mentioned confirm an already established finding in the literature: the complexity of the cardiac surgical procedure is positively and strongly correlated with prolonged ventilation times and delayed extubation. Therefore, isolated CABG and isolated valve surgery are more likely to successfully achieve early extubation, in contrast to more complex procedures, such as the combined ones, the implantation of ventricular assist device or extracorporeal membrane oxygenation, and the heart and/or lung transplantation. Moreover, aortic surgery has an expected greater risk of bleeding and thus may not be the best scenario when implementing a "fast-track" extubation. Hence, protocols for early extubation should certainly be encouraged in patients undergoing isolated CABG or isolated valve surgery, if the risk of perioperative complications (i.e., bleeding) is deemed reasonable and not particularly increased. For instance, a study published in 2002 on patients undergoing cardiac surgery for coronary artery disease found that early extubation does not increase postoperative complication rates after CABG with cardiopulmonary bypass (CPB), thus establishing it as a reproducible and safe procedure [8].

Apart from being linked to more complex procedures, there are several other pathophysiological reasons why a longer CPB time may negatively influence the decision to perform fast-track extubation for the potential repercussions on the metabolic, hemodynamic, and respiratory function [9, 10]. The necessity to maintain the heart arrested in diastole with cardioplegia for prolonged periods results in greater myocardial stunning and higher likelihood of using high doses of inotropes and vasopressors when coming off CPB. The need for mechanical assistance is also more likely to happen in such cases (i.e., the intra-aortic balloon pump). Moreover, prolonged intraoperative time implies that greater doses of sedatives and analgesics are administered with the risk of greater accumulation. In this context, the type of drugs administered and the patient's hepatic and renal function are crucial determinants. Furthermore, the risk of delirium is higher with prolonged procedures. Not only the cardiovascular and neurological functions are conditioned by prolonged CPB time, but also other organs are affected. Indeed, the coagulation pathway may experience platelet dysfunction with increasing the risk of bleeding, the respiratory function is usually conditioned with worsening gas exchanges [11], and the renal function may deteriorate with well-known consequences. Also, the number of blood product transfusions may be considered as it increases the risk of lung damage, and "fast-track" approach is safer in patients with good gas exchanges and lower risk of perioperative pulmonary complications. Under conditions of prolonged CPB, greater cardiovascular support, and worse lung function, a more watchful approach in the first few hours may be in the patient's best interest, ensuring that cardiovascular stability is achieved, bleeding risk is contained, and gas exchanges are optimized.

Regarding the surgical techniques that can influence early extubation strategies in cardiac surgery, the use of beating heart techniques and of minimally invasive surgery must certainly be mentioned. The elimination of CPB may theoretically reduce the need for prolonged postoperative ventilation [12], though this had not been clearly demonstrated [13–15]. However, it is possible that off-pump procedures, when restricted to patients with simpler coronary anatomy and targets experience shorter intraoperative time and have a faster recovery of cardiovascular function, will reduce the need of postoperative ventilation. Minimally invasive approaches may favor "fast-track" extubation, not only because they are intrinsically adopted for more simpler cases (i.e., isolated valve surgery, single-vessel CABG), but also because the management of postoperative pain could be simpler, especially with the implementation of locoregional anesthesia.

From intraoperative anesthesiological perspectives, several factors can be of interest. Among others, the use of time-directed extubation protocol and low-dose opioid anesthesia has been intensively studied and summarized in a Cochrane literature review [16]. In this systematic review, the authors reported no differences in the risk of 1-year mortality nor of postoperative complications after cardiac surgery between a time-directed extubation protocol and usual care. Moreover, a time-directed extubation protocol seemed to reduce time to extubation (variable from approximately 4–9 h, 16 trials, over 2000 participants) and length of stay in the intensive care unit (reduction of approximately 4–10 h, 13 trials, almost 1900 participants). Although with high heterogeneity, low-dose opioid anesthesia was associated with lower time to extubation (approximately with a reduction from 4 to 10 h, 14 trials, almost 2500 patients) and shorter stay in the ICU (approximately with a reduction from 0.4 to 7 h, 12 trials, almost 1400 participants). However, all these findings were burdened from low level of evidence.

Notably, if a fast-track extubation is planned preoperatively, this decision is usually brought forward in case of a smooth intraoperative course and absence of early postoperative complications. Conversely, it is possible in some cases that the intraoperative course suggests a more cautious approach, as could be in the case of greater than expected CPB time, cardiovascular instability with need of high doses of vasopressors, bleeding, and other complications.

Hence, the preoperative plan may change due to complications in the intraoperative period. Of course, such complications (bleeding, cardiovascular instability and increased lactate levels, oliguria and metabolic derangements, poor gas exchanges, and impaired lung function to name the most common ones) may occur also in the first postoperative hours and may refrain the ICU doctors from pushing forward the plan for "fast-track" extubation.

19.2.3 Postoperative Factors

The postoperative factors that may influence the decision to undertake fast-track extubation usually are a consequence of the preoperative evaluation and of the intraoperative course and finally complete a clinical picture confirming or not the preoperative suggestion to undertake "fast-track" extubation.

Apart from the patients' characteristics and the intraoperative variables, another important concept, is the safety of performing extubation in the late afternoon or in the evening. This issue is certainly linked to lower resources in terms of staffing overnight and possibly to a lower staff reactivity. Extubation during nighttime hours has indeed raised concerns due to potential differences in staffing levels and the availability of experienced personnel. Hence, some studies have evaluated the feasibility of performing overnight extubation, and this is relevant to this chapter as any patient returning to the ICU after being scheduled as afternoon case is extremely likely to have the 6-h window falling after 7.00 or 8.00 pm. The decision whether it is feasible to perform nighttime extubation should be left to the single group of cardiac ICU physicians, depending on local factors. However, three studies showed no increased risk of performing nighttime extubation as compared to daytime [17–19].

The first study analyzed almost 40,000 patients and aimed to investigate the impact of overnight extubation in a statewide, multicenter Society of Thoracic Surgeons database [17]. The primary objective was to determine whether overnight extubation was associated with increased risks of reintubation, mortality, or composite morbidity-mortality. Patients were stratified to three groups according to extubation time: 06:00–18:00, 18:00–24:00, and 24:00–06:00. Overnight extubation was performed in over half of the patients (52.1%) although these were slightly older and with a longer duration of ventilation. There were no differences in operative mortality, reintubation, and composite morbidity-mortality. This was confirmed also by risk adjustment analysis. However, a subgroup analysis showed that those extubated between 24:00 and 06:00 had increased composite morbidity-mortality (OR 1.18) but no difference in reintubation or mortality. A second and smaller study performed on over 2200 patients (less than one-third extubated in the nighttime period) showed interesting findings [18]. Indeed, the likelihood of reintubation was significantly lower for the nighttime than for daytime extubation even after multivariable adjustment (OR = 0.5), with a similar trend for the outcome of reintubation within 72 h (OR = 0.7, though the p value did not reach statistical significance, $p = 0.07$). The ICU length of stay was significantly shorter for the nighttime, but this is likely the result of greater likelihood of discharging to the cardiac surgery ward in the morning. A third retrospective cohort single-center study analyzed over 2200 patients [19], hence with similar numbers to the previous one. However, in this study, the percentage of patients extubated overnight was much smaller (lower than 10%). The authors found that rates of reintubation were similar between groups, though nighttime extubation was associated with shorter duration of mechanical ventilation and ICU stay and hospital LOS. The evidence from these studies suggests that routine overnight extubation in cardiac surgery patients is probably safe, though the slight increase in composite morbidity-mortality for very-late-night extubation suggested by the largest study warrants attention. Another consideration that clinicians should balance is the fact that usually patients scheduled for operation in the afternoon may suffer from prolonged fasting and more impactful consequences from metabolic and hemodynamic perspectives [20]. However, the literature is conflictual in this regard, with studies suggesting both an increase or not in the mortality and morbidity of patients scheduled in the afternoon as compared to those operated in the morning [21–24].

Overall, the above findings support the practice of not delaying extubation purely based on the time of day, provided that patients meet the necessary clinical criteria.

However, there are several clinical implications:

1. Staffing and training: Adequate staffing levels and availability of experienced personnel during nighttime hours must be ensured to manage potential complications promptly.
2. Monitoring and support: Robust monitoring and protocols must be implemented to quickly identify and address any adverse events occurring after extubation, regardless of the time of the day.

3. Individualized care: Decisions on extubation timing should be individualized based on patient-specific factors, clinical stability, and readiness for extubation rather than strictly adhering to a daytime extubation policy.

Having said that overnight extubation seems safe, it is also worth suggesting that a publication bias may be present when looking at the literature from this perspective. Indeed, studies with a positive message are more likely to get published as compared to others with more negative findings. Moreover, there could be some fear from authors in reporting a negative result from their institution. In this interesting retrospective data analysis paper, Gutsche et al. tried to increase early extubation rates by redesigning patient care processes using Lean principles to remove barriers and facilitate early extubation with guideline management [25]. Using Lean methodologies, the care process for cardiac surgery patients was analyzed from the preoperative period to postoperative extubation. A value stream analysis identified waste and root causes of delays, including hypothermia upon ICU admission, prolonged weaning using arterial blood gas results, and equipment delays. Lean work design principles were implemented to address these issues. Post-intervention, the rate of extubation within 6 h significantly increased from 27% to 50%. The median length of intubation significantly decreased from approximately 10–6 h. Factors predicting extubation within 6 h included age, renal failure, and gender. This project demonstrates the effectiveness of using Lean principles to improve clinical processes and outcomes in cardiac surgery patients. We summarize the most frequent complications that may occur in the first postoperative hours and delay the decision to extubate, as follows:

- Worsening cardiovascular instability with increase in pharmacological and/or mechanical support.
- Deterioration in gas exchanges or reduction in lung compliance with increase in the ventilatory support.
- Decrease in the urine output and/or increase in the catabolites and other markers of organ hypoperfusion (lactates, venous oxygen saturation, venoarterial carbon dioxide gap, etc.)
- Increased output from chest drains as sign of possible defects in hemostasis and/or signs of ongoing coagulopathy.

19.3 Strategies to Achieve Early Extubation

Although success of early extubation is strictly correlated with patients' selection, also physicians' management and strategies can importantly influence it. In fact, the success of fast-track extubation depends on various clinical interventions and strategies, and many of these are anesthesia related. This paragraph examines the factors associated with early extubation in cardiac surgery, with a particular focus on findings from recent research and a consensus statement by ITACTAIC [26].

The role of anesthesiologists is pivotal in performing fast-track cardiac surgery, as most interventions associated with extubation within 6 h post-surgery relate to anesthesia strategies. In this regard, the above mentioned consensus evaluated among others which anesthesia-related approaches are associated with shorter periods of mechanical ventilation in randomized controlled trials, highlighting several potentially effective approaches that are hereby summarized.

1. General anesthesia: (a) The use of dexmedetomidine in theater in elective patients and as a postoperative sedation strategy in the ICU seems to be associated with reduced duration of endotracheal intubation. (b) Opioid-sparing approaches: enhanced recovery and quicker respiratory recovery are associated with the use of low-dose and short-acting opioids.
2. Monitoring: In patients undergoing general anesthesia, anesthesia depth monitoring with either processed EEG or halogenated end tidal concentration is associated with fast-track extubation.
3. Locoregional anesthesia: locoregional anesthesia for pain management has shown promises in promoting fast-track extubation.

Techniques such as the parasternal block, particularly if performed postoperatively, and the erector spinae plane block have demonstrated efficacy in pain management and support fast-track protocols.
4. Adaptive support ventilation is an emerging technology that automates ventilatory adjustments to meet the patient's respiratory needs. Studies have shown that adaptive support ventilation can significantly shorten time to extubation compared to conventional ventilation methods.
5. Surgical techniques: Minimally invasive surgical access is associated with fast-track extubation.

The above-summarized consensus provides actionable insights for daily clinical practice, emphasizing the role of careful selection of drugs and dosages, hence suggesting the use of precision medicine approaches with anesthesia depth monitoring. The shift towards implementation of fascial blocks in cardiac surgery patients is "unstoppable" and rapidly evolving with improvements in the strategies for pain management of these patients. Future studies should focus on refining fast-track extubation protocols, particularly the roles of specific fascial blocks like serratus (no RCT performed) and parasternal blocks, the two most commonly used peripheral blocks in cardiac surgery.

One more technique that should be performed by al physicians is patient educational: psychological readiness in fact plays a crucial role. Patients who are well-informed about the procedure and the post-operative care process, including the expectations for early extubation, tend to experience less anxiety and better overall outcomes.

19.4 Criteria for Safe Extubation in Postoperative Cardiac Surgery Patients

Safe extubation in cardiac surgery patients is a critical component of postoperative care. It requires a careful assessment of specific criteria to ensure if the patient is ready for extubation. Strategies such as the use of appropriate anesthetic agents, meticulous control of hemodilution, and vigilant postoperative monitoring are essential for achieving early and safe extubation. Adhering to these criteria and strategies minimizes the risk of complications and promotes a smoother recovery process for cardiac surgery patients [17, 18].

Unless extubation takes place in the operating room, at the end of each cardiac surgery procedure, the patient is transported to the ICU for postoperative monitoring and organ support whenever needed. The decision to extubate is based on a thorough assessment of the patient's clinical status. The key criteria for extubation can be summarized in:

1. Consciousness: On sedation hold, the patient must be fully conscious and able to follow commands. This indicates adequate neurological function and recovery from anesthesia. This ensures that the patient can protect their airway and participate actively in respiratory recovery.
2. Pain should be well controlled.
3. Normothermia: The patient must have achieved stable and normal body temperature. Among others, hypothermia can affect metabolic, coagulation pathway and cardiovascular function, making early extubation risk.
4. Hemodynamic stability: The patient must be hemodynamically stable, meaning that blood pressure and heart rate are within normal or acceptable range without the need for excessive pharmacological support (the use of the inotropic score may be a good option with a cutoff considered by each institution) and that such support is in decalage or stable rather than on the rise. The hemodynamic stability, whenever possible, should be checked using echocardiography evaluation. Hemodynamic stability suggests a lower risk of adverse events upon extubation.
5. Absence of active bleeding: There must be no suspicion that the patient is experiencing bleeding with an adequate monitoring of the output from the chest drains. Active bleeding

can lead to hemodynamic instability and complicate the extubation process.
6. Good gas exchanges: The patient must demonstrate adequate respiratory function with no compromise when ventilation is downgraded to a support mode (most typically in pressure support), including sufficient oxygenation and ventilation. This is typically assessed by blood gas analysis and clinical evaluation of respiratory mechanics. A chest X-ray was usually performed after surgery and checked before extubation.
7. Adequate metabolic conditions: The patient's condition should suggest that organ perfusion is adequate, for instance showing that lactate levels are not on the rise, and that renal function is appropriate with a normal urine output.

Once the above conditions are met, it can be clinically judged that the patient may continue the pathway of fast track as preventively and adequately planned. Conversely, if any of the above criteria are not satisfactorily met, it can be risky to push for an early extubation without addressing the ongoing alterations and discrepancies.

19.5 Conclusion

Nowadays, early extubation by the sixth postoperative hour seems to be a crucial goal for the cardiac anesthesiologist, and it is likely to become a standard practice for certain categories of patients. However, the adequate selection of the candidates to early extubation remains a challenge as it depends on patient's demographics data and comorbidities, type of surgical intervention, and a regular intra- and postoperative course. Moreover, local factors play an important role and should be considered by each team.

Patients adequately selected as appropriate for early extubation should receive targeted interventions within a fast-track protocol, favoring a speedy recovery. For instance, regional anesthesia techniques and opioid-sparing strategies offer advantages in this regard. However, patients may not proceed further towards early extubation if the intra- and postoperative course is not smooth.

It seems clear that early extubation in cardiac surgery patients is facilitated not only by a combination of advance in surgical and anesthesia techniques but also by an hospital systematic approach that can favour this approach. Ongoing research and consensus efforts continue to refine these protocols, aiming to enhance patient recovery and optimize healthcare resources.We envisage that the proportion of patients undergoing early extubation will gradually increase. However, large studies and possibly databases are needed to provide clinicians with the tools to select the patients for early extubation. Artificial intelligence may play a role with machine learning from large datasets and could help in creating prediction models applicable at the bedspace.

References

1. Engelman DT, Ben Ali W, Williams JB, Perrault LP, Reddy VS, Arora RC, et al. Guidelines for perioperative care in cardiac surgery: enhanced recovery after surgery society recommendations. JAMA Surg. 2019;154(8):755–66.
2. Nguyen Q, Coghlan K, Hong Y, Nagendran J, MacArthur R, Lam W. Factors associated with early extubation after cardiac surgery: a retrospective single-center experience. J Cardiothorac Vasc Anesth. 2021;35(7):1964–70.
3. Arom KV, Emery RW, Petersen RJ, Schwartz M. Cost-effectiveness and predictors of early extubation. Ann Thorac Surg. 1995;60(1):127–32.
4. Bezanson JL, Deaton C, Craver J, Jones E, Guyton RA, Weintraub WS. Predictors and outcomes associated with early extubation in older adults undergoing coronary artery bypass surgery. Am J Crit Care. 2001;10(6):383–90.
5. Kurki TS, Kataja M. Preoperative prediction of postoperative morbidity in coronary artery bypass grafting. Ann Thorac Surg. 1996;61(6):1740–5.
6. Brandt M, Harder K, Walluscheck KP, Schöttler J, Rahimi A, Möller F, et al. Severe obesity does not adversely affect perioperative mortality and morbidity in coronary artery bypass surgery. Eur J Cardiothorac Surg. 2001;19(5):662–6.
7. Kiessling AH, Huneke P, Reyher C, Bingold T, Zierer A, Moritz A. Risk factor analysis for fast track protocol failure. J Cardiothorac Surg. 2013;8:47.
8. Reis J, Mota JC, Ponce P, Costa-Pereira A, Guerreiro M. Early extubation does not increase complication rates after coronary artery bypass graft surgery with

cardiopulmonary bypass. Eur J Cardiothorac Surg. 2002;21(6):1026–30.
9. Sanfilippo F, Chiarenza F, Cassisi C, Santonocito C, Tsoutsouras T, Trivella M, et al. The effects of on-pump and off-pump coronary artery bypass surgery on metabolic profiles in the early postoperative period. J Cardiothorac Vasc Anesth. 2016;30:909.
10. Chiarenza F, Tsoutsouras T, Cassisi C, Santonocito C, Gerry S, Astuto M, et al. The effects of on-pump and off-pump coronary artery bypass surgery on respiratory function in the early postoperative period. J Intensive Care Med. 2019;34(2):126–32.
11. Sanfilippo F, Palumbo GJ, Bignami E, Pavesi M, Ranucci M, Scolletta S, et al. Acute respiratory distress syndrome in the perioperative period of cardiac surgery: predictors, diagnosis, prognosis, management options, and future directions. J Cardiothorac Vasc Anesth. 2022;36(4):1169–79.
12. Mack MJ. Beating heart surgery: does it make a difference? Am Heart Hosp J. 2003;1(2):149–57.
13. Lamy A, Devereaux PJ, Prabhakaran D, Taggart DP, Hu S, Paolasso E, et al. Off-pump or on-pump coronary-artery bypass grafting at 30 days. N Engl J Med. 2012;366(16):1489–97.
14. Legare JF, Buth KJ, King S, Wood J, Sullivan JA, Hancock Friesen C, et al. Coronary bypass surgery performed off pump does not result in lower in-hospital morbidity than coronary artery bypass grafting performed on pump. Circulation. 2004;109(7):887–92.
15. Diegeler A, Borgermann J, Kappert U, Breuer M, Boning A, Ursulescu A, et al. Off-pump versus on-pump coronary-artery bypass grafting in elderly patients. N Engl J Med. 2013;368(13):1189–98.
16. Wong WT, Lai VK, Chee YE, Lee A. Fast-track cardiac care for adult cardiac surgical patients. Cochrane Database Syst Rev. 2016;9(9):Cd003587.
17. Krebs ED, Hawkins RB, Mehaffey JH, Fonner CE, Speir AM, Quader MA, et al. Is routine extubation overnight safe in cardiac surgery patients? J Thorac Cardiovasc Surg. 2019;157(4):1533–42.
18. Tischenkel BR, Gong MN, Shiloh AL, Pittignano VC, Keschner YG, Glueck JA, et al. Daytime versus nighttime extubations: a comparison of reintubation, length of stay, and mortality. J Intensive Care Med. 2016;31(2):118–26.
19. Gershengorn HB, Wunsch H, Hua M, Bavaria JE, Gutsche J. Association of overnight extubation with outcomes after cardiac surgery in the intensive care unit. Ann Thorac Surg. 2019;108(2):432–42.
20. Santonocito C, Cassisi C, Chiarenza F, Caruso A, Murabito P, Maybauer MO, et al. Morning or afternoon scheduling for elective coronary artery bypass surgery: influence of longer fasting periods from metabolic and hemodynamic perspectives. Ann Card Anaesth. 2024;27(2):136–43.
21. Ranucci M, Casalino S, Frigiola A, Diena M, Parolari A, Boveri S, et al. The importance of being the morning case in adult cardiac surgery: a propensity-matched analysis. Eur J Cardiothorac Surg. 2023;63(6)
22. Nemeth S, Schnell S, Argenziano M, Ning Y, Kurlansky P. Daytime variation does not impact outcome of cardiac surgery: results from a diverse, multi-institutional cardiac surgery network. J Thorac Cardiovasc Surg. 2021;162(1):56–67.e44.
23. Montaigne D, Marechal X, Modine T, Coisne A, Mouton S, Fayad G, et al. Daytime variation of perioperative myocardial injury in cardiac surgery and its prevention by rev-Erbα antagonism: a single-centre propensity-matched cohort study and a randomised study. Lancet (London, England). 2018;391(10115):59–69.
24. du Fay de Lavallaz J, Puelacher C, Lurati Buse G, Bolliger D, Germanier D, Hidvegi R, et al. Daytime variation of perioperative myocardial injury in non-cardiac surgery and effect on outcome. Heart. 2019;105(11):826–33.
25. Gutsche JT, Erickson L, Ghadimi K, Augoustides JG, Dimartino J, Szeto WY, et al. Advancing extubation time for cardiac surgery patients using lean work design. J Cardiothorac Vasc Anesth. 2014;28(6):1490–6.
26. Silvetti S, et al. Recommendations for fast-track extubation in adult cardiac surgery patients: a consensus statement. Minerva Anestesiol. 2024;90(11):957–68.

20 Post-operative Implications

Simona Silvetti, Tommaso Aloisio, and Pietro Bertini

20.1 Respiratory Management

Effective respiratory management is essential for achieving early extubation and successful recovery in the context of ERACS protocols for cardiac patients. This section details strategies for evaluating respiratory function, supporting respiration post-extubation, and managing potential respiratory complications.

Continuous respiratory rate and oxygen saturation monitoring are crucial in assessing the patient's spontaneous breathing and oxygenation levels. Safe extubation typically requires a respiratory rate of 12–20 breaths per minute and an $SpO_2 > 92\%$ on minimal or no supplemental oxygen [1]. Arterial blood gas analysis is also essential, providing critical data on the patient's ability to maintain adequate gas exchange independently. Parameters such as a PaO_2/FiO_2 ratio above 200 and an average acid-base balance indicate readiness for extubation [2].

Measuring inspiratory muscle strength is another essential step. This involves assessing the functionality of the diaphragmatic and respiratory muscles, with a negative inspiratory force stronger than −20 cmH_2O generally supporting extubation readiness [3]. Additionally, chest X-rays ensure no acute changes that might complicate extubation, such as new infiltrates, pneumothorax, or significant atelectasis [4]. A spontaneous breathing trial assesses the patient's ability to breathe unassisted. Successfully passing a spontaneous breathing trial, which often involves 30–120 min of breathing without assistance, indicates potential extubation [5].

For patients at high risk of extubation failure, noninvasive ventilation may be used immediately post-extubation to support ventilation and prevent re-intubation [6]. High-flow nasal cannula is another strategy that provides heated and humidified oxygen at high flow rates, improving comfort and maintaining airway hydration and patency, which is particularly beneficial after extubation [7]. Chest physiotherapy, including percussion, vibration, and postural drainage, facilitates secretion clearance and improves lung compliance [8].

Incentive spirometry and early and regular mobilization prevent or treat atelectasis [9], a common issue post-cardiac surgery. Vigilance for signs of pneumonia is critical, with aggressive treatment involving antibiotics and supportive care initiated promptly upon diagnosis [10].

S. Silvetti
Department of Cardiac Anesthesia and Intensive Care, Cardiovascular Network, IRCCS Ospedale Policlinico San Martino, Genoa, Italy

T. Aloisio
Department of Cardiothoracic and Vascular Anesthesia and Intensive Care Unit (ICU), Istituto di Ricovero e Cura a Carattere Scientifico (IRCCS) Policlinico San Donato, San Donato Milanese, Milan, Italy
e-mail: tommaso.aloisio@grupposandonato.it

P. Bertini (✉)
Department of Anesthesia and Intensive Care, Casa di Cura San Rossore, Pisa, Italy

G. Sepolvere, S. Silvetti (eds.), *Fast-Track in Cardiac Anesthesia*,
https://doi.org/10.1007/978-3-031-70899-2_20

Should respiratory distress occur, criteria for re-intubation are clearly defined within ERAS protocols, and timely re-intubation is critical to patient outcomes. Re-intubation criteria typically include the presence of signs such as severe respiratory distress, inability to maintain adequate oxygenation or ventilation despite noninvasive support, and hemodynamic instability. These criteria are based on objective measures, including a drop in oxygen saturation below a critical threshold (often $SpO_2 < 90\%$ on high-flow oxygen), a significant increase in respiratory rate (e.g., >35 breaths per minute), or the development of hypercapnia with acidosis indicated by arterial blood gas analysis (elevated $PaCO_2$ and low pH).

The decision to re-intubate should be made swiftly to prevent further deterioration. Delays in re-intubation can lead to severe hypoxemia, cardiac arrest, or other life-threatening complications. The process involves quickly assessing the patient's respiratory status and ensuring that all necessary equipment and personnel are available for the procedure. Once the decision is made, the re-intubation process must be executed efficiently to minimize patient discomfort and complications.

Timely re-intubation also allows for the stabilization of respiratory and hemodynamic parameters, reducing the risk of subsequent complications such as ventilator-associated pneumonia. This proactive approach aligns with the goals of ERAS protocols, which emphasize minimizing patient discomfort and optimizing outcomes through early identification and management of complications. By adhering to these protocols, healthcare providers can ensure that patients receive the best possible care during the critical postoperative period, thereby enhancing recovery and overall outcomes [11].

20.2 Pain Management

The pain from cardiac surgery reaches a peak in the first 2 days. Causes of pain include surgery, operative positioning, and invasion of medical presidia such as chest tubes and endotracheal tubes. ERACS recommends effective perioperative pain control to improve patient outcomes, alleviate suffering, gain early mobilization after surgery, reduce hospital stay, and improve patient satisfaction and functional recovery [12]. Optimal analgesia control is crucial for successful early extubation after cardiac surgery. Poor pain management during the early post-cardiac surgery period results in deleterious side effects on lung (atelectasis, pneumonia, and bronchial secretion stasis) and cardiovascular (increased oxygen consumption and tachycardia) and musculoskeletal (muscle weakness and disuse) systems that can lead to re-intubation.

This section discusses the strategies employed to manage pain following cardiac surgery, particularly in the context of early extubation.

20.2.1 Pharmacological Approaches

To obtain adequate analgesia control and simultaneously opioid sparing, these needed to be replaced with something else. As a solution, ERACS recommends multimodal analgesia and recommends consideration of regional analgesia in all patients who underwent cardiac surgery procedures [13, 14].

20.2.1.1 Opioids

Opioid-based anesthesia and analgesia were traditional components of perioperative care for cardiac surgery patients. The growing enthusiasm for enhanced recovery programs coupled with evidence of potential harm associated with high-dose opioids suggests that we reconsider the role of opioids in cardiac surgery. While it is effective, the use of opioids is minimized in the context of early extubation to avoid respiratory depression. Short-acting opioids are preferred for their quick onset and ease of titration during the postoperative period.

Recently, an interdisciplinary North American panel of experts defined a consensus recommendations for optimal pain management and opioid stewardship for cardiac surgery patients [15]. The process resulted in six statements regarding analgesia strategy, focused on avoiding high-dose opioids and encouraging ERACS protocol application, such as using multimodal analgesia and locoregional anesthesia, patient education, and structured system-level opioid prescription practices.

The recommendations for cardiac surgery patients are the following:

1. Against the routine use of high-dose opioid anesthesia or analgesia (grade: strong; level of evidence [LOE]: B).
2. Implementation of perioperative opioid stewardship (grade: robust; LOE: B).
3. Use of multimodal non-opioid analgesics (grade: strong; LOE: C).
4. Consider using regional techniques (grade: weak; LOE C).
5. Patients and healthcare providers receive formal education on perioperative analgesia, including pain management expectations, analgesic options, and potential side effects (grade: strong; LOE: B).
6. Development of program-specific multidisciplinary pathways for perioperative pain management (grade: strong; LOE: B).

20.2.1.2 Non-opioid Analgesics

The "fast-track" approach first demonstrated the effectiveness of an opioid-sparing strategy in improving cardiac surgical outcomes. ERACS guidelines are cited as follows: "Multimodal analgesia has emerged as an essential component of all ERAS pathways since concurrent use of primarily non-opioid analgesics can have additive, if not synergistic, analgesic effect" [14].

Using multiple agents and techniques that each target a different pain pathway, modern multimodal cardiac surgical protocols hope to create a synergy to improve pain control and decrease opioid dependence [12]. Further, the goal is to use lower doses of each agent and decrease the incidence of side effects.

Table 20.1 summarizes the typical non-opioid drugs and dosage used after cardiac surgery procedures.

An essential element of multimodal pain management is preemptive analgesic dosing rather than reactive medication use. Analgesics are started preoperatively and intraoperatively, and some agents are administered at scheduled times during the postoperative period. This preemptive approach can achieve improved analgesia management with decreased opioid use [16, 17]. Regional anesthesia for cardiac surgery is also a promising adjunct.

Table 20.1 Pharmacological multimodal analgesia strategies

Drug	Dosage
Acetaminophen	500–1000 mg IV every 6 h
Gabapentin	100–300 mg IV every 8 h
Pregabalin	Preoperative 50–150 mg IV–postoperative 50–150 mg IV every 8 h
Ketamine	0.1–1 mg/kg IV
Dexmedetomidine	0.5–1 γ/kg/h infusion
NSAID	Every 6–8 h
Lidocaine	1 mg/kg IV bolus, then infusion 0.5–2 mg/kg/h

20.2.1.3 Regional Anesthesia

Several studies investigating neuraxial analgesia, as either thoracic epidural analgesia or spinal analgesia, reported reduced perioperative opioid consumption, improved pain control, earlier extubation, and possibly reduced cardiopulmonary complications [18, 19].

Having now passed the era of neuraxial blocks (epidural and paravertebral block) due to the well-known side effects such as epidural hematoma and pneumothorax or due to concerns related to anticoagulation, cardiac anesthesia is oriented towards new regional techniques that can have the desired pain control as a final result.

Many studies have recently been published about fascial blocks in cardiac surgery. The most studied blocks are parasternal superficial block (PSB), pectoral block (PECS) (described for the first time by Blanco et al. for breast surgeries), and erector spinae plane (ESP) block, and because these are all superficial blocks, they have significantly lower side effects and risk of hematoma formation [20].

A randomized controlled trial (RCT) published in 2018 by Kumar et al. [21] analyzed 40 adult patients undergoing coronary artery bypass grafting or valve surgeries through midline sternotomy. Group 1 patients did not receive Pecs block, whereas group 2 patients received bilateral Pecs block postoperatively. As a result, Pecs group patients required a lesser duration of ventilator support ($P < 0.0001$) than the control group. Pain scores at rest and cough were significantly low in the Pecs group at 0, 3, 6, 12, and 18 h from extubation ($P < 0.05$). Furthermore, 34 episodes of rescue analgesia were given in the control group, whereas in the Pecs group, there were only 4 episodes of rescue analgesia.

A more recent RCT by Zang et al. [22] investigated the effect of bilateral pectoral-intercostal fascial block in 108 patients undergoing open cardiac surgery allocated to either receive or have no nerve block. This study concluded that the nerve block provides adequate analgesia and accelerates recovery (in terms of time of extubation, ICU stay, and hospital length of stay) in patients undergoing open cardiac surgery.

A meta-analysis published by Dost et al. [23] analyzed the effects of regional anesthesia on postoperative opioid consumption in patients undergoing open cardiac surgery. This study concluded that all the regional anesthesia techniques evaluated significantly reduced postoperative opioid consumption at 24 h and that the ESP block was the most effective treatment.

A similar finding was published in another recent Li J et al. meta-analysis. The authors evaluated ultrasound-guided PSB and found a decrease in opioid consumption, other than improvement in clinical outcomes, such as mechanical ventilation time, total length of ICU stay, and hospital days [24].

Several fascial blocks, at the moment, are still challenging to determine which is better, given the lack of studies available in the literature. With this evidence, we can conclude that regional anesthesia is a crucial pain technique in this new era of cardiac surgery, as it induces opioid sparing, reduces hemodynamic impact without interfering with the coagulative status of the patient, and enables a prompt fast track.

20.3 Cognitive and Psychological Outcomes

The impact of early extubation on cognitive and psychological outcomes in postoperative cardiac surgery patients is significant and multifaceted. Implementing early extubation protocols within the ERAS framework requires careful consideration of both potential benefits and associated cognitive and psychological health risks.

Early extubation has been shown to potentially reduce the incidence of delirium, a common complication associated with prolonged sedation and mechanical ventilation. Delirium, characterized by acute confusion and cognitive dysfunction, can significantly affect patient recovery and long-term outcomes. Shorter durations of mechanical ventilation are crucial in mitigating factors contributing to postoperative cognitive dysfunction. Studies, such as those conducted by Girard et al. [25], have demonstrated that reducing the time patients spend on mechanical ventilation can lower the incidence of delirium. This reduction is particularly beneficial for elderly patients, who are more susceptible to cognitive decline and delirium due to their age and the invasive nature of cardiac surgery [26].

There is ongoing debate about whether early extubation contributes to long-term cognitive decline. While the early removal of the endotracheal tube can potentially reduce exposure to anesthetics and sedatives, which might negatively impact cognitive function, this approach must be balanced with the patient's physiological readiness and the potential for hemodynamic instability. Research by Pandharipande et al. [27] suggests that minimizing sedative use can help maintain cognitive function postoperatively. However, it is critical to carefully assess each patient to ensure that the benefits of early extubation outweigh the risks. This selective approach helps balance achieving cognitive benefits and avoiding complications arising from premature extubation.

Psychologically, early extubation can significantly alleviate feelings of anxiety and distress associated with prolonged mechanical ventilation. The psychological benefits of reducing the duration of mechanical ventilation include alleviating the sensations of breathlessness and claustrophobia, which can substantially reduce anxiety levels. Patients often report a sense of regained control and normalcy, which benefits their mental health and overall recovery. Studies such as those by Jubran et al. [28] highlight that early extubation can foster a sense of control and normalcy, contributing to reduced anxiety and improved mental health outcomes.

Patient satisfaction tends to be higher with early extubation. Allowing for earlier communication, nutrition, and mobilization significantly contributes to a sense of progress and recovery. Patients extubated earlier often report higher satisfaction levels due to increased comfort and reduced time spent in the ICU. Research by Fiest et al. [29] supports these findings, indicating that patient satisfaction is closely linked to the timing of extubation, with those extubated earlier reporting a better overall recovery experience.

Comfort is another critical aspect impacted by early extubation. The early removal of the endotracheal tube generally improves patient comfort, significantly affecting the overall recovery experience. Comfort is vital to patient care, influencing physical recovery and psychological well-being. Thompson et al. [30] emphasize that enhanced patient comfort through early extubation leads to better recovery outcomes, as patients are more likely to engage in necessary postoperative activities, such as mobilization and respiratory exercises, which are essential for recovery.

The careful management of cognitive and psychological aspects in the postoperative care of cardiac surgery patients is essential. As part of a comprehensive ERACS protocol, early extubation can potentially enhance the recovery experience by addressing these critical outcomes. However, individual assessments and tailored approaches are crucial to optimize patient-specific protocols. By focusing on each patient's individual needs, healthcare providers can ensure that early extubation is implemented safely and effectively, maximizing the cognitive and psychological benefits while minimizing the associated risks.

20.4 Protocols for Postoperative Care

Postoperative care protocols aligned with early extubation strategies under ERAS protocols are essential for optimizing recovery in cardiac surgery patients. These protocols involve an interdisciplinary approach, encompassing adjustments in anesthesia, surgical practices, and nursing care. Effective postoperative care begins with closely monitoring vital signs, fluid balance, and electrocardiographic changes immediately after surgery. This vigilant monitoring ensures that deviations from standard recovery patterns are promptly identified and addressed. Continuous surveillance allows healthcare providers to address issues such as hemodynamic instability, arrhythmias, or respiratory distress promptly, which are common in the immediate postoperative period. For instance, continuous ECG monitoring can detect arrhythmias early, allowing immediate intervention to prevent further complications. Similarly, regular fluid balance assessment helps avoid dehydration and fluid overload, which are critical in maintaining hemodynamic and respiratory stability.

Early mobilization, patient education, and nursing care adjustments further support recovery, leading to shorter hospital stays and better overall outcomes for cardiac surgery patients. This comprehensive, patient-centered approach ensures a smooth transition through the different phases of postoperative recovery [31].

Pain management is a cornerstone of postoperative care, particularly in the context of early extubation. Implementing multimodal pain management strategies, including regional anesthesia, helps minimize opioid use and facilitates early mobilization. Adequate pain control enhances patient comfort, improves respiratory mechanics, and reduces the risk of complications such as atelectasis and pneumonia. Studies have shown that multimodal analgesia, which may include acetaminophen, NSAIDs, gabapentinoids, and local anesthetics, can significantly reduce pain and opioid consumption, supporting early extubation goals. Opioid-sparing strategies are essential as they reduce the risk of side effects like respiratory depression, which can delay extubation and recovery. The combination of various analgesics targets different pain pathways, providing effective relief while minimizing the use of any single medication. This approach, supported by evidence from Kehlet and Wilmore

(2008), enhances patient recovery and reduces hospital stays. Multimodal pain management strategies are particularly effective in reducing opioid reliance, ensuring that patients experience less discomfort and recover more swiftly. By minimizing opioid use and employing diverse analgesic techniques, healthcare providers can significantly improve postoperative outcomes and facilitate earlier extubation in cardiac surgery patients [32].

Respiratory support is another critical component of postoperative care, especially for patients undergoing early extubation. Techniques such as incentive spirometry, noninvasive positive-pressure ventilation, and other respiratory therapies support lung function and oxygenation. These interventions help maintain adequate ventilation and prevent respiratory complications, crucial for patients transitioning from mechanical ventilation to independent breathing. Incentive spirometry encourages deep breathing and helps prevent atelectasis, a common complication following surgery. Noninvasive ventilation methods like CPAP or BiPAP provide necessary respiratory support, ensuring that patients maintain adequate oxygenation and ventilation without the risks associated with re-intubation. This aspect of care is essential in the immediate post-extubation period, promoting smoother transitions and reducing the likelihood of respiratory distress. These respiratory support methods are vital for maintaining lung function post-extubation, ensuring that patients breathe effectively and recover swiftly. By employing these techniques, healthcare providers can significantly improve postoperative outcomes, facilitating early extubation and enhancing overall recovery in cardiac surgery patients [33].

Fluid and nutrition management are vital in postoperative care. Early initiation of enteral nutrition supports healing by providing necessary nutrients, while careful fluid management prevents complications such as pulmonary edema, which can impair respiratory function and delay recovery.

Maintaining this balance is crucial for optimal hydration and nutritional status, essential for overall recovery. Early enteral nutrition aids the healing process, and monitoring fluid intake and output helps avoid volume overload. This approach ensures that patients receive adequate nutrition without risking fluid-related complications, promoting smoother recovery, and reducing the likelihood of issues such as pulmonary edema. Proper fluid and nutrition management are critical to supporting patients' overall recovery and preventing further complications in the postoperative period [34].

Early mobilization is crucial for preventing postoperative complications like deep vein thrombosis and pulmonary embolism. Encouraging patients to move as soon as possible after surgery improves circulation, muscle strength, and pulmonary function. Studies have shown that early mobilization significantly reduces the risk of complications and promotes faster recovery. This proactive approach helps shorten hospital stays and enhance overall functional recovery. Collaboration among healthcare team members, including physical therapists, nurses, and physicians, is essential to create a safe and effective mobilization plan tailored to each patient's needs. By prioritizing early mobilization, healthcare providers can ensure better outcomes and a smoother recovery process for cardiac surgery patients [35].

Patient education is crucial for ensuring understanding and cooperation with postoperative care protocols. Educating patients about the goals of care, including the benefits and process of early extubation, helps them understand the importance of participating in recovery. Effective education can reduce anxiety, improve compliance with rehabilitation protocols, and enhance patient outcomes. Patient education is a critical component of postoperative care [36].

Nursing care adjustments are integral to supporting the early extubation process. Nurses frequently assess pain, respiratory distress, and signs of neurological changes to detect any complications early. They collaborate closely with respiratory therapists to wean patients from the ventilator according to established criteria. Proper management of surgical incisions, including appropriate dressings and monitoring for signs of infection, is also an essential aspect of nursing care. Teaching patients effective coughing and deep breathing techniques is essential to maintain airway clearance post-extubation. Providing reassurance and psychological support helps address anxiety or discomfort associated with early extubation and recovery, which is vital for patient well-being. Nursing care adjustments are essential for supporting the complex needs of postoperative patients [37].

These protocols and adjustments are designed to support the early extubation process, minimize the risk of complications, and ensure a smooth transition through the different phases of postoperative recovery. A comprehensive approach that covers all aspects of patient care, from physiological monitoring to emotional support, is crucial for facilitating a successful recovery for cardiac surgery patients. By employing an interdisciplinary and patient-centered approach, healthcare providers can optimize outcomes and enhance the overall recovery experience for patients undergoing cardiac surgery.

20.5 Long-Term Outcomes and Resource Utilization

Implementing early extubation practices in cardiac surgery within the ERACS protocols profoundly impacts resource utilization and long-term outcomes. These practices are designed to optimize ICU and overall hospital resources while assessing their cost-effectiveness and improving patient outcomes. Early extubation removes the endotracheal tube within 6 h post-surgery, facilitating earlier patient recovery and reducing the need for prolonged ICU stays.

First, early extubation has been shown to reduce the incidence of long-term complications associated with prolonged mechanical ventilation. Studies have indicated that prolonged ventilation increases the risk of chronic respiratory issues, muscle weakness, and other long-term health problems [25]. By reducing the duration of mechanical ventilation, early extubation can mitigate these risks and promote better long-term health outcomes for patients.

Second, the psychological benefits of early extubation also play a critical role in long-term recovery. Reduced anxiety and discomfort associated with shorter ventilation times and quicker ICU discharges can lead to better mental health outcomes. Patients who are extubated early often report higher levels of satisfaction and well-being, which can positively influence their overall recovery trajectory [28]. This enhanced psychological state can reduce the likelihood of post-traumatic stress disorder and other long-term psychological issues that are sometimes associated with prolonged ICU stays.

Another significant aspect of early extubation is its role in facilitating early mobilization. Early mobilization is a critical component of the ERAS protocols and is associated with numerous benefits, including improved cardiovascular function, enhanced pulmonary mechanics, and reduced risk of deep vein thrombosis and pulmonary embolism. Encouraging patients to ambulate as soon as possible after surgery helps improve circulation and lung function, accelerating recovery and reducing hospital stays.

This proactive approach requires collaboration among the healthcare team, including physical therapists, nurses, and physicians, to create a safe and effective mobilization plan tailored to each patient's needs.

From a long-term perspective, the benefits of early extubation extend beyond immediate cost savings and resource optimization. Early extubation, mobilization, and fewer complications contribute to a quicker return to normal activities and work, positively impacting patients' quality of life and economic productivity. Patients who recover faster are more likely to return to their daily routines and professional responsibilities sooner, which can positively impact their mental health and overall well-being. This aspect of recovery is crucial for working-age adults who may face economic pressures and responsibilities [38].

Finally, by facilitating earlier weaning from mechanical ventilation, patients can be transferred out of the ICU to less intensive levels of care more rapidly. This frees up critical ICU beds for other patients in need and reduces the workload and staffing demands in these high-acuity areas [31]. Reducing ICU occupancy translates to decreased utilization of monitoring equipment, ventilators, and other specialized ICU resources. This cascading effect allows for more efficient allocation of hospital resources, impacting various aspects of hospital operations, from the pharmacy to ancillary services such as laboratory and radiology departments [39].

Moreover, early extubation is associated with improved patient outcomes, further contributing to cost-effectiveness by potentially reducing readmission rates and the need for post-discharge long-term care facilities [27].

The cost-effectiveness of early extubation is evident when considering the reduction in ICU-related costs. Shorter ICU stays decrease expenses related to staffing, equipment use, and high cost of intensive care. Additionally, early extubation can lead to considerable cost savings by reducing the potential for ventilator-associated complications, which often result in extended hospital stays and additional treatments [40].

References

1. Motes A, Singh T, Vinan Vega N, Nugent K. A focused review of the initial management of patients with acute respiratory distress syndrome. J Clin Med. 2023;12:4650.
2. Ellis MF, Pena H, Cadavero A, Farrell D, Kettle M, Kaatz AR, et al. Reducing intubation time in adult cardiothoracic surgery patients with a fast-track extubation protocol. Crit Care Nurse. 2021;41:14–24.
3. Chatwin M, Ross E, Hart N, Nickol AH, Polkey MI, Simonds AK. Cough augmentation with mechanical insufflation/exsufflation in patients with neuromuscular weakness. Eur Respir J. 2003;21:502–8.
4. Cantinotti M. The importance and ways of exploring the entire chest before and after cardiac surgery: chest radiography, lung ultrasonography, and computed tomography. J Thorac Cardiovasc Surg. 2018;155:2041–2.
5. Boles J-M, Bion J, Connors A, Herridge M, Marsh B, Melot C, et al. Weaning from mechanical ventilation. Eur Respir J. 2007;29:1033–56.
6. Jabri G, Alotaibi F, Ahmed AM, Jose J, Alenezi FZ, Sadat M, et al. Noninvasive ventilation in critically ill patients with severe acute respiratory infections. Respir Care. 2024;69:1138.
7. Spoletini G, Alotaibi M, Blasi F, Hill NS. Heated humidified high-flow nasal oxygen in adults: mechanisms of action and clinical implications. Chest. 2015;148:253–61.
8. Ntoumenopoulos G, Presneill JJ, McElholum M, Cade JF. Chest physiotherapy for the prevention of ventilator-associated pneumonia. Intensive Care Med. 2002;28:850–6.
9. Stiller K. Physiotherapy in intensive care: an updated systematic review. Chest. 2013;144:825–47.
10. Kollef MH, Shorr A, Tabak YP, Gupta V, Liu LZ, Johannes RS. Epidemiology and outcomes of health-care-associated pneumonia: results from a large US database of culture-positive pneumonia. Chest. 2005;128:3854–62.
11. Girard TD, Alhazzani W, Kress JP, Ouellette DR, Schmidt GA, Truwit JD, et al. An official american thoracic society/american college of chest physicians clinical practice guideline: liberation from mechanical ventilation in critically ill adults. Rehabilitation protocols, ventilator liberation protocols, and cuff leak tests. Am J Respir Crit Care Med. 2017;195:120–33.
12. Wick EC, Grant MC, Wu CL. Postoperative multimodal analgesia pain management with nonopioid analgesics and techniques: a review. JAMA Surg. 2017;152:691–7.
13. Barr LF, Boss MJ, Mazzeffi MA, Taylor BS, Salenger R. Postoperative multimodal analgesia in cardiac surgery. Crit Care Clin. 2020;36:631–51.
14. Engelman DT, Lother S, George I, Funk DJ, Ailawadi G, Atluri P, et al. Adult cardiac surgery and the COVID-19 pandemic: aggressive infection mitigation strategies are necessary in the operating room and surgical recovery. J Thorac Cardiovasc Surg. 2020;160:447–51.
15. Grant MC, Chappell D, Gan TJ, Manning MW, Miller TE, Brodt JL, et al. Pain management and opioid stewardship in adult cardiac surgery: joint consensus report of the PeriOperative quality initiative and the enhanced recovery after surgery cardiac society. J Thorac Cardiovasc Surg. 2023;166:1695–706.
16. Doleman B, Read D, Lund JN, Williams JP. Preventive acetaminophen reduces postoperative opioid consumption, vomiting, and pain scores after surgery: systematic review and meta-analysis. Reg Anesth Pain Med. 2015;40:706–12.
17. Nir R-R, Nahman-Averbuch H, Moont R, Sprecher E, Yarnitsky D. Preoperative preemptive drug administration for acute postoperative pain: a systematic review and meta-analysis. Eur J Pain. 2016;20:1025–43.
18. Blanco R, Fajardo M, Parras MT. Ultrasound description of Pecs II (modified Pecs I): a novel approach to breast surgery. Rev Esp Anestesiol Reanim. 2012;59:470–5.
19. Landoni G, Isella F, Greco M, Zangrillo A, Royse CF. Benefits and risks of epidural analgesia in cardiac surgery. Br J Anaesth. 2015;115:25–32.
20. Caruso TJ, Lawrence K, Tsui BCH. Regional anesthesia for cardiac surgery. Curr Opin Anaesthesiol. 2019;32:674–82.
21. Kumar KN, Kalyane RN, Singh NG, Nagaraja PS, Krishna M, Babu B, et al. Efficacy of bilateral pectoralis nerve block for ultrafast tracking and postopera-

tive pain management in cardiac surgery. Ann Card Anaesth. 2018;21:333–8.
22. Zhang Y, Gong H, Zhan B, Chen S. Effects of bilateral pecto-intercostal fascial block for perioperative pain management in patients undergoing open cardiac surgery: a prospective randomized study. BMC Anesthesiol. 2021;21:175.
23. Dost B, De Cassai A, Balzani E, Tulgar S, Ahiskalioglu A. Effects of ultrasound-guided regional anesthesia in cardiac surgery: a systematic review and network meta-analysis. BMC Anesthesiol. 2022;22:409.
24. Li J, Lin L, Peng J, He S, Wen Y, Zhang M. Efficacy of ultrasound-guided parasternal block in adult cardiac surgery: a meta-analysis of randomized controlled trials. Minerva Anestesiol. 2022;88:719–28.
25. Girard TD, Jackson JC, Pandharipande PP, Pun BT, Thompson JL, Shintani AK, et al. Delirium as a predictor of long-term cognitive impairment in survivors of critical illness. Crit Care Med. 2010;38:1513–20.
26. Inouye SK, Westendorp RGJ, Saczynski JS. Delirium in elderly people. Lancet. 2014;383:911–22.
27. Pandharipande PP, Pun BT, Herr DL, Maze M, Girard TD, Miller RR, et al. Effect of sedation with dexmedetomidine vs lorazepam on acute brain dysfunction in mechanically ventilated patients: the MENDS randomized controlled trial. JAMA. 2007;298:2644–53.
28. Jubran A, Grant BJB, Duffner LA, Collins EG, Lanuza DM, Hoffman LA, et al. Effect of pressure support vs unassisted breathing through a tracheostomy collar on weaning duration in patients requiring prolonged mechanical ventilation: a randomized trial. JAMA. 2013;309:671–7.
29. Fiest KM, Soo A, Hee Lee C, Niven DJ, Ely EW, Doig CJ, et al. Long-term outcomes in ICU patients with delirium: a population-based cohort study. Am J Respir Crit Care Med. 2021;204:412–20.
30. Thompson DR, Hamilton DK, Cadenhead CD, Swoboda SM, Schwindel SM, Anderson DC, et al. Guidelines for intensive care unit design. Crit Care Med. 2012;40:1586–600.
31. Reich DL, Bodian CA, Krol M, Kuroda M, Osinski T, Thys DM. Intraoperative hemodynamic predictors of mortality, stroke, and myocardial infarction after coronary artery bypass surgery. Anesth Analg. 1999;89:814–22.
32. Kehlet H, Wilmore DW. Evidence-based surgical care and the evolution of fast-track surgery. Ann Surg. 2008;248:189–98.
33. Brochard L, Mancebo J, Wysocki M, Lofaso F, Conti G, Rauss A, et al. Noninvasive ventilation for acute exacerbations of chronic obstructive pulmonary disease. N Engl J Med. 1995;333:817–22.
34. Casaer MP, Mesotten D, Hermans G, Wouters PJ, Schetz M, Meyfroidt G, et al. Early versus late parenteral nutrition in critically ill adults. N Engl J Med. 2011;365:506–17.
35. Fisher SR, Kuo Y, Graham JE, Ottenbacher KJ, Ostir GV. Early ambulation and length of stay in older adults hospitalized for acute illness. Arch Intern Med. 2010;170:1942–3.
36. Livingston DS, Krishnan V. Nurses' perceptions of intensive care unit orientation patient education pamphlet. ATS Sch. 2023;4:332–43.
37. Balas MC, Vasilevskis EE, Burke WJ, Boehm L, Pun BT, Olsen KM, et al. Critical care nurses' role in implementing the "ABCDE bundle" into practice. Crit Care Nurse. 2012;32:35–47.
38. Pashikanti L, Von Ah D. Impact of early mobilization protocol on the medical-surgical inpatient population: an integrated review of literature. Clin Nurse Spec. 2012;26:87–94.
39. Tiganila R, McCoy C, Gilbert R, Raco J. The safety of immediate extubation, and factors associated with delayed extubation, in cardiac surgical patients receiving fast-track cardiac anesthesia: an integrative review. Can J Respir Ther. 2023;59:8–19.
40. Barnett NM, Liesman DR, Strobel RJ, Wu X, Paone G, DeLucia A, et al. The association of intraoperative and early postoperative events with risk of pneumonia following cardiac surgery. J Thorac Cardiovasc Surg. 2023.;S0022-5223(23)00882-6; https://doi.org/10.1016/j.jtcvs.2023.09.056.

Haemodynamic Considerations 21

Ciprian Nita, Antonio Rubino, Fabio Sangalli, and Gianluca Paternoster

21.1 Importance of Haemodynamic Management in ERAS

A wealth of data is available regarding the pre-, intra- and post-operative anaesthetic priorities for optimization of haemodynamic function, with the emergence of concepts such as goal-directed therapy (GDT) management and goal-directed perfusion (GDP). Improvement of cardiovascular parameters by means of GDT has been showed to improve outcomes such as in-hospital mortality, hospital length of stay, postsurgical acute kidney injury (AKI) and transfusions [1, 2].

GDP, while an attractive concept, aimed at targeting optimal oxygen delivery to tissues (DO_2), has met with mixed responses and uptake by high-volume centres. A recent joint consensus statement on ERAS in cardiothoracic surgery has graded the level of evidence towards employing GDP as a means of reducing end-organ injury as low [3].

The same consensus attributes a moderate level of evidence towards using goal-directed fluid and haemodynamic therapy as guides to perioperative resuscitation and prevention of post-operative organ injury.

ERAS protocols for specific cardiovascular parameters are not routinely employed outside standardized care which includes monitoring, and targets include adequate blood pressure, cardiac rhythm, haemoglobin levels, urine output, lactate levels, and central venous oxygen saturation ($ScVO_2$).

While a common-sense approach looking at normal levels of lactate, maintaining $ScVO_2$ as a surrogate for tissue oxygenation, urine output, etc. is often employed, a deeper focus on measures that may improve quality indices is needed.

We suggest considering these goals as an essential part of a successful early extubation strategy.

21.2 Preoperative Haemodynamic Optimization

For optimization of haemodynamic function, a preoperative assessment is required, one that for our purposes focuses on cardiac, respiratory, renal and haematological status. It has been documented that in contemporary cardiac surgery, the risk of poor outcomes lies more frequently

C. Nita · A. Rubino
Cardiothoracic Anaesthesia and Intensive Care, Royal Papworth Hospital, Cambridge, UK

F. Sangalli
Anaesthesia and Intensive Care, ASST Valtellina e Alto Lario, Milan, Italy

G. Paternoster (✉)
Department of Health Science Anaesthesia and ICU School of Medicine, University of Basilicata San Carlo Hospital, Potenza, Italy

G. Sepolvere, S. Silvetti (eds.), *Fast-Track in Cardiac Anesthesia*,
https://doi.org/10.1007/978-3-031-70899-2_21

with the patient rather than the surgical procedure itself [4]. As such, identifying high-risk patients and establishing appropriate optimization strategies become imperative.

Out of the cumulus of comorbidities associated with worse outcomes, of importance to haemodynamic status are factors such as age >65, arterial or pulmonary hypertension, peripheral arterial disease, cardiac failure, coronary artery disease, impaired ventricular function, severe valvular pathology, abnormal cardiac rhythm, presence of permanent pacemaker and anaemia [5].

This preoperative evaluation as well as haemodynamic optimization is also pivotal in selecting patients suitable for an early extubation strategy.

21.3 Anaesthetic Management

The anaesthetic management plays a fundamental role in an early extubation strategy, particularly in fragile patients.

A multimodal approach seems to be best suited to ERAS as well as for patients who are candidates for early extubation.

The preoperative assessment should help the clinician orientate towards an anaesthesiological conduct that includes a cautious induction and intraoperative management that respects targets for blood pressure, heart rate, ECG changes, etc.

The choice of anaesthetic drugs should be made in concordance with their impact to haemodynamic stability and also to ensure an adequate depth of anaesthesia. There is no universally accepted recipe for cardiac anaesthesia, with multiple agents being able to achieve adequate operating conditions.

Generally speaking, the choice of agents and their doses needs to be selected based on their effects on a patient that might have one or multiple cardiac conditions that will lead to cardiovascular collapse. As a rule of thumb, careful anaesthesia with upward titrated doses of induction agents and simultaneous use of vasopressor and inotropic agents as needed to maintain cardiac output and perfusion pressure [6]. Frequently, high dose of opioids are employed due to their conferral of haemodynamic stability and simultaneous sparing of other anaesthetic agents [7].

Special attention needs to be given to patients with severely impaired left ventricular ejection fraction, critical valvular lesions or coronary artery disease involving the left main stem and right ventricular impairment/pulmonary hypertension. In such cases, there is a greater risk for cardiovascular collapse, and a good strategy is to commence infusions with cardiovascular support agents prior to induction and to avoid significant changes in blood pressure and heart rate (Table 21.1).

Other essential consideration needs to be given to the patient's comorbid conditions that may modify accepted pharmacokinetics and pharmacodynamics, this in conjecture with the effects of cardiopulmonary bypass and hypothermia. Factors such as hypoalbuminemia and altered plasma protein binding, haemodilution, hypotension, modified global and regional perfusion in addition to hypothermia and heparin administration may have a significant impact on the effect of the doses of anaesthetic agents used and as such also on haemodynamic profiles [8].

Whether patients deemed at moderate or high risk of perioperative morbidity or mortality should receive intraoperative transoesophageal echocardiography (TEE) monitoring even for isolated coronary artery bypass grafting (CABG) is still disputed. While there is evidence that the use of TEE in high-risk patients is associated with lower mortality and more unplanned valvular surgery [9], there is also considerable extra risk to patients of major complications (1 in 1300) with a high (40%) mortality in such events [10]. Studies dedicated to the impact of TEE specifically on CABG surgeries underline its significance. These studies highlight TEE's role in improving procedural success and patient outcomes. Analysis of TEE-integrated CABG procedures indicates a correlation with reduced mortality rates and lowered post-operative complications. These findings emphasize the instrumental role of TEE in enhancing surgical outcomes, suggesting that its benefits may outweigh the risks for certain patient populations.

Table 21.1 Haemodynamic goals

	Preload	Heart rate	Rhythm	Contractility	SVR
Aortic stenosis	Up	60–80	SR	Maintain	Maintain or increase
Aortic regurgitation	Increase	60–80	SR	Increase	Low
Mitral stenosis	Increase	60–80	SR	Maintain	Avoid increase
Mitral regurgitation	Maintain	80–100	SR preferable (often is in AF)	Increase	Support
HOCM	Increase	60–80	SR	Maintain—avoid inotropes	Maintain or increase
Dilated cardiomyopathy	Avoid overfilling	Avoid tachycardia	SR	Maintain inotropic support	Maintain or slight decrease
Restrictive cardiomyopathy	Increase	80–100—fixed SV	SR	Maintain inotropic support	Maintain—fixed SV
Pericardial tamponade	Up	Fast	SR	Increase—will cause high BP after release of tamponade	Maintain
Pulmonary hypertension/ right-heart failure	Avoid overfilling	80–100	SR	Increase	Maintain—consideration to PVR
Reduced LVEF	Maintain—slight increase	80–100	SR	Increase	Support

SVR systemic vascular resistance, *SR* sinusal rhythm, *PVR* pulmonary vascular resistance, *SV* stroke volume, *AF* atrial fibrillation

Using raw or processed EEG signal monitors may help guide with dosing infusions during CPB and thus help with reducing cardiovascular pharmacological support levels; however, the benefit behind such monitoring devices has been disputed [11, 12].

EEG monitoring during CPB can provide real-time insights into the patient's cerebral function, potentially allowing for more precise adjustments of anaesthetic and an overall reduction in drug dosages. This tailored approach could minimize the risk of under- or overmedication, stabilizing haemodynamics more effectively and reducing the need for additional cardiovascular pharmacological interventions.

Despite these theoretical advantages, the efficacy of EEG signal monitors in this context remains controversial. Some studies suggest that the use of these monitors can significantly enhance patient outcomes by enabling more accurate management of drug infusions, which in turn may lead to a decrease in post-operative complications and a shorter duration of hospital stay. However, other research has questioned the practical benefits, citing a lack of substantial evidence to support improved outcomes.

21.4 Postoperative Haemodynamic Management

Maintaining hemodynamic stability is crucial for the success of early extubation protocols in cardiac surgery patients.

21.4.1 Monitoring Techniques

(a) Invasive Blood Pressure Monitoring: Continuous arterial line monitoring provides real-time data on blood pressure and is essential for immediate detection of hypotensive or hypertensive episodes post-extubation.
(b) Central Venous Pressure monitoring often started during surgery, help assess right ventricular function and fluid status, guiding fluid and diuretic therapy to manage preload conditions.
(c) Pulmonary Artery Catheterization: while not universally used due to invasiveness, pulmonary artery catheters can provide comprehensive data including pulmonary artery pressures and cardiac output, particularly useful in patients with complex cardiac conditions.

(d) Echocardiography: Bedside transthoracic or transesophageal echocardiography plays a critical role in assessing ventricular function, valvular performance, and overall cardiac function after extubation.
(e) Continuous Cardiac Output Monitoring Systems: Devices like the FloTrac system or PiCCO provide continuous insight into cardiac output and other hemodynamic variables, aiding in dynamic assessment post-extubation.

21.4.2 Vasoactive Medication

Cardiovascular support remains one of the crucial management priorities in patients scheduled to ERAS process and early extubation. This is mostly achieved with the administration of vasopressors and inotropes throughout the perioperative course but may also include cardiac pacing and mechanical circulatory support.

The choice of pharmacological agents depends on the haemodynamic targets that are considered appropriate for each case, clinician's familiarity with the agent, comorbidities and cost [13]. However, there is little robust evidence to suggest one agent or a combination of agents over others [14]. The most important factor is the patient's cardiovascular status, and a key insight is that the low cardiac output (LCO) state is likely multifactorial and careful attention needs to be given in order to optimize preload, afterload, rate and metabolic disturbances simultaneously.

Knowledge of various agents' mechanisms of action and effects is needed in order to adequately treat underlying causes of LCO and titrate doses to the desired effect. In cases of refractory LCO, multiple lines of inotropes and vasopressor can be employed, with different mechanisms of action. Antidiuretic hormone (ADH) can often achieve SVR targets that noradrenaline or phenylephrine fails to with increasingly higher doses [13] (Table 21.2).

21.4.3 Management of Hemodynamic Fluctuations

(a) Fluid Management: Judicious administration of fluids to manage preload and ensure adequate stroke volume without causing fluid overload, which can exacerbate pulmonary issues and affect breathing post-extubation.

Table 21.2 Effects of different vasoactive agents

Medication	Usual doses	Receptor				Haemodynamic effect
		α_1	β_1	β_2	Other	
Vasopressor/inotropes						
Dopamine	0.5–2 μg/kg/min	–	+	–	Dopamine+++	↑CO
	5–10 μg/kg/min	+	+++	+	Dopamine++	↑↑CO, ↑SVR
	10–10 μg/kg/min	+++	++	–	Dopamine++	↑CO, ↑SVR
Adrenaline	0.01–0.5 μg/kg/min	++++	++++	+++	–	↑↑CO, ↑↑SVR
Phenylephrine	0.1–10 μg/kg/min					↑↑SVR
Noradrenaline	0.05–0.4 μg/kg/min	++++	++	+	–	↑CO, ↑↑SVR
Vasopressin	0.02–0.04 U/min	–	–	–	V1 receptors in smooth muscle	↑↑SVR, ↔PVR
Inodilators						
Dobutamine	2.5–20 μg/kg/min	+	++++	++	–	↑↑CO, ↓SVR, ↓PVR
Isoproterenol	2.0–20 μg/min	–	++++	+++	–	↑↑CO, ↓SVR, ↓PVR
Milrinone	0.125–0.75 μg/kg/min				PD3 inhibitor	↑CO, ↓SVR, ↓PVR
Enoximone	2–10 μg/kg/min				PD3 inhibitor	↑CO, ↓SVR, ↓PVR
Levosimendan	0.05–0.2 μg/kg/min				Ca^{2+} sensitizer, PD3 inhibitor	↑CO, ↓SVR, ↓PVR

CO cardiac output, *SVR* systemic vascular resistance, *PVR* pulmonary vascular resistance, *PD3* phosphodiesterase-3 inhibitor

(b) Adjusting Cardiac Medications: Titration of medications to stabilize blood pressure and heart rate without compromising cardiac output.
(c) Rapid Response to Arrhythmias: Immediate management of new or worsening arrhythmias with antiarrhythmics or cardioversion if necessary, as arrhythmias can compromise hemodynamic stability.
(d) Postural Adjustments: Simple measures such as adjusting the bed position can help manage orthostatic hypotension observed in some patients post-extubation.

A significant amount of research is around goal-directed therapy, where by means of fluid resuscitation and inotrope/vasopressor optimization in the intraoperative and post-operative period, the patient achieves targeted parameters like stroke volume, cardiac index, SVR/SVRI, $ScVO_2$, DO_2 or SVV.

Indeed, there is evidence that GDT as part of ERAS reduces the incidence of AKI when aiming to maximize stroke volume in the first 8 h post-admission to ICU [1, 15]. Other benefits of perioperative GDT have been repeatedly demonstrated in multiple studies and systematic reviews, such as reduced time to extubation and reduced ICU and hospital length of stay [16, 17], but also improvement in biomarkers such as lactate, BNP and neutrophil gelatinase-lipocalin [16]. At the same time, it does not seem that applying GDT leads to an increase in the incidence of adverse effects as pulmonary oedema, arrhythmias or other outcomes as mortality [18].

21.5 Outcomes and Future Directions

While outcomes in cardiac surgery have steadily improved over the past decades, despite an increasingly older population and more complicated procedures [19], the focus on results is shifting towards qualitative outcomes—duration of ICU/hospital stay, patient satisfaction and prevention of adverse events. As always, innovation is required, both in techniques and devices, but also in philosophy of practice and organizational structure. Haemodynamic monitoring and management have the potential to contribute significantly to ERAS and success of early extubation and are also an area that lends itself to modern medical concepts.

One of the most interesting developments in recent years has been that of machine learning and applying artificial intelligence principles to haemodynamic monitoring. Employing such principles implies better haemodynamic profiles by means of prediction of high risk of hypotension and prevention/quick reaction, compared to the traditional reactive strategies widely used in anaesthesia. While it has been shown that periods of hypotension are correlated directly to adverse outcomes in non-cardiac surgery [20], it stands to reason that similar results may be expected in cardiac surgery.

Anaesthesia as a field of practice, and especially cardiac anaesthesia, is an ideal area for development in ML/AI due to its large, often digitally recorded data sets and its lengthy procedures.

The applications of interest in cardiac anaesthesia have been described and include predicting events and risk, haemodynamic monitoring, automation of echocardiography, overcoming alarm fatigue and developing better early warning scores [21, 22].

21.6 Conclusion

Effective hemodynamic monitoring and management play pivotal roles in the safe implementation of early extubation protocols. By ensuring stability in these parameters, clinicians can improve the likelihood of successful outcomes and reduce the risk of complications associated with instability post-extubation. This integrated approach facilitates not only a faster recovery but also a reduction in the duration of intensive care and overall hospital stay.

It is becoming increasingly evident that pursuing adequate cardiovascular targets needs to happen not only during the operative phase, but also during preoperative preparation and continuing into the post-operative ICU admission, in order to mitigate the deleterious effects of the huge stress on the patient exerted by cardiac surgery and cardiopulmonary bypass.

While there is a clear signal of the benefit of haemodynamic targets for ERAS, there is significant heterogeneity in current studies, and it is unclear if an individualized approach or a universal one with clear targets for certain parameters should be employed.

As such, further research is needed, not only into haemodynamic targets for ERAS, but also in the complex interplay between different paths that have shown positive effects and potential innovative technology, like software power by artificial intelligence, all the while focusing on patient-centred results.

References

1. Osawa EA, Rhodes A, Landoni G, Galas FRBG, Fukushima JT, Park CHL, et al. Effect of perioperative goal-directed hemodynamic resuscitation therapy on outcomes following cardiac surgery: a randomized clinical trial and systematic review. Crit Care Med. 2016;44:724–33.
2. Povero M, Pradelli L. Comparison between traditional and goal directed perfusion in cardiopulmonary by-pass. A differential cost analysis in US. Farmeconomia. 2015;16:77–86.
3. Grant MC, Crisafi C, Alvarez A, Arora RC, Brindle ME, Chatterjee S, et al. Perioperative care in cardiac surgery: a joint consensus statement by the Enhanced Recovery After Surgery (ERAS) Cardiac Society, ERAS International Society, and The Society of Thoracic Surgeons (STS). Ann Thorac Surg. 2024;117:669–89.
4. Fleisher LA, Beckman JA, Brown KA, Calkins H, Chaikof E, Fleischmann KE, et al. ACC/AHA 2007 guidelines on perioperative cardiovascular evaluation and care for noncardiac surgery: a report of the American College of Cardiology/American Heart Association Task Force on Practice Guidelines (Writing Committee to Revise the 2002 Guidelines on Perioperative Cardiovascular Evaluation for Noncardiac Surgery): developed in collaboration with the American Society of Echocardiography, American Society of Nuclear Cardiology, Heart Rhythm Society, Society of Cardiovascular Anesthesiologists, Society for Cardiovascular Angiography and Interventions, Society for Vascular Medicine and Biology, and Society for Vascular Surgery. Circulation. 2007;116:e418–99.
5. Cornelissen H, Arrowsmith JE. Preoperative assessment for cardiac surgery. Continuing Educ Anaesth Crit Care Pain. 2006;6:109–13.
6. Alwardt CM, Redford D, Larson DF. General anesthesia in cardiac surgery: a review of drugs and practices. J Extra Corpor Technol. 2005;37:227–35.
7. Edward L, Phillips H, Levine Frederick H, Daggett Willard M, Gerald AW, Laver Myron B. Cardiovascular response to large doses of intravenous morphine in man. N Engl J Med. 1969;281:1389–93.
8. Mets B. The pharmacokinetics of anesthetic drugs and adjuvants during cardiopulmonary bypass. Acta Anaesthesiol Scand. 2000;44:261–73.
9. Metkus TS, Thibault D, Grant MC, Badhwar V, Jacobs JP, Lawton J, et al. Transesophageal echocardiography in patients undergoing coronary artery bypass graft surgery. J Am Coll Cardiol. 2021;78:112–22.
10. Ramalingam G, Choi S-W, Agarwal S, Kunst G, Gill R, Fletcher SN, et al. Complications related to perioperative transoesophageal echocardiography—a one-year prospective national audit by the Association of Cardiothoracic Anaesthesia and Critical Care. Anaesthesia. 2020;75:21–6.
11. Lee KH, Egan TD, Johnson KB. Raw and processed electroencephalography in modern anesthesia practice: a brief primer on select clinical applications. Korean J Anesthesiol. 2021;74:465–77.
12. Dhawan R. EEG in cardiac surgery—moving past the obvious. J Cardiothorac Vasc Anesth. 2022;36:3526–8.
13. DiMarco RF. Postoperative care of the cardiac surgical patient. Surg Intensive Care Med. 2010:535–66.
14. Uhlig K, Efremov L, Tongers J, Frantz S, Mikolajczyk R, Sedding D, et al. Inotropic agents and vasodilator strategies for the treatment of cardiogenic shock or low cardiac output syndrome. Cochrane Database Syst Rev. 2020;11(11):CD009669. https://doi.org/10.1002/14651858.CD009669.pub4/full.
15. Thomson R, Meeran H, Valencia O, Al-Subaie N. Goal-directed therapy after cardiac surgery and the incidence of acute kidney injury. J Crit Care. 2014;29:997–1000.
16. Kapoor PM, Magoon R, Rawat R, Mehta Y. Perioperative utility of goal-directed therapy in high-risk cardiac patients undergoing coronary artery bypass grafting: 'a clinical outcome and biomarker-based study'. Ann Card Anaesth. 2016;19:638–82.
17. Li P, Qu L-P, Qi D, Shen B, Wang Y-M, Xu J-R, et al. Significance of perioperative goal-directed hemodynamic approach in preventing postoperative complications in patients after cardiac surgery: a meta-analysis and systematic review. Ann Med. 2017;49:343–51.
18. Arulkumaran N, Corredor C, Hamilton MA, Ball J, Grounds RM, Rhodes A, et al. Cardiac complications associated with goal-directed therapy in high-risk surgical patients: a meta-analysis. Br J Anaesth. 2014;112:648–59.
19. Grant SW, Kendall S, Goodwin AT, Cooper G, Trivedi U, Page R, et al. Trends and outcomes for cardiac surgery in the United Kingdom from 2002 to 2016. JTCVS Open. 2021;7:259–69.
20. Vincent J-L, Nielsen ND, Shapiro NI, Gerbasi ME, Grossman A, Doroff R, et al. Mean arterial pressure and mortality in patients with distributive shock: a retrospective analysis of the MIMIC-III database. Ann Intensive Care. 2018;8:107.
21. Myatra SN, Jagiasi BG, Singh NP, Divatia JV. Role of artificial intelligence in haemodynamic monitoring. Indian J Anaesth. 2024;68:93–9.
22. Rellum SR, Schuurmans J, van der Ven WH, Eberl S, Driessen AHG, Vlaar APJ, et al. Machine learning methods for perioperative anesthetic management in cardiac surgery patients: a scoping review. J Thorac Dis. 2021;13:6976–93.

Part V

Future Considerations in Cardiac Surgery

22 Ultrafast-Track Extubation

Giuseppe Sepolvere, Loredana Cristiano, Dorela Haxhiademi, and Simona Silvetti

22.1 Introduction

Enhanced Recovery After Surgery (ERAS) is a multimodal, multidisciplinary approach to the care of patient throughout their perioperative period aiming at the early restoring of preoperative status [1].

ERAS protocols are associated with reductions of complications and length of stay (LOS), improved patient satisfaction, and cost-effectiveness [2]. Enhanced recovery cardiac anesthesia procedures, labeled "fast-track cardiac surgery," have been used since the early 1980s–1990s involving an early extubation, use of short-acting hypnotic or reduced doses of drugs and opioids, and use of antifibrinolytics and drugs to prevent atrial fibrillation [3–5]. Through a review of meta-analyses, randomized clinical trials, large non-randomized studies, and reviews, in 2019, a cardiac surgery recommendations study was first published by an expert consensus and then endorsed by the ERAS Society providing evidence-based protocols for perioperative care, improvement in clinical outcomes, and cost saving for optimal management of cardiac surgery patients [6].

As widely shown in the previous chapters, prolonged intubation and mechanical ventilation after cardiac surgery have been associated with increased hospital and intensive care unit (ICU) LOS due to the higher risk of atelectasis, intrapulmonary shunting, pneumonia [7] and many other complications. In contrast, ERAS procedures aim at early extubation which is divided into a fast-track extubation currently used to describe extubation within 6 h after the end of the surgery and ultrafast-track extubation (UFT) which is defined to describe extubation in the operating room (ORE) or within 1 postoperative hour [8, 9]. The concept of fast-track extubation was first published around 40 years ago marking a turning point in anesthesia management, and over the years, anesthetic techniques contextually evolved with the advances in cardiovascular surgery providing new strategies to achieve and improve the early extubation [10–14]. Despite evidences that these strategies optimize care processes and shorten ICU and hospital stays, to date, there is no standardized protocol for ultra-fast-track extubation after cardiac surgery

G. Sepolvere (✉) · L. Cristiano
Department of Anesthesia and Cardiac Surgery Intensive Care Unit, San Michele Hospital, Maddaloni, Caserta, Italy

D. Haxhiademi
Department of Anesthesia and Intensive Care Unit, Heart Hospital "G. Pasquinucci", National Research Council-Tuscany Foundation "G. Monasterio", Massa, Italy
e-mail: Dorela@ftgm.it

S. Silvetti
Department of Cardiac Anesthesia and Intensive Care, Cardiovascular Network, IRCCS Ospedale Policlinico San Martino, Genoa, Italy

G. Sepolvere, S. Silvetti (eds.), *Fast-Track in Cardiac Anesthesia*,
https://doi.org/10.1007/978-3-031-70899-2_22

remaining usually reserved for a selected group of patients and surgeries also depending on the individual anesthesiologic expertise and skills [15]. Through randomized controlled trials and expert consensus, it is mandatory to assess which types of surgery and category of patients are eligible for ultrafast-track extubation.

22.2 From Fast Track to Ultrafast Track

The first attempt of enhanced recovery program and early extubation in cardiac surgery was suggested in a 1980 study with promising results in terms of reduced administration of morphine and diazepam and lower risk of pulmonary complications [11]. The "fast-track protocol" in 1994 was one of the first multimodal approaches consisting of eight key points decreasing the endotracheal intubation time from 22 to 15 h: (1) preoperative education; (2) early extubation; (3) methylprednisolone; (4) prophylactic digitalization, metoclopramide HCl, docusate sodium, and ranitidine HCl; (5) accelerated rehabilitation; (6) early discharge; (7) a dedicated fast-track coordinator to perform both daily telephone contact and a 1-week postoperative examination; and (8) a routine 1-month postoperative visit. In 1997, Reyes et al. demonstrated the feasibility and benefits of fast-track cardiac anesthesia, achieving success in these key measures. Over the time, systematic reviews of fast-track cardiac anesthesia have consistently demonstrated the methodology to be safe and effective [16]. Fast track extubation is now a well-accepted and widely utilized approach to post-operative cardiac surgical care and the main studies focused on UFT and ORE. In 2024 the joint Consensus Statement by ERAS Cardiac Society was published and UFT achieved one statement that cite "highly selective intraoperative or immediate postoperative extubation may be appropriate for patients undergoing low-risk cardiac surgery" with low grade of evidence due to the limited availability of data directly comparing intraoperative with early extubation [17]. Hawkins et al. in 2024 [18] compare the outcomes of ORE versus fast-track extubation within 6 hours in patients undergoing nonemergent cardiac surgery from 2011 to 2021. They concluded that ORE is associated with a higher postoperative risk of reintubation and reoperation due to bleeding, but lower resource utilization. Differently Teman et al. in 2024 [19] published the results on their analysis conducted on 669,099 patients across 1069 hospitals included 36,298 ORE patients in 296 hospitals. The authors concluded defined ORE safe and effective in a selected patient population and associated with superior outcomes in coronary artery bypass, aortic valve replacement, and mitral valve replacement. The different results from these two studies are explained by Michael C. Grant [20]: Teman et al analyzed only a selective group of patients, for example they excluded from the analysis al patients undergoing heart failure surgery such as transplant or left ventricular assist device (LVAD) placement; furthermore they excluded all patients undergoing ORE in centers performing this maneuver infrequently (defined as less than ten ORE over the 2017-2022 period). The fast-track pathway protocols led to the development of new paradigms of cardiac anesthesiology philosophies as new short-acting intravenous anesthesia agents and opiate administration and the use of chest wall blocks.

22.3 Predictors of Ultrafast-Track Extubation Failure and Success

Some authors identified the patients characteristics associated with UFT. Rodriguez-Blanco et al. observed that arterial hypertension, left ventricular ejection fraction ≥30%, off-pump heart surgery, and shorter duration of surgery increased the rate of successful extubation in the operating room [21]. Cuerda et al. in 2015 have identified the following risk factors for failed UFT:

NYHA preoperative functional classes III–IV.
Acute myocardial infarction within 2 days of surgery.

Intra-aortic balloon pump, urgent or emergency surgery.
Intraoperative transfusion of platelets.
Intraoperative inotropes and vasopressor support.
Urgent or emergency surgery.
Use of antiplatelet or anticoagulant agents within 24 h of surgery.
Permanent pacemaker or implantable cardioverter-defibrillator.
Glomerular filtration rate (GFR) <65 mL/min/BSA [22].

A more recent retrospective study published in 2017 by Subramaniam et al. [23] and conducted on 1518 cardiac surgery patients reported that the likelihood of ORE was statistically associated with the following demographic factors: younger age, lower body mass index, absence of chronic lung disease and diabetes, and preoperative albumin levels. Moreover, the authors identified also factors associated with surgical plan, and in this regard, the factors favoring the early extubation were surgical approaches other than full sternotomy, isolated coronary artery bypass grafting (CABG), and elective operational status. Notably, this study is interesting as the authors conducted a multivariate logistic regression model analysis along with intraoperative factors primarily related to surgical technique. Based on all the above-mentioned factors, they proposed a scale that results in a score where higher positive values correlate with greater likelihood of ORE, whilst scores near zero or even negative values correlate with low likelihoods of early extubation.

22.4 Perioperative Pathway

Patients eligible for ultrafast-track extubation should follow an appropriate and scheduled pathway aimed at optimizing their perioperative conditions. A societal guidelines and consensus statement should be created. The conditions for UFT could be divided into a preoperative, intraoperative, and postoperative phase (Table 22.1).

22.4.1 Preoperative Phase

Structured and complete preoperative information should be provided by anesthesiologists, surgeons, and nurses to patients and relatives as the first step towards the early extubation. Although the timing and duration of preoperative nutrition are still unidentified [24], it is ascertained that the optimization of nutritional status has the potential to improve patient outcomes, reduce the surgical site infection, improve wound healing, reduce mechanical ventilation times, shorten ICU stay, decrease hospital readmissions, and lower mortality [25]. In addition, cardiac prehabilitation should be considered to reduce both the incidence and severity of postoperative compli-

Table 22.1 Perioperative pathway strategies for early extubation

Perioperative pathway	Strategies for early extubation	
Preoperative phase	Intraoperative phase	Postoperative phase
• Nursing, anesthesia, and surgical preoperative assessment • Cardiac prehabilitation including optimizing perioperative nutrition • Carbohydrate preloading preoperatively in select patients	• Reduced doses of opioids or the use of ultrashort-acting opioids • Reserved use of short-acting benzodiazepines rather than long-acting benzodiazepines • Lung-protective ventilation: Low tidal volumes (6–8 mLkg_1 of predicted body weight) associated with higher positive end-expiratory pressure (PEEP), limitation of fraction of inspired oxygen (FiO_2) • Recruitment maneuvers before weaning from cardiopulmonary bypass • Multimodal analgesia	• Avoidance of postoperative hypothermia (<36 °C) • Monitoring and reversal of muscle paralysis • Postoperative nurse-led weaning and extubation protocol with protective ventilation strategy • Screening and active preemptive management of delirium • Chest fascial blocks

cations [26] through aerobic exercises and respiratory muscle training, smoking cessation, alcohol consumption decreasing, sleep pattern improving, weight control, medical comorbidity optimization, and psychosocial assessment [24].

22.4.2 Intraoperative Phase

Opioid-sparing protocols or the use of ultrashort-acting opioids and benzodiazepines added to propofol or volatile anesthesia is the main strategy of the intraoperative phase. Muscle paralysis should be maintained, and insulin, antifibrinolytic agent, and ionotropic and vasoactive medications should be administered when needed [27]. Compared to fentanyl or sufentanil during general anesthesia, remifentanil showed favorable properties reducing time to extubation, length of stay, and risk of mortality [28]. Intraoperative lung-protective ventilation strategies are mandatory with a view to the ultrafast-track extubation, and they are associated with lower pulmonary high complications. The major components of protective ventilatory management include assist-controlled mechanical ventilation with low tidal volumes (6–8 mL/kg of predicted body weight) associated with modified driving pressure (peak inspiratory pressure, PEEP) <16 cm H_2O and PEEP 5 cm H_2O, limitation of fraction of inspired oxygen (FiO_2), and finally recruitment maneuvers to prevent atelectasis. In particular, PEEP is necessary to reduce the risk of atelectasis due to low-volume ventilation [29, 30]. The ERAS Cardiac recommendations suggest the chest wall regional anesthesia as an effective component of a multimodal approach to perioperative pain management reducing reliance on opioid-based analgesia and allowing an early extubation in selected patients [17]. They were born in the hands of Rafael Blanco and have been growing faster and faster starting as analgesic techniques and becoming anesthetic procedures allowing the management of critically ill respiratory cardiac surgery patients in spontaneous breathing avoiding general anesthesia and intubation.

22.4.3 Postoperative Phase

Extubation was attempted in the operating room if the following requirements were met: response to verbal commands, spontaneous breathing with $SatO_2 > 95\%$ and $FiO_2 < 0.5$, stable blood pressure (mean arterial pressure > 65 mmHg), body temperature > 36 °C, and adequate arterial blood gases (pH >7.30, PaO_2 > 60–70 mmHg, and $PaCO_2$ < 45 mmHg). The postoperative ERAS models include early intake of oral fluids and solids, ambulation, early mobilization, pain management, patient reorientation, cognitive stimulation, removal of drains, and promotion of normal sleep-wake circadian patterns. Delirium in the postoperative period can be particularly problematic, affecting between 20% and 80% of patients [31]. Delirium increases complication rates, duration of mechanical ventilation, morbidity, and mortality and has been associated with long-term cognitive changes [32]. Current guidelines recommend that nonbenzodiazepine sedatives (either propofol or dexmedetomidine) are preferable to benzodiazepine sedatives (either midazolam or lorazepam) because of improved short-term outcomes, such as ICU LOS, duration of mechanical ventilation, and delirium [33]. Published guidelines recommend routinely screening patients for known risk factors (frailty, genetics, lifestyle, underlying diseases, drug therapy, surgical trauma, anesthesia management (including the use of benzodiazepines), venous congestion, and pain management). The postoperative pain management should follow the ERAS opioid-sparing model within a multimodal approach including regional anesthesia in the form of ultrasound chest wall blocks. The latter allow a safe and effective pain relief aiming at early extubation (operating room or ICU) avoiding the several side effects related to opioid administration [34] (Figs. 22.1 and 22.2).

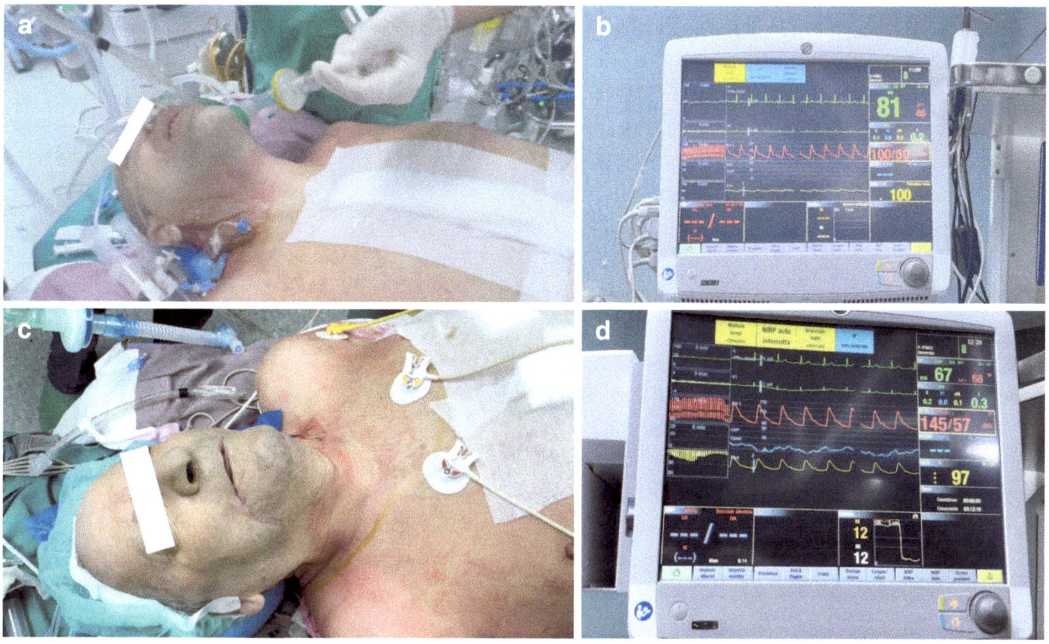

Fig. 22.1 Ultrafast-track extubation in operating room after receiving chest wall blocks. (**a**) Single coronary artery bypass grafting through median sternotomy. (**c**) Single coronary artery bypass grafting through left mini-thoracotomy. (**b**, **d**) Post-extubation hemodynamic and respiratory stability

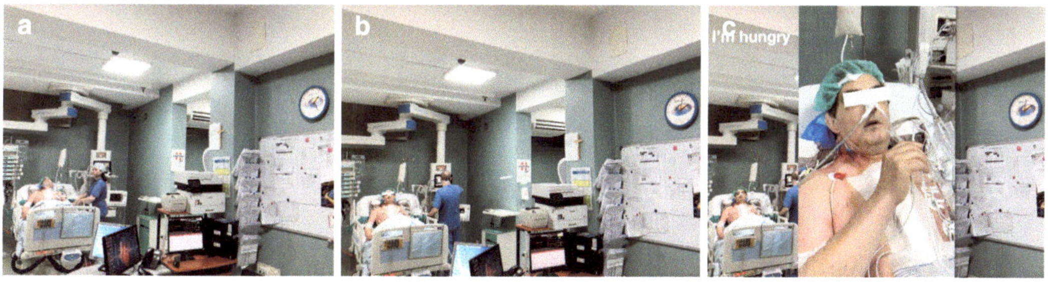

Fig. 22.2 Ultrafast-track extubation within the first post-operative hour. (**a**) Patient admission at 13.25. (**b**) Extubation at 14.00. (**c**) The patient reported to be hungry immediately after the extubation. No postoperative nausea and vomiting

22.5 Conclusion

Ultrafast-track extubation after cardiovascular surgery is still rarely performed. Despite limited to the single-center experience or described by the analysis of small and selected surgical population, ORE may be feasible in selected adult patients undergoing cardiovascular surgery. Although the extubation in operating room appears to be attractive and promising, some limitations should be taken and the success rate of this practice depends on three main factors that we could reassume as follow: first, a properly identifying patients as suitable candidates for extubation ahead of time is paramount; second, ORE to be effective must be common practice and a greater institutional experience is essencial, it's success is strictly related to the surgeon's and anesthesiologist's expertise and skills; finally, a protocolization and programmatic culture is necessary: a multidisciplinary protocols including preoperative optimization programs, goal directed anesthetics, and intensive care processes that support patients through their initial high-risk postextubation periods is needed. Chest wall blocks play a key role in the immediate postoperative pain control and extubation in operating room reducing both the use and the side effects of opioid administration. Ultrasound regional anesthesia in cardiac surgery represents the new wave in the regional anesthesia panorama. On this basis, more randomized controlled trials are needed to provide higher and stronger level of evidence whose results could be generalized to the entire adult cardiac surgery population.

References

1. Ljungqvist O. The enhanced recovery after surgery in cardiac surgery revolution. JAMA Surg. 2019;154(8):767. https://doi.org/10.1001/jamasurg.2019.1154.
2. Ljungqvist O, Scott M, Fearon KC. Enhanced recovery after surgery: a review. JAMA Surg. 2017;152(3):292–8. https://doi.org/10.1001/jamasurg.2016.4952.
3. Engelman RM, Rousou JA, Flack JE 3rd, Deaton DW, Humphrey CB, Ellison LH, Allmendinger PD, Owen SG, Pekow PS. Fast-track recovery of the coronary bypass patient. Ann Thorac Surg. 1994;58(6):1742–6. https://doi.org/10.1016/0003-4975(94)91674-8.
4. Myles PS, Daly DJ, Djaiani G, Lee A, Cheng DC. A systematic review of the safety and effectiveness of fast-track cardiac anesthesia. Anesthesiology. 2003;99(4):982–7. https://doi.org/10.1097/00000542-200310000-00035.
5. Reyes A, Vega G, Blancas R, Morató B, Moreno JL, Torrecilla C, Cereijo E. Early vs conventional extubation after cardiac surgery with cardiopulmonary bypass. Chest. 1997;112(1):193–201. https://doi.org/10.1378/chest.112.1.193.
6. Engelman DT, Ben Ali W, Williams JB, Perrault LP, Reddy VS, Arora RC, Roselli EE, Khoynezhad A, Gerdisch M, Levy JH, Lobdell K, Fletcher N, Kirsch M, Nelson G, Engelman RM, Gregory AJ, Boyle EM. Guidelines for perioperative care in cardiac surgery: enhanced recovery after surgery society recommendations. JAMA Surg. 2019;154(8):755–66. https://doi.org/10.1001/jamasurg.2019.1153.
7. Reddy SL, Grayson AD, Griffiths EM, Pullan DM, Rashid A. Logistic risk model for prolonged ventilation after adult cardiac surgery. Ann Thorac Surg. 2007;84(2):528–36. https://doi.org/10.1016/j.athoracsur.2007.04.002.
8. Parody Cuerda G, Jiménez Del Valle JR, Fernández López AR, Barquero Aroca JM. Ultra-fast track extubation protocol following cardiovascular surgery: predictors of failure and outcomes. Rev Esp Anestesiol Reanim (Engl Ed). 2023;70(5):259–68. https://doi.org/10.1016/j.redare.2023.05.002.
9. Wong WT, Lai VK, Chee YE, Lee A. Fast-track cardiac care for adult cardiac surgical patients. Cochrane Database Syst Rev. 2016;9(9):CD003587:CD003587. https://doi.org/10.1002/14651858.CD003587.pub3.
10. Prakash O, Jonson B, Meij S, Bos E, Hugenholtz PG, Nauta J, Hekman W. Criteria for early extubation after intracardiac surgery in adults. Anesth Analg. 1977;56(5):703–8. https://doi.org/10.1213/00000539-197709000-00019.
11. Quasha AL, Loeber N, Feeley TW, Ullyot DJ, Roizen MF. Postoperative respiratory care: a controlled trial of early and late extubation following coronary-artery bypass grafting. Anesthesiology. 1980;52(2):135–41.
12. Foster GH, Conway WA, Pamulkov N, Lester JL, Magilligan DJ Jr. Early extubation after coronary artery bypass: brief report. Crit Care Med. 1984;12(11):994–6. https://doi.org/10.1097/00003246-198411000-00017.
13. Higgins TL. Pro: early endotracheal extubation is preferable to late extubation in patients following coronary artery surgery. J Cardiothorac Vasc Anesth. 1992;6(4):488–93. https://doi.org/10.1016/1053-0770(92)90019-4.
14. Cheng DC, Karski J, Peniston C, Raveendran G, Asokumar B, Carroll J, David T, Sandler A. Early tracheal extubation after coronary artery bypass graft surgery reduces costs and improves resource use. A prospective, randomized, controlled trial. Anesthesiology. 1996;85(6):1300–10. https://doi.org/10.1097/00000542-199612000-00011.
15. Grocott HP. Early extubation after cardiac surgery: the evolution continues. J Thorac Cardiovasc Surg. 2017;154(5):1654–5. https://doi.org/10.1016/j.jtcvs.2017.07.025.
16. Zhu F, Lee A, Chee YE. Fast-track cardiac care for adult cardiac surgical patients. Cochrane Database Syst Rev. 2012;10:CD003587. https://doi.org/10.1002/14651858.CD003587.pub2.
17. Grant MC, Crisafi C, Alvarez A, Arora RC, Brindle ME, Chatterjee S, Ender J, Fletcher N, Gregory AJ, Gunaydin S, Jahangiri M, Ljungqvist O, Lobdell KW, Morton V, Reddy VS, Salenger R, Sander M, Zarbock A, Engelman DT. Perioperative care in cardiac surgery: a joint consensus statement by the Enhanced Recovery After Surgery (ERAS) cardiac society, ERAS International Society, and The Society of Thoracic Surgeons (STS). Ann Thorac Surg. 2024;117(4):669–89. https://doi.org/10.1016/j.athoracsur.2023.12.006.
18. Hawkins AD, Strobel RJ, Mehaffey JH, Hawkins RB, Rotar EP, Young AM, Yarboro LT, Yount K, Ailawadi G, Joseph M, Quader M, Teman NR. Operating

room versus intensive care unit extubation within 6 hours after on-pump cardiac surgery: early results and hospital costs. Semin Thorac Cardiovasc Surg. 2024;36(2):195–208. https://doi.org/10.1053/j.semtcvs.2022.09.013.
19. Teman NR, Strobel RJ, Bonnell LN, Preventza O, Yarboro LT, Badhwar V, Kaneko T, Habib RH, Mehaffey JH, Beller JP. Operating room extubation for patients undergoing cardiac surgery: a national society of thoracic surgeons database analysis. Ann Thorac Surg. 2024;118(3):692–9. https://doi.org/10.1016/j.athoracsur.2024.05.033.
20. Grant MC. Extubation after cardiac surgery: it's better early, if often. Ann Thorac Surg. 2024;118(3):699–700. https://doi.org/10.1016/j.athoracsur.2024.06.026.
21. Rodriguez Blanco YF, Candiotti K, Gologorsky A, Tang F, Giquel J, Barron ME, Salerno TA, Gologorsky E. Factors which predict safe extubation in the operating room following cardiac surgery. J Card Surg. 2012;27(3):275–80. https://doi.org/10.1111/j.1540-8191.2012.01434.x.
22. Youssefi P, Timbrell D, Valencia O, Gregory P, Vlachou C, Jahangiri M, Edsell M. Predictors of failure in fast-track cardiac surgery. J Cardiothorac Vasc Anesth. 2015;29(6):1466–71. https://doi.org/10.1053/j.jvca.2015.07.002.
23. Subramaniam K, DeAndrade DS, Mandell DR, Althouse AD, Manmohan R, Esper SA, Varga JM, Badhwar V. Predictors of operating room extubation in adult cardiac surgery. J Thorac Cardiovasc Surg. 2017;154(5):1656–65. https://doi.org/10.1016/j.jtcvs.2017.05.107.
24. Gregory AJ, Grant MC, Manning MW, Cheung AT, Ender J, Sander M, Zarbock A, Stoppe C, Meineri M, Grocott HP, Ghadimi K, Gutsche JT, Patel PA, Denault A, Shaw A, Fletcher N, Levy JH. Enhanced recovery after cardiac surgery (ERAS cardiac) recommendations: an important first step-but there is much work to be done. J Cardiothorac Vasc Anesth. 2020;34(1):39–47. https://doi.org/10.1053/j.jvca.2019.09.002.
25. Stoppe C, Goetzenich A, Whitman G, Ohkuma R, Brown T, Hatzakorzian R, Kristof A, Meybohm P, Mechanick J, Evans A, Yeh D, McDonald B, Chourdakis M, Jones P, Barton R, Tripathi R, Elke G, Liakopoulos O, Agarwala R, Lomivorotov V, Nesterova E, Marx G, Benstoem C, Lemieux M, Heyland DK. Role of nutrition support in adult cardiac surgery: a consensus statement from an international multidisciplinary expert group on nutrition in cardiac surgery. Crit Care. 2017;21(1):131. https://doi.org/10.1186/s13054-017-1690-5.
26. Arthur HM, Daniels C, McKelvie R, Hirsh J, Rush B. Effect of a preoperative intervention on preoperative and postoperative outcomes in low-risk patients awaiting elective coronary artery bypass graft surgery. A randomized, controlled trial. Ann Intern Med. 2000;133(4):253–62. https://doi.org/10.7326/0003-4819-133-4-200008150-00007.
27. Fitch ZW, Debesa O, Ohkuma R, Duquaine D, Steppan J, Schneider EB, Whitman GJ. A protocol-driven approach to early extubation after heart surgery. J Thorac Cardiovasc Surg. 2014;147(4):1344–50. https://doi.org/10.1016/j.jtcvs.2013.10.032.
28. Greco M, Landoni G, Biondi-Zoccai G, Cabrini L, Ruggeri L, Pasculli N, Giacchi V, Sayeg J, Greco T, Zangrillo A. Remifentanil in cardiac surgery: a meta-analysis of randomized controlled trials. J Cardiothorac Vasc Anesth. 2012;26(1):110–6. https://doi.org/10.1053/j.jvca.2011.05.007.
29. Lellouche F, Delorme M, Bussières J, Ouattara A. Perioperative ventilatory strategies in cardiac surgery. Best Pract Res Clin Anaesthesiol. 2015;29(3):381–95. https://doi.org/10.1016/j.bpa.2015.08.006.
30. Neto AS, Hemmes SN, Barbas CS, Beiderlinden M, Fernandez-Bustamante A, Futier E, Gajic O, El-Tahan MR, Ghamdi AA, Günay E, Jaber S, Kokulu S, Kozian A, Licker M, Lin WQ, Maslow AD, Memtsoudis SG, Reis Miranda D, Moine P, Ng T, Paparella D, Ranieri VM, Scavonetto F, Schilling T, Selmo G, Severgnini P, Sprung J, Sundar S, Talmor D, Treschan T, Unzueta C, Weingarten TN, Wolthuis EK, Wrigge H, Amato MB, Costa EL, de Abreu MG, Pelosi P, Schultz MJ. PROVE network investigators. Association between driving pressure and development of postoperative pulmonary complications in patients undergoing mechanical ventilation for general anaesthesia: a meta-analysis of individual patient data. Lancet. Respir Med. 2016;4(4):272–80. https://doi.org/10.1016/S2213-2600(16)00057-6.
31. Ely EW, Shintani A, Truman B, Speroff T, Gordon SM, Harrell FE Jr, Inouye SK, Bernard GR, Dittus RS. Delirium as a predictor of mortality in mechanically ventilated patients in the intensive care unit. JAMA. 2004;291(14):1753–62. https://doi.org/10.1001/jama.291.14.1753.
32. Nomura Y, Nakano M, Bush B, Tian J, Yamaguchi A, Walston J, Hasan R, Zehr K, Mandal K, LaFlam A, Neufeld KJ, Kamath V, Hogue CW, Brown CH 4th. Observational study examining the association of baseline frailty and postcardiac surgery delirium and cognitive change. Anesth Analg. 2019;129(2):507–14. https://doi.org/10.1213/ANE.0000000000003967.
33. Devlin JW, Skrobik Y, Gélinas C, Needham DM, Slooter AJC, Pandharipande PP, Watson PL, Weinhouse GL, Nunnally ME, Rochwerg B, Balas MC, van den Boogaard M, Bosma KJ, Brummel NE, Chanques G, Denehy L, Drouot X, Fraser GL, Harris JE, Joffe AM, Kho ME, Kress JP, Lanphere JA, McKinley S, Neufeld KJ, Pisani MA, Payen JF, Pun BT, Puntillo KA, Riker RR, Robinson BRH, Shehabi Y, Szumita PM, Winkelman C, Centofanti JE, Price C, Nikayin S, Misak CJ, Flood PD, Kiedrowski K, Alhazzani W. Executive summary: clinical practice guidelines for the prevention and management of pain, agitation/sedation, delirium, immobility, and sleep disruption in adult patients in the ICU. Crit Care

Med. 2018;46(9):1532–48. https://doi.org/10.1097/CCM.0000000000003259.
34. DAS-Taskforce 2015, Baron R, Binder A, Biniek R, Braune S, Buerkle H, Dall P, Demirakca S, Eckardt R, Eggers V, Eichler I, Fietze I, Freys S, Fründ A, Garten L, Gohrbandt B, Harth I, Hartl W, Heppner HJ, Horter J, Huth R, Janssens U, Jungk C, Kaeuper KM, Kessler P, Kleinschmidt S, Kochanek M, Kumpf M, Meiser A, Mueller A, Orth M, Putensen C, Roth B, Schaefer M, Schaefers R, Schellongowski P, Schindler M, Schmitt R, Scholz J, Schroeder S, Schwarzmann G, Spies C, Stingele R, Tonner P, Trieschmann U, Tryba M, Wappler F, Waydhas C, Weiss B, Weisshaar G. Evidence and consensus based guideline for the management of delirium, analgesia, and sedation in intensive care medicine. Revision 2015 (DAS-Guideline 2015)—short version. Ger Med Sci. 2015;13:Doc19. https://doi.org/10.3205/000223.

Awake Surgery

23

Giuseppe Sepolvere, Valeria Rita Scialdone, and Fabrizio Di Zazzo

23.1 Introduction

General anesthesia was reasonably considered for years the "gold standard" technique used for cardiac surgery both with on-pump and off-pump techniques. In the era of Enhanced Recovery After Surgery (ERAS), with the improvement of the anesthesia procedures, general anesthesia could be safely associated with locoregional techniques to manage the perioperative pain reducing both the opioid administration and time of intubation or ventilatory support. The high thoracic epidural anesthesia (TEA) as an adjunct to general anesthesia and the paravertebral block have been widely described providing pain relief after cardiac surgery and have shown many potentially favorable effects throughout the perioperative period, such as thoracic sympathicolysis with subsequent improvement of coronary and mammary artery perfusion, reduced risk of perioperative arrhythmia with a decreased heart rate and less endogenous stress response, reduced risk for myocardial ischemia, more hemodynamic stability, and improved pulmonary compliance. A further stage in cardiac anesthesia was the use of TEA without general anesthesia as the only anesthetic technique in patients undergoing off-pump coronary artery bypass graft (CABG) by minithoracotomy producing high satisfaction in a wide number of selected patients. Despite the potential use of TEA in cardiac anesthesia, there is still an ongoing discussion about the potential risks of epidural hematoma and subsequent adverse neurologic sequelae related to this anesthetic technique, discouraging many anesthesiologists from using TEA in these patients. With the advent of the emerging chest wall fascial blocks, performable regardless of the coagulation status, a fair number of critically ill respiratory patients result as eligible for awake cardiac surgery avoiding the side effects of opioid administration, prolonged orotracheal intubation, and neurologic injuries. Actually, the most performed chest wall blocks in awake and spontaneous breathing patients are represented by the parasternal, serratus anterior plane, and interpectoral plane (PECS)-pectoserratus plane (PECS II) blocks to manage sternal dehiscence, sternal wound debridement, rib fractures, chest tube insertion for pneumothorax, pacemaker and subcutaneous implantable cardioverter defibrillator (S-ICD) implantation, and transcatheter aortic valve implantation (TAVI). It is noteworthy that only few case reports describing selected awake patients undergoing cardiac surgery performed both with neuraxial anesthesia and chest fascial blocks are reported. Even if awake cardiac surgery became of increasing interest to surgeons and anesthesiologists in terms of minimally invasive treatment, locoregional anesthesia could be

G. Sepolvere (✉) · V. R. Scialdone · F. Di Zazzo
Department of Anesthesia and Cardiac Surgery Intensive Care Unit, San Michele Hospital, Maddaloni, Caserta, Italy

G. Sepolvere, S. Silvetti (eds.), *Fast-Track in Cardiac Anesthesia*,
https://doi.org/10.1007/978-3-031-70899-2_23

applied on the basis of the personal expertise also evaluating the risks and the benefits for the patients. To date, more randomized controlled trials are needed to validate the efficacy and the safety of these techniques.

23.2 The Role of Thoracic Paravertebral Block and Epidural Anesthesia in Awake Cardiac Surgery

The ultrasound thoracic paravertebral block in cardiac surgery represents a locoregional technique mostly used as analgesic procedure to ensure an adequate perioperative pain management added to general anesthesia to provide a fast extubation within the 6 postoperative hours. To date, no studies or case reports are reported to describe its use in awake cardiac surgery [1–3]. In contrast, the use of high landmark-based epidural thoracic anesthesia was described as few case reports or single-center study with low sample sizes in particular for off-pump CABG surgery in patients with severely impaired pulmonary function reducing the complications associated with general anesthesia. In 2014, TEA was defined as the future of awake cardiac surgery improving analgesia, reducing ventilation time, improving pulmonary function, reducing incidence of renal failure and myocardial infarction, providing coronary vasodilation or cardioprotection, lowering stress response, improving cardiac function, and reducing psychological morbidity. Additional benefits are represented by the reduction of atrial fibrillation, costs, and length of stay [4]. Aybek et al. enrolled 35 patients undergoing off-pump CABG via median sternotomy with high TEA kept awake during the surgery stating that this approach could be considered safe and feasible for high-risk patients [5]. Through the use of high TEA, Watanabe et al. describe the use of subxiphoid CABG using right epiploic gastric artery in awake patients avoiding sternotomy and opening of the pleura. High TEA provides visceral coronary arteries and internal mammary artery vasodilatation, sympathetic nerve efferent fiber block, heart rate reduction during beating heart CABG, and reduction of plasma level of adrenal-corticotropic hormone, cortisol, epinephrine, norepinephrine, and glucose [6, 7]. Given that general anesthesia remains a risk in patients who have severe carotid artery stenosis before surgery, as well as in those with a history of severe cerebral infarction or respiratory failure, the use of only epidural anesthesia was found to be a promising modality for ultra-minimally invasive cardiac surgery through totally endoscopic robotic cardiac surgery [8]. An additional approach avoiding general anesthesia and endotracheal intubation for minimally invasive coronary artery bypass surgery beating heart procedures is represented by the continuous epidural infusion of local anesthetics at levels T2–T3 to manage intra- and postoperative analgesia with less need for intensive care unit monitoring and faster mobilization and recovery [9]. The technological advances in cardiac surgery procedures allow minimally invasive surgical techniques such as robotic and endoscopic cardiac surgery avoiding median sternotomy. Thus, mitral valve plasty, atrial septal defect closure, multivessel minimally invasive direct coronary artery bypass grafting, and CABG can be totally endoscopic in awake patients under the use of epidural anesthesia [10]. In his study, Aybek et al. placed a thoracic epidural catheter at levels of T2–T3 the day before the CABG through median sternotomy keeping the patient conscious throughout the whole 12 enrolled procedures without complications showing the feasibility and safety of the protocol [11]. Kessler et al. enrolled 20 patients undergoing awake and spontaneous breathing CABG placing a thoracic epidural catheter at the level of T1/2 or T2/3 and stating that the use of this technique was feasible and safe for CABG via median sternotomy or through minimally invasive direct coronary artery bypass grafting technique [12–14]. Kirali et al. performed a high thoracic epidural anesthesia 1 h before the bilateral internal mammary artery grafts through median sternotomy and off-pump technique in four awake patients without complications concluding that this approach allows for complete revascularization when general anesthesia is contraindicated [15]. Although some studies have demonstrated the feasibility of performing cardiac surgery in awake patients with consciousness and spontaneous breathing with epidural anesthesia, several significant concerns limit its use and discourage anesthesiologists from using TEA due to the possibility of severe complications such as epidural hematoma and neurological permanent injury hampering the development of this approach. On the other hand, only few patients were enrolled, and randomized controlled trials with a higher sample size are needed to state the role of TEA alone in awake cardiac surgery. On this basis, with the advent of the ultrasound chest wall blocks, the use of TEA in standard and awake cardiac surgery is not recommended.

23.3 The Role of Chest Wall Fascial Blocks in Awake Cardiac Surgery

The introduction of minimally invasive cardiac techniques as endoscopic, robotic, or less invasive surgery approaches performed through ministernotomy or minithoracotomy has improved less invasive cardiac anesthesia strategies. As shown in the previous chapters, ultrasound locoregional anesthesia in the form of chest wall fascial blocks could be used for both analgesic and anesthetic needs. They were born as sole analgesic procedures [16], but, over the time, they became anesthetic techniques for cardiac surgery procedures in the management of critically ill patients affected by pulmonary diseases but also for minor surgery in patients with different comorbidities in spontaneous breathing avoiding the general anesthesia and the administration of opioids. Actually, the most performed chest wall blocks in awake and spontaneous breathing patients are represented by the parasternal, serratus anterior plane, and interpectoral plane (IPP-PECS I)-pectoserratus plane (PSP-PECS II) blocks and rectus sheath block (RSB) to manage sternal dehiscence, sternal wound debridement, rib fractures, chest tube insertion for pneumothorax, pacemaker and S-ICD implantation, and TAVI. Sepolvere et al. used the superficial parasternal block to manage the sternal dehiscence and sternal wire removal in two different patients affected by severe pulmonary disease (Chap. 25, clinical case n. 25.5). The first patient was laryngectomized 30 years before, and, in the postoperative CABG period, he reported a sternal dehiscence for which a general anesthesia was avoided performing a superficial parasternal block in spontaneous breathing under dexmedetomidine sedation (Fig. 23.1). The second patient was a severe chronic obstructive pulmonary disease (COPD) affected by postoperative sternal wire infection, and a superficial parasternal block was used to remove the wires in spontaneous breathing under total intravenous propofol infusion avoiding the potential side effects of further orotracheal intubation [17]. Toscano et al. described a case of a 75-year-old frail patient who underwent mediastinal revision via subxiphoid access due to the sternal wire infections. Through a combination of pectoralis intercostal and rectus sheath blocks, both the wound revision and the subxiphoid drainage were managed keeping the patient conscious, and no complications were reported [18]. The ultrasound superficial parasternal block was successfully adopted to fix the sternum in a patient with C2 vertebral fracture, and conscious sedation in spontaneous breathing was obtained through the administration of midazolam and remifentanil infusion. No complications were reported, and the patient was discharged on the first postoperative day [19]. Sternal dehiscence occurred in a severe COPD patient who underwent CABG and who presented a postoperative pneumothorax that lasted for about 30 days, which was treated with Heimlich valve (Chap. 25 clinical case n. 25.11). The sternal fixation was managed with superficial parasternal block, avoiding orotracheal intubation and potential further pneumothorax, in spontaneous breathing and dexmedetomidine intravenous sedation without any complications (Fig. 23.2). The chest wall blocks may also be used for critically ill patients with difficult-to-predict airway management as described by Costa et al. who performed a superficial parasternal block for sternotomy debridement in awake and spontaneous breathing

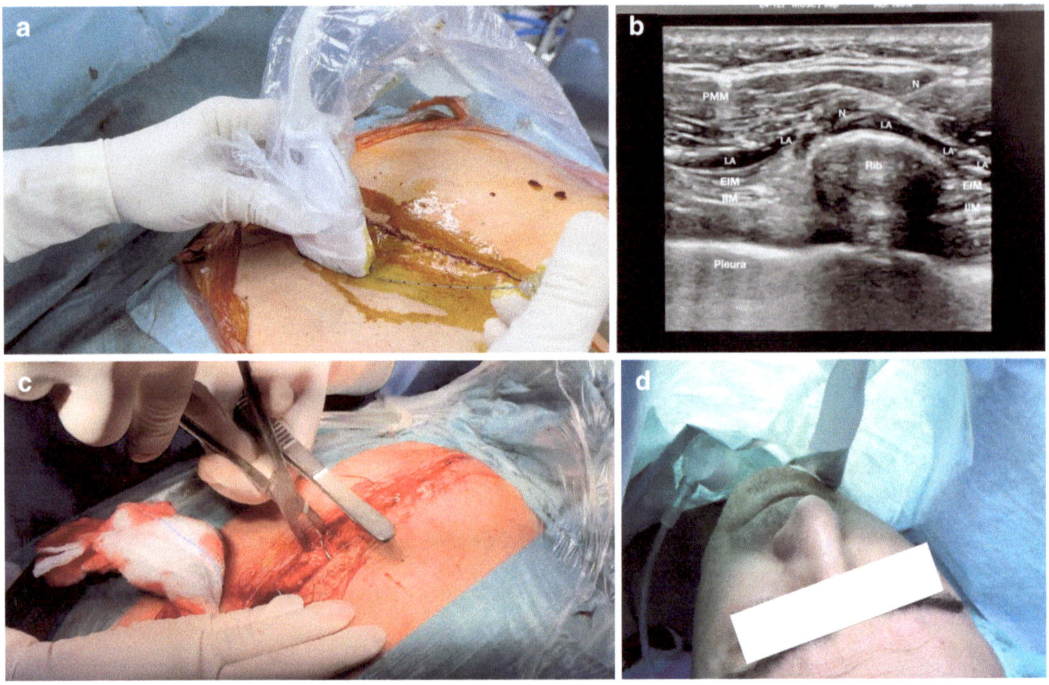

Fig. 23.1 Sternal resynthesis in spontaneous breathing. (**a**) Patient and probe position. (**b**) Modified superficial parasternal block. The local anesthetic is injected between the pectoralis major and external intercostal muscles. (**c**) Sternal resynthesis. (**d**) Spontaneous breathing. *PMM* pectoralis major muscle, *EIM* external intercostal muscle, *IIM* internal intercostal muscle, *Rib* rib, *N* needle, *LA* local anesthetic

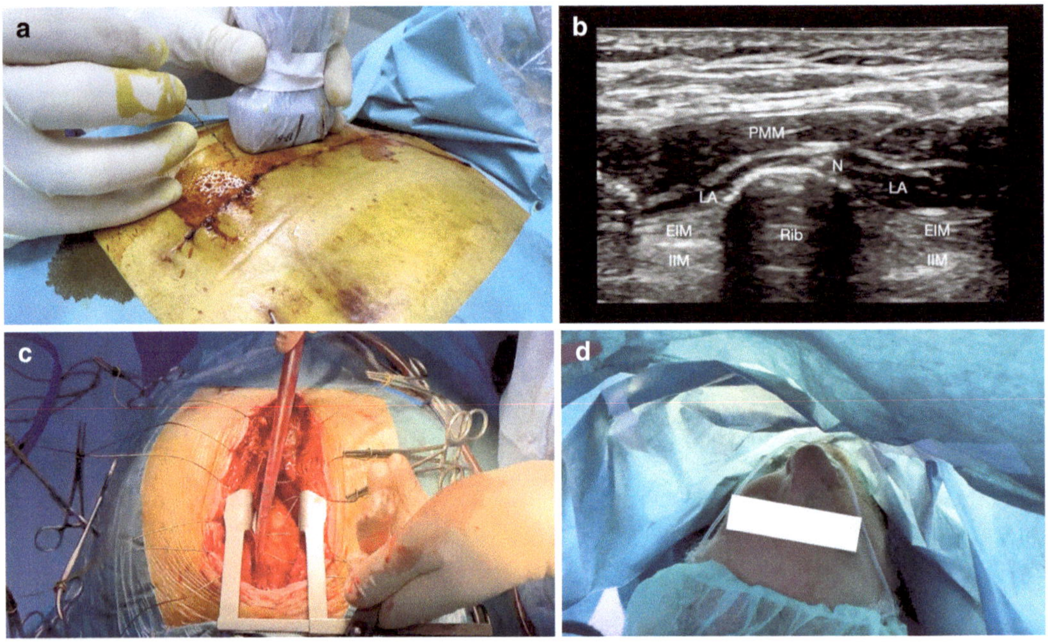

Fig. 23.2 Parasternal block and sternal resynthesis in spontaneous breathing. (**a**) Patient and probe position. (**b**) Modified superficial parasternal block. The local anesthetic is injected between the pectoralis major and external intercostal muscles. (**c**) Sternal wire insertion. (**d**) Spontaneous breathing. *PMM* pectoralis major muscle, *EIM* external intercostal muscle, *IIM* internal intercostal muscle, *Rib* rib, *N* needle, *LA* local anesthetic

patients [20]. IPP-PECS I and PSP-PECS II plane blocks alone or combined with serratus anterior plane block are widely and routinely used for pacemaker [21–23] and S-ICD implantation in patients with severe comorbidity and respiratory failures both providing analgesia and anesthesia, a good hemodynamic profile, and opioid sparing and reducing the complications related to general anesthesia and orotracheal intubation [24–26] (Chap. 25, clinical case n.25.7 and 25.14). Single-shot or continuous serratus anterior plane block may be safely performed in the emergency department to manage multiple rib fracture pain or chest tube insertion for spontaneous or postoperative pneumothorax (Chap. 25, clinical case n. 25.2 and 25.8), hematic pleural effusion, rib metastasis ablation through light sedation, and spontaneous breathing avoiding the admission to intensive care unit [27–30]. Berthoud et al. described a case of transcatheter aortic valve replacement performed in awake patients and ketamine sedation approached via left minithoracotomy through single-shot serratus plane block without complications [31].

23.4 Conclusion

Awake cardiac surgery represents an appealing methodology among anesthesiologists due to the need to avoid the wide number of side effects and complications deriving from general anesthesia, orotracheal intubation, and opioid administration in critically ill patients affected by serious pulmonary disease and comorbidity. To date, despite the description of using the thoracic epidural anesthesia, the risk of spinal hematoma remains the main obstacle among anesthesiologists and no randomized controlled trials with large sample size are published in the scientific panorama. On this basis, the use of thoracic epidural anesthesia is not recommended. In contrast, chest wall blocks may be performed regardless of the coagulation status and no neuraxial bleeding is reported. In addition, chest fascial blocks may be considered highly safe and effective in the treatment of serious respiratory patients kept conscious and in spontaneous breathing as an alternative to general anesthesia avoiding further pulmonary complications. The limits of fascial blocks are represented both by the uncovering of visceral pain and the few awake surgery application fields but represent an interesting growing research sector. The future of awake cardiac surgery is projected towards the implementation and development of randomized controlled trial with large sample size to discover the whole potential of these techniques.

References

1. El Shora HA, El Beleehy AA, Abdelwahab AA, Ali GA, Omran TE, Hassan EA, Arafat AA. Bilateral paravertebral block versus thoracic epidural analgesia for pain control post-cardiac surgery: a randomized controlled trial. Thorac Cardiovasc Surg. 2020;68(5):410–6. https://doi.org/10.1055/s-0038-1668496.
2. Neuburger PJ, Ngai JY, Chacon MM, Luria B, Manrique-Espinel AM, Kline RP, Grossi EA, Loulmet DF. A prospective randomized study of paravertebral blockade in patients undergoing robotic mitral valve repair. J Cardiothorac Vasc Anesth. 2015;29(4):930–6. https://doi.org/10.1053/j.jvca.2014.10.010.
3. Pujara J, Singh G, Prajapati M, Ninama S, Rajesh VSP, Trivedi V, Pandya H. Thoracic paravertebral versus interpleural catheter for post-thoracotomy pain control in minimally invasive cardiac surgery. Asian Cardiovasc Thorac Ann. 2023;31(3):202–9. https://doi.org/10.1177/02184923231154497.
4. Chakravarthy M. Future of awake cardiac surgery. J Cardiothorac Vasc Anesth. 2014;28(3):771–7. https://doi.org/10.1053/j.jvca.2013.03.005.
5. Aybek T, Kessler P, Dogan S, Neidhart G, Khan MF, Wimmer-Greinecker G, Moritz A. Awake coronary artery bypass grafting: utopia or reality? Ann Thorac Surg. 2003;75(4):1165–70. https://doi.org/10.1016/s0003-4975(02)04710-0.
6. Watanabe G, Yamaguchi S, Tomiya S, Ohtake H. Awake subxyphoid minimally invasive direct coronary artery bypass grafting yielded minimum invasive cardiac surgery for high risk patients. Interact Cardiovasc Thorac Surg. 2008;7:910–2. https://doi.org/10.1510/icvts.2007.173377.
7. Tacconi F, Pompeo E, Sellitri F, Mineo TC. Experimental surgical stress hormones response is reduced after awake videothoracoscopy. Interactive CardioVascular Thorac Surg. 2010;10:666–71. https://doi.org/10.1510/icvts.2009.224139.
8. Ishikawa N, Watanabe G. Ultra-minimally invasive cardiac surgery: robotic surgery and awake CABG. Surg Today. 2015;45:1–7. https://doi.org/10.1007/s00595-014-0961-x.

9. Aybek T, Dogan S, Kessler P, Neidhart G, Khan MF, Wimmer-Greinecker G, Moritz A. Complete arterial surgical revascularization through median sternotomy in awake patients. Z Kardiol. 2002;91:238–42. © Steinkopff Verlag 2002
10. Ishikawa N, Watanabe G. Ultra-minimally invasive cardiac surgery: robotic surgery and awake CABG. Surg Today. 2015;45(1):1–7. https://doi.org/10.1007/s00595-014-0961-x.
11. Aybek T, Dogan S, Neidhart G, Kessler P, Matheis G, Wimmer-Greinecker G, Moritz A. Coronary artery bypass grafting through complete sternotomy in conscious patients. Heart Surg Forum. 2002;5(1):17–20.
12. Kessler P, Neidhart G, Lischke V, Bremerich DH, Aybek T, Dogan S, Byhahn C. Koronare Bypassoperation mit kompletter medianer Sternotomie am wachen Patienten in hoher thorakaler Periduralanästhesie [coronary bypass operation with complete median sternotomy in awake patients with high thoracic peridural anesthesia]. Anaesthesist. 2002;51(7):533–8. https://doi.org/10.1007/s00101-002-0337-2.
13. Kessler P, Neidhart G, Bremerich DH, Aybek T, Dogan S, Lischke V, Byhahn C. High thoracic epidural anesthesia for coronary artery bypass grafting using two different surgical approaches in conscious patients. Anesth Analg. 2002;95(4):791–7. https://doi.org/10.1097/00000539-200210000-00002.
14. Aybek T, Kessler P, Khan MF, Dogan S, Neidhart G, Moritz A, Wimmer-Greinecker G. Operative techniques in awake coronary artery bypass grafting. J Thorac Cardiovasc Surg. 2003;125(6):1394–400. https://doi.org/10.1016/s0022-5223(02)73607-6.
15. Kirali K. Composite bilateral internal thoracic artery grafts via standard sternotomy for lateral wall revascularization in conscious patients. Heart Surg Forum. 2005;8(6):E473–7. https://doi.org/10.1532/HSF98.20051164.
16. Sepolvere G, Tedesco M, Fusco P, Scimia P, Cristiano L. Fascial plane blocks in cardiac surgery: a future to discover. Minerva Anestesiol. 2021;87(3):382–3. https://doi.org/10.23736/S0375-9393.20.15271-4.
17. Sepolvere G, Tedesco M, Cristiano L. Ultrasound parasternal block as a novel approach for cardiac sternal surgery: could it be the safest strategy? J Cardiothorac Vasc Anesth. 2020;34(8):2284–6. https://doi.org/10.1053/j.jvca.2020.03.014.
18. Toscano A, Balzani E, Capuano P, Vaninetti A, Perrucci C, Simonato E, Rinaldi M, Brazzi L. Awake cardiac surgery using the novel pectoralis-intercostal-rectus sheath (PIRS) plane block and subxiphoid approach. J Card Surg. 2022;37(9):2923–6. https://doi.org/10.1111/jocs.16658.
19. Dost B, Taflan MG, Kaya C, Gurz S, Tulgar S. Awake sternal fixation using the ultrasound-guided superficial parasternal intercostal plane block in a patient with cervical spine fracture. Cureus. 2022;14(8):e28618. https://doi.org/10.7759/cureus.28618.
20. Costa F, Caruso S, Pascarella G, Nenna A, Grande S, Sarubbi D, Chello M, Agrò FE. Sternotomy debridement in critical patient with difficult predicted airway: can regional anesthesia be the labyrinth exit? Minerva Anestesiol. 2020;86(4):462–3. https://doi.org/10.23736/S0375-9393.19.14133-8.
21. Bozyel S, Yalnız A, Aksu T, Guler TE, Genez S. Ultrasound-guided combined pectoral nerve block and axillary venipuncture for the implantation of cardiac implantable electronic devices. Pacing Clin Electrophysiol. 2019;42(7):1026–31. https://doi.org/10.1111/pace.13725.
22. Mavarez AC, Ripat CI, Suarez MR. Pectoralis plane block for pacemaker insertion: a successful primary anesthetic. Front Surg. 2019;6:64. https://doi.org/10.3389/fsurg.2019.00064.
23. Elhaddad AM, Hefnawy SM, El-Aziz MA, Ebraheem MM, Mohamed AK. Pectoral nerve blocks for transvenous subpectoral pacemaker insertion in children: a randomized controlled study. Korean J Anesthesiol. 2023;76(5):424–32. https://doi.org/10.4097/kja.22681.
24. Droghetti A, Fusco P, Marini M, Harizai F, Scimia P. Ultrasound guided serratus anterior plane block and parasternal block in cooperative sedation for S-ICD implantation. Pacing Clin Electrophysiol. 2019;42(7):1076–8. https://doi.org/10.1111/pace.13727.
25. Droghetti A, Basso Ricci E, Scimia P, Harizai F, Marini M. Ultrasound-guided serratus anterior plane block combined with the two-incision technique for subcutaneous ICD implantation. Pacing Clin Electrophysiol. 2018;41(5):517–23. https://doi.org/10.1111/pace.13318.
26. Ziacchi M, Bisignani G, Palmisano P, Scalone A, Martignani C, Elvira Mocavero P, Caravati F, Della Cioppa N, Mazzuero A, Pecora D, Vicentini A, Landolina ME, Debonis S, Scimia P, Lovecchio M, Valsecchi S, Diemberger I, Droghetti A. Serratus anterior plane block in subcutaneous implantable cardioverter defibrillator implantation: a case-control analysis. J Cardiovasc Electrophysiol. 2020;31(1):144–9. https://doi.org/10.1111/jce.14293.
27. Paul S, Bhoi SK, Sinha TP, Kumar G. Ultrasound-guided serratus anterior plane block for rib fracture-associated pain management in emergency department. J Emerg Trauma Shock. 2020;13(3):208–12. https://doi.org/10.4103/JETS.JETS_155_19.
28. Gorecha M, Menon A, Woodford E, Yahia S, Marimuthu K. Early serratus plane block for rib fracture management could avoid intensive care unit admission. Indian J Crit Care Med. 2020;24(10):995. https://doi.org/10.5005/jp-journals-10071-23631.
29. Fusco P, Scimia P, Di Carlo S, Testa A, Luciani A, Petrucci E, Marinangeli F. Ultrasound-guided serratus plane block and fast-track tracheal extubation in the operating room for thoracic trauma patients: a case report. A A Case Rep. 2017;9(11):305–7. https://doi.org/10.1213/XAA.0000000000000600.
30. Fusco P, Vespasiano M, Di Carlo S, Scimia P, Petrucci E, Marinangeli F. Ultrasound-guided serratus plane

block and image-guided microwave ablation of a rib metastasis. Minerva Anestesiol. 2018;84(12):1426–7. https://doi.org/10.23736/S0375-9393.18.12938-5.

31. Berthoud V, Ellouze O, Bièvre T, Konstantinou M, Jazayeri S, Bouchot O, Girard C, Bouhemad B. Serratus anterior plane block for apical TAVR in an awake patient. J Cardiothorac Vasc Anesth. 2018;32(5):2275–7. https://doi.org/10.1053/j.jvca.2017.12.042.

24 Costs and Length of Stay in Cardiac Surgery

Daniele Marianello, Cesare Biuzzi, Federico Franchi, and Sabino Scolletta

24.1 What Influences Costs in the Context of Cardiac Surgery?

24.1.1 Preoperative Evaluation

The pathway of each surgical intervention begins with a detailed and comprehensive preoperative assessment. A key component of this initial phase is the anesthesiology evaluation, whose primary goal is to examine in depth the patient's overall health history and the starting medical condition. This evaluation typically involves a variety of laboratory and diagnostic tests. These tests may include echocardiography to assess heart function, chest radiography, coronary angiography, as well as other specific diagnostic procedures that may be required based on the individual patient's health condition. In this phase, it's essential to thoroughly review the patient's medical history in order to identify any pre-existing medical conditions and medications that could have repercussions during the intraoperative and postoperative periods. An inadequate preoperative assessment can lead to underestimating risk conditions, resulting in foreseeable complications that can sometimes be managed preventively. After a good preoperative evaluation, the healthcare team is able to design a highly individualized care plan and anticipate, as much as possible, potential complications that could prolong the hospital stay and increase costs.

24.1.2 Surgical Procedure

The type and complexity of the surgical procedure play a major role in determining overall costs. From coronary artery bypass graft to valve repair or replacement, each procedure brings with it a range of associated expenses. These include the costs of surgical supplies, the use of specialized equipment, and the time required in the operation room, all of which can vary significantly depending on the complexity of the operation. Among the various procedures, the repair of atrial or ventricular defects tends to have the lowest average hospitalization costs. This is followed by coronary artery bypass graft (CABG) and valve replacements, particularly involving aortic or mitral valves. However, costs rise significantly for more complex procedures, such as the Bentall

D. Marianello · F. Franchi
Department of Medical Science, Surgery and Neurosciences, Cardiothoracic and Vascular Anesthesia and Intensive Care Unit, University Hospital of Siena, Siena, Italy

S. Scolletta (✉)
Department of Medical Science, Surgery and Neurosciences, Anesthesia and Intensive Care Unit, University Hospital of Siena, Siena, Italy
e-mail: sabino.scolletta@dbm.unisi.it

C. Biuzzi
Department of Emergency-Urgency, Anesthesia and Intensive Care Unit, University Hospital of Siena, Siena, Italy

G. Sepolvere, S. Silvetti (eds.), *Fast-Track in Cardiac Anesthesia*,
https://doi.org/10.1007/978-3-031-70899-2_24

procedure or replacement of the ascending aorta. At the top end of the cost range, the highest average hospitalization expenses are associated with patients who undergo a combination of multiple procedures, such as aortic valve replacement + mitral valve replacement + coronary artery bypass grafting, all performed during the same operation [1]. In addition to the type of surgery, other intraoperative factors can impact postoperative management, influencing both the duration of hospital stay and the overall costs. These factors include the techniques used for myocardial protection during surgery and the strategies employed to control blood loss. Managing these variables effectively can help reduce complications and optimize recovery, ultimately influencing the total cost of care.

24.1.3 Post-Operative Care: Intensive Care Unit (ICU) Admission

The postoperative phase is equally critical and is marked by several factors that influence the total hospitalization cost. After undergoing cardiac surgery, all patients are typically transferred to the intensive care unit (ICU) for close monitoring and weaning from mechanical ventilation. The duration and intensity of this monitoring can vary significantly depending on the patient's condition and outcomes of the surgery. ICUs represent the largest portion of hospital expenditure, often accounting for up to 60% of the total costs. Additionally, these units tend to utilize disproportionate amount of resources for a limited number of patients, which can further drive up overall healthcare costs [2]. Several factors can negatively impact total healthcare expenses during the postoperative phase. For example, prolonged sedation time, extendend oro-tracheal intubation and mechanical ventilation time can lead to increase costs. The latter exposes the patient to a higher risk of ventilator-associated pneumonia, which not only necessitates additional treatment but also often results in a longer hospital stay. Research by Salhiyyah et al has shown that promoting a faster recovery process in the recovery unit following cardiac surgery can decrease the intensive care length of stay in the ICU as well as the total duration of intubation [3].

Therefore, when surgical outcomes and patient's condition permit, it is advisable to initiate early awakening and extubation to facilitate a more efficient recovery process and ultimately reduce overall health care costs. These premises are one hinge of ERAS.

24.1.4 Complications and Readmissions

Complications that occur after cardiac surgery can lead to a substantial increase in health care costs, often requiring additional resources and resulting in prolonged hospital stay. These complications may include arrhythmias and reduced cardiac function, both of which require the use of specific and often expensive medications and sometimes also mechanical support, to manage the patient's condition effectively. Infectious complications are a possible occurrence in ICUs. Issues as wound infections or pneumonia can arise, posing serious risk to recovery. The increasingly prevalence of bacterial resistance to commonly used antibiotics can complicate treatment, sometimes requiring the use of extremely expensive next-generation drugs. Moreover, these infections tend to lengthen hospital stays, further contributing to rising healthcare costs. During the hospitalization period, it is also important to consider the costs related to the use of albumin, specific solutions for volume expansion, and various products used to correct hemostatic disorders such as fibrinogen and coagulation factors [1]. Delirium represents another complication that can significantly increase hospitalization costs. This condition is associated with various negative outcomes, such as self-extubation, as well as increased healthcare expenses and increased morbidity [4].

Finally, readmissions to the ICU due to complications create additional strain on healthcare resources and incur costs that could be otherwise avoided. Addressing these complications proactively is essential for managing overall expenses and improving patient's outcome in the postoperative care setting.

24.1.5 Progress

Over the years, advancements in technology and surgical techniques have significantly revolutionized the field of cardiac surgery, leading to improve patient's outcomes and shorter recovery times. The introduction of minimally invasive techniques has been a major breakthrough, allowing surgeons to perform complex procedures with less trauma to the body. For instance, minimally invasive approaches can also be used in cardiac surgery, for example, in the treatment of mitral valve disease, offering patients a less invasive alternative with potentially faster recovery. Additionally, in some cases of ischemic heart disease, off-pump surgery can be utilized, which avoid the need for cardiopulmonary bypass, thereby reducing the risks and complications associated with this technique. Despite the many benefits of these innovative approaches, their adoptions come with high costs. The advanced equipment, specialized training and extended preparation required for minimally invasive and off-pump surgery can drive up the overall costs of the procedures. As a result, while these techniques improve patients outcomes and reduce recovery times, they also have a considerable impact on the total financial burden associated with cardiac surgery. Differently, all new anesthesiological approach proposed by ERASC society, as locoregional anesthesia and opioids sparing or early extubation, are low cost or zero cost and, if performed in a good manner, they are able to improve patients outcomes.

24.2 What Are the Determinants of Length of Stay?

24.2.1 Patient-Related Factors

Patient age, overall health status, the presence of comorbidities, and adherence to preoperative instructions are critical factors in determining the length of hospital stay following cardiac surgery. Patients who have multiple comorbidities or are at higher risk for postoperative complications generally require prolonged hospitalization to ensure proper monitoring and recovery. For example, many variables were identified to be independent predictors of ICU length of stay: increased age, chronic obstructive pulmonary disease, renal failure, atrial fibrillation, New York Heart Association class III-IV, previous cardiac surgery and inotropes support [5]. Meadows et al., using the European System for Cardiac Operative Risk Evaluation, have demonstrated that the length of stay can be accurately predicted based on these factors. Excellent prediction of prolonged ICU stay can be achieved by using Society of Thoracic Surgeons data as demonstrated by Rotar and colleagues [6]. Being able to predict a patient's stay in ICU offers numerous advantages. For the patients, it allows for more precise postoperative care planning, ensuring that necessary resources and interventions are in place. For healthcare organizations, it helps in optimizing resource allocation, improving efficiency, and ensuring better use of ICU beds and staff, ultimately enhancing the overall management of healthcare services [7].

24.2.2 Surgical Intervention

Complex surgical procedures inevitably lead to extend hospital stays due to the need for comprehensive postoperative monitoring and management. Zarrizi et al shown that having more than two chest tubes, occurrence of atelectasis and occurrence of atrial fibrillation after CABG were risk factors associated with longer ICU length of stay [8]. Following such procedures, patients often require specialized care in ICU, which may include the use of the mechanical ventilation, hemodynamic support, or other advanced interventions to stabilize their condition and aid recovery. These critical care needs contribute significantly to the prolonged length of stay in the ICU, as they ensure the patient is closely monitored and managed to prevent complications, ultimately increasing the overall duration of hospitalization.

24.2.3 Complications

As previously discussed, the occurence of complications, such as infections, bleeding, or organ dysfunction, can greatly extend the duration of hospitalization. These complications require additional medical interventions and close monitoring, which inevitably delay the patient's recovery and prolongs their stay in hospital. Another factor that affects the length of stay is the recovery of functional independence. The time it takes for a patient to regain the ability to perform daily activities without assistance and achieve optimal recovery plays a crucial role in determining when they are ready for discharge. Patients who recover their independence more quickly can often be discharged earlier, whereas those needing more time for rehabilitation and support may experience longer hospital stays.

24.3 What Strategies Can Optimise Costs and Length of Stay?

An important strategy for optimizing both cost and hospital stay is the implementation of Enhanced Recovery After Surgery (ERAS) protocols. These protocols when applied in cardiac surgery, promote standardized preoperative care pathways designed to minimize surgical stress, optimize organ function and accelerate recovery times. By following ERAS guidelines, healthcare teams can streamline care process, reduce variability and improve patient outcomes. Collaboration among multidisciplinary teams, which include surgeons, anesthesiologists, nurses, and other healthcare professionals, is crucial in ensuring comprehensive patient care. This collaborative approach allows for the early detection of potential complications that could lead to increased costs and prolonged hospital stays, ensuring timely intervention. A key component of this strategy is patient education. By educating patients about their condition, available treatment options, and the perioperative process, they become more engaged and actively involved in their care journey. This not only empowers patients but also improve adherence to care plans, which can enhance recovery and reduce the need for extended hospitalization. Data analysis plays a vital role in identifying areas for improvement and establishing best practices in perioperative management. Through continuous monitoring and evaluation of patient outcomes, healthcare institutions can implement targeted interventions aimed at optimizing costs and minimizing the length of hospital stays. In conclusion, managing costs and hospital stay in cardiac surgery demands a multifactorial approach that integrates clinical expertise, technological advances, and personalized patient care. By optimizing resource utilization, minimizing complications, and promoting early recovery, healthcare professionals can achieve the best optimal outcomes for patients while ensuring efficient use of healthcare resources.

References

1. Thelogou S, Konstantakopoulou O, Vozikis A. Factors increasing hospitalization cost in adult patients post cardiac surgery. Int J Caring. 2020;13:1752–61.
2. Aung YN, Nur AM, Ismail A, Aljunid S. Determining the cost and leght of stay at intensive care unit and factors influencing them in a teaching hospital in Malaysia. Value Health Regional Issues. 2020;13:149–56.
3. Salhiyyah K, Elsobky S, Raja S, Attia R, Brazier J, Cooper GJ. A clinical and economic evaluation of fast-track recovery after cardiac surgery. Heart Surg Forum. 2011;14(6):E330–4. https://doi.org/10.1532/HSF98.20111029. PMID: 22167756.
4. Milbrandt EB, Deppen S, Harrison PL, Shintani AK, Speroff T, Stiles RA. Costs associated with delirium in mechanically ventilated patients". Crit Care Med. 2004;32(4):955–62.
5. Almashrafi A, Elmontsri M, Aylin P. Systematic review of factors influencing length of stay in ICU after adult cardiac surgery BMC Health Services Research. 2016;16:318.
6. Rotar EP, Beller JP, Smolkin ME, Chancellor WZ, Ailawadi G, Yarboro LT, Hulse M, Ratcliffe SJ, Teman NR. Prediction of prolonged intensive care unit length of stay following cardiac surgery Semin Torac Cardiovasc Surg. 2022;34(1):172–9.
7. Meadows K, Gibbens R, Gerrard C, Vuylsteke A. Prediction of patient length of stay on the intensive care unit following cardiac surgery: a logistic regression analysis based on the cardiac operative mortality risk calculator, EuroSCORE J Cardiothorac Vasc Anesth. 2018;32(6):2676–82.
8. Zarrizi M, Paryad E, Khanghah AG, Leili EK, Faghani H. Predictors of length of stay in ICU after coronary artery bypass grafting: development a risk scoring system Braz J Cardiovasc Surg. 2021;36(1):57–63.

Part VI

Clinical Cases

25 Clinical Cases

Giuseppe Sepolvere

25.1 Introduction

The most asked question about the perioperative management of critically ill patients or in case of emergency conditions regards the appropriate anesthetic technique matching with the surgical needs. The main criteria for choosing the proper anesthetic approach are focused on the acquisition of the basic notions of standard and ultrasound anatomy, patient's conditions, type of surgery, and individual anesthetic skills. Further doubts are related both to the local anesthetic or adjuvant dosages and volumes and concentrations used while performing a regional technique. The description of several clinical cases aims at providing a fast-decision-making model to all beginner and experienced anesthesiologists who are looking for innovative techniques for fast-track daily practice. The below-described associative visualization model, showing the main fascial blocks and their anatomical and dermatomal regions, may result useful for a quick evaluation of a proper chest wall block and its relationship with the surgical site [1] (Fig. 25.1).

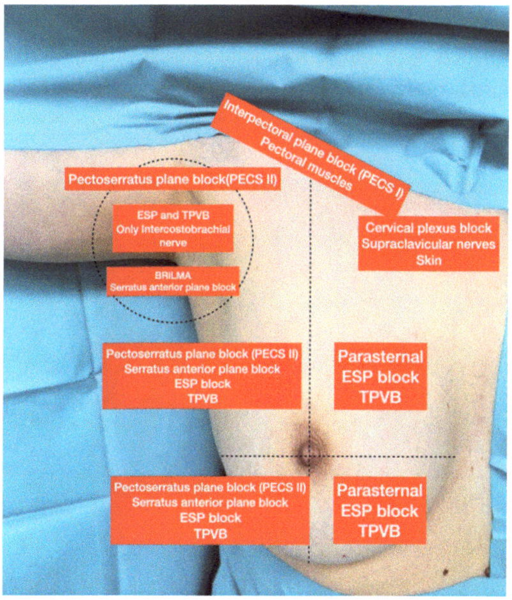

Fig. 25.1 Associative visualization model, showing the main fascial blocks and their anatomical and dermatomal regions, useful for a quick evaluation of a proper chest wall block depending on the surgical site. *ESP* erector spinae block, *TPVB* thoracic paravertebral block, *BRILMA blocking the* cutaneous branches of intercostal nerves in the middle axillary line

G. Sepolvere (✉)
Department of Anesthesia and Cardiac Surgery
Intensive Care Unit, San Michele Hospital,
Maddaloni, Caserta, Italy

G. Sepolvere, S. Silvetti (eds.), *Fast-Track in Cardiac Anesthesia*,
https://doi.org/10.1007/978-3-031-70899-2_25

25.2 Deep Serratus Anterior Plane Block for a Pleural Drainage Insertion in Awake Patient After Left Pneumothorax

A severe chronic obstructive pulmonary disease patient was admitted to emergency room mildly dyspneic with a spontaneous left pneumothorax [2] (Fig. 25.2).

Medical history: 76 Years old, previous coronary artery bypass grafting, on therapy with acetyl salicylic acid, ASA 2.

Anesthetic technique: Left single-shot deep serratus anterior plane block (BRILMA) performed with a high-frequency linear probe on the midaxillary line at the level of the fifth rib and a 100 mm 21G needle inserted through an in-plane approach (Fig. 25.3).

Local anesthetic: Mepivacaine 1% (chosen for the short-term anesthesia and analgesia in the tube insertion region).

Volume and dosage: 30 mL (300 mg of Mepivacaine 1%).

Adjuvant: None.

Intraoperative sedation: None.

Airway management: Spontaneous breathing with nasal goggles (O_2 3 L/m) (Fig. 25.4).

Intraoperative monitoring: ECG, HR, NIBP, SpO_2.

Postoperative pain: NRS 0.

Postoperative analgesia: None.

Perioperative complications or adverse events: None.

Patient satisfaction level: Excellent.

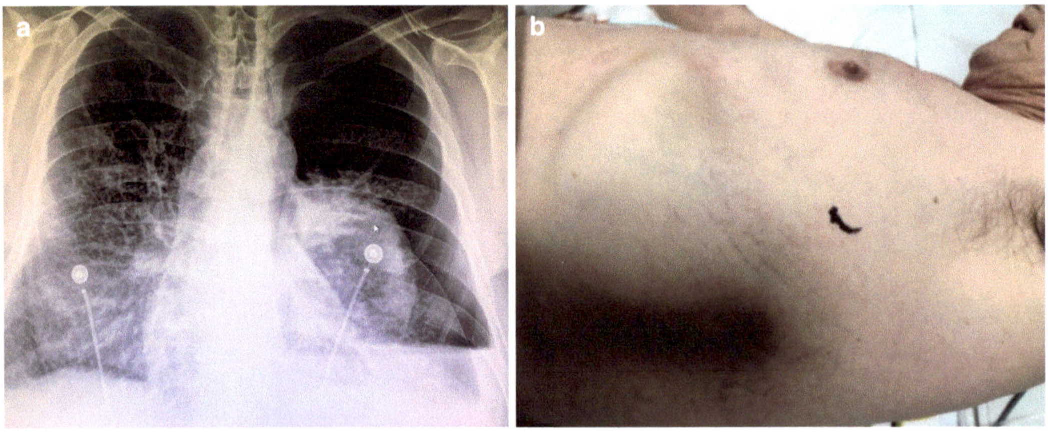

Fig. 25.2 (**a**) X-ray left pneumothorax. (**b**) Tube insertion site

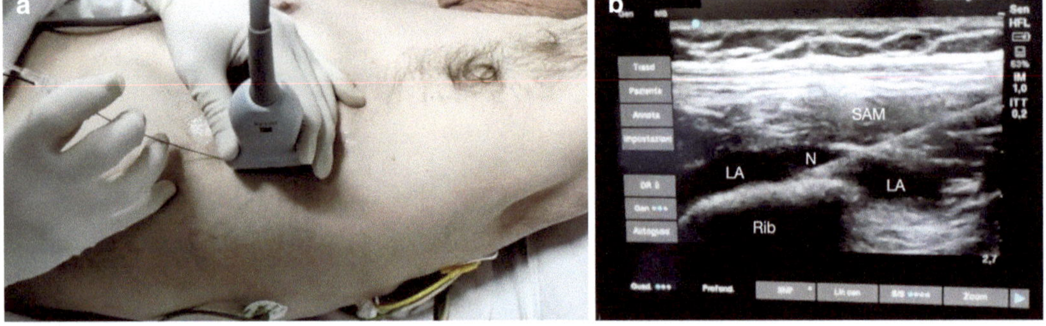

Fig. 25.3 Deep serratus plane block for chest tube insertion. (**a**) Patient and probe position. The patient is placed in right lateral position, and the probe is on the midaxillary lane. The needle is inserted in a caudal-to-cranial direction. (**b**) The tip of the needle is placed on the rib surface, and the local anesthetic is injected below the serratus anterior muscle. *SAM* serratus anterior muscle, *N* needle, *Rib* rib, *LA* local anesthetic

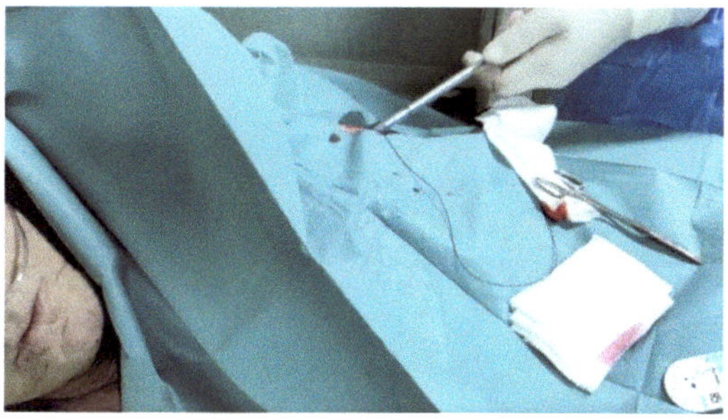

Fig. 25.4 Chest tube insertion and spontaneous breathing

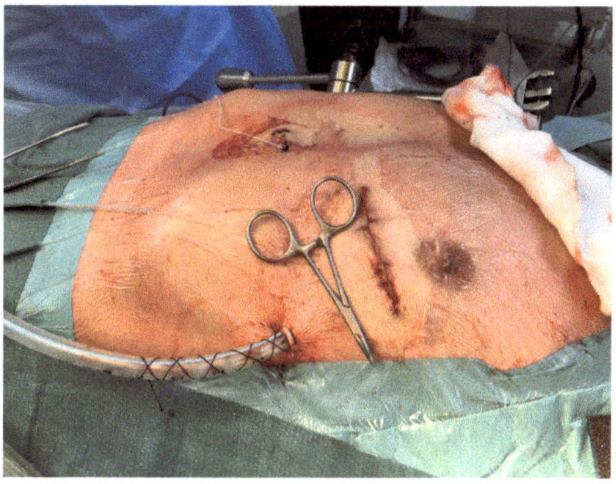

Fig. 25.5 Coronary artery bypass grafting through left minithoracotomy. The drainage tube is inserted into the VI left intercostal space

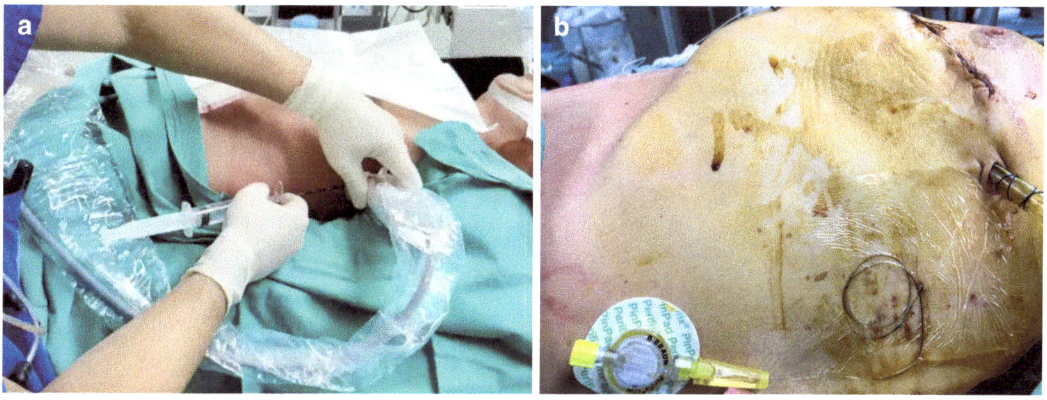

Fig. 25.6 Continuous deep serratus anterior plane block. (**a**) Patient and probe position. (**b**) Catheter insertion and medication

25.3 Continuous Deep Serratus Anterior Plane Block for Postoperative Analgesia in a Patient Undergoing Coronary Artery Bypass Surgery Through Left Minithoracotomy

The following patient was scheduled for coronary artery bypass grafting through left minithoracotomy. A continuous deep serratus anterior plane block was performed to manage the postoperative pain and allow the fast-track extubation and the early pulmonary rehabilitation [3] (Fig. 25.5).

Medical history: 67 Years old, blood hypertension, dyslipidemia, allergy to paracetamol, ASA 3.

Anesthesiological technique: Left deep continuous serratus anterior plane block (BRILMA) performed with a high-frequency linear probe on the midaxillary line at the level of the fifth rib and a 100 mm 22 G needle Tuohy inserted through an in-plane approach below the serratus anterior muscle (Figs. 25.6 and 25.7).

Local anesthetic: 30 mL of levobupivacaine 0.375% (112.5 mg) as single shot allowing the catheter insertion; continuous infusion of levobupivacaine 0.125% (10 mL/h) used for the postoperative pain management.

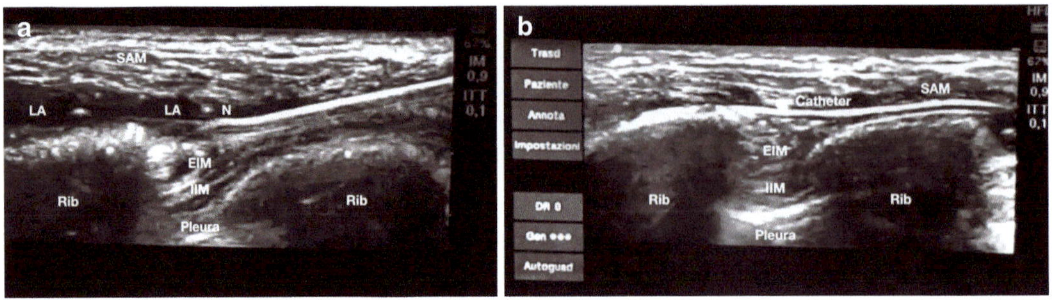

Fig. 25.7 Continuous deep serratus anterior plane block. (**a**) Local anesthetic is injected below the serratus anterior muscle. (**b**) The catheter is placed between the serratus anterior muscle and ribs. *SAM* serratus anterior muscle, *EIM* external intercostal muscle, *IIM* internal intercostal muscle, *Rib* rib, *Pleura* pleura, *LA* local anesthetic, *N* needle, *Catheter* catheter

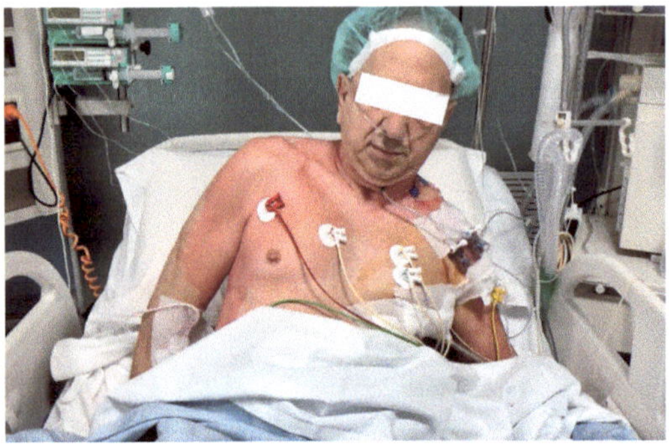

Fig. 25.8 The patient is able to move independently in bed to get a comfortable position without feeling pain

Adjuvant: None.

Intraoperative sedation: General anesthesia through 1.5–2 ng/mL propofol and remifentanil target controlled infusion (TCI).

Airway management: Orotracheal intubation.

Intraoperative monitoring: ECG, HR, IBP, SpO_2; $ETCO_2$; temperature.

Postoperative analgesia: Continuous infusion of ketorolac 150 mg over 48 h; continuous infusion of levobupivacaine 0.125% (5 mL/h). Infusion stopped 48 h after surgery, and the catheter removed on the fourth postoperative day.

Postoperative pain: NRS between 0 and 4.

Perioperative complications or adverse events: None.

Patient satisfaction: Excellent (Fig. 25.8).

25.4 Postoperative Pacemaker Implantation in a Patient Undergoing Mitral Valve Replacement

On the third postoperative day, the patient developed a third-degree atrioventricular block, and a pacemaker was implanted [4, 5].

Medical history: Woman, 70 years old, blood hypertension, severe mitral valve insufficiency, atrial fibrillation treated with warfarin, ASA 4.

Anesthetic technique: Interpectoral plane (PECS I) block performed with a high-frequency linear probe and a 100 mm 21G needle inserted through a lateral to medial direction and in-plane approach between the pectoralis major and minor muscles (Fig. 25.9).

Local anesthetic: Levobupivacaine 0.5% 15 mL (75 mg).

Adjuvant: Dexamethasone 4 mg.

Intraoperative sedation: Midazolam 5 mg.

Airway management: Spontaneous breathing with nasal goggles (O_2 5 L/m).

Intraoperative monitoring: ECG, HR, NIBP, SpO_2.

Postoperative analgesia: None.

Postoperative pain: NRS 0.

Perioperative complications or adverse events: None.

Patient satisfaction level: Excellent.

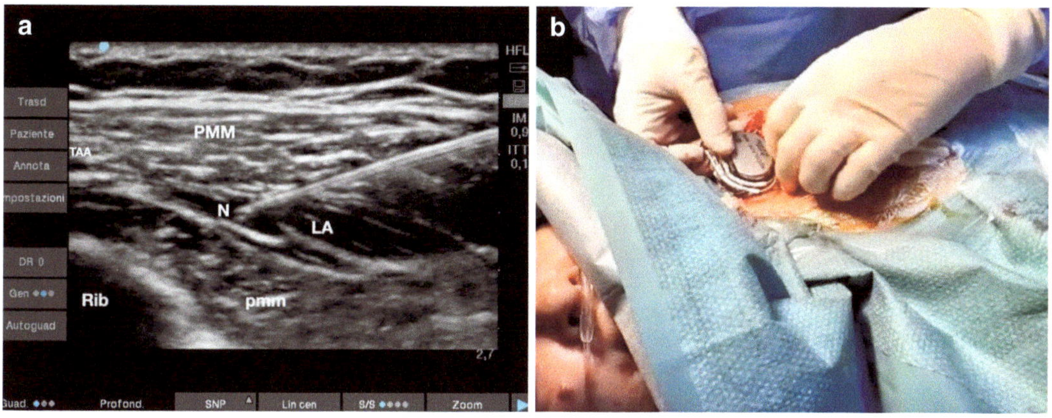

Fig. 25.9 (**a**) Interpectoral plane (PECS I) block. (**b**) Pacemaker implantation and spontaneous breathing. *PMM* pectoralis major muscle, *pmm* pectoralis minor muscle, *N* needle, *LA* local anesthetic, *Rib* rib, *TAA* thoracoacromial artery

25.5 Bilateral Modified Superficial Parasternal Block for Sternal Resynthesis in Awake Patient

The following is the case of a sternal resynthesis in awake laryngectomee patient suffering from serious respiratory diseases [6–10].

Medical history: Man, 73 years old, previous laryngectomy for a laryngeal cancer, severe chronic obstructive pulmonary disease, home oxygen therapy, underwent coronary artery bypass grafting surgery 10 days before, on therapy with acetyl salicylic acid, ASA 3.

Anesthetic technique: Bilateral modified superficial parasternal block performed with a high-frequency linear probe and a 100 mm 21G needle inserted at the level of second and fourth ribs through an in-plane approach and caudal-to-cranial direction. Two injections for each side for a total of four injections (Fig. 25.10a, b).

Local anesthetic: Levobupivacaine 0.375%. 15 mL (56.25 mg of levobupivacaine 0.375%) for each side and a total of 112.5 mg of levobupivacaine 0.375% and a volume of 30 mL.

Adjuvants: Dexmedetomidine 1 mcg/kg (60 mcg) mixed with the anesthetic solution.

Intraoperative sedation: Intravenous dexmedetomidine starting at 0.8 mcg/kg in 20 min and then at 0.6 mcg/kg/h.

Airway management: Spontaneous breathing with oxygen 5 L/m through tracheotomy tube.

Intraoperative monitoring: ECG, HR, NIBP, SpO_2.

Postoperative analgesia: Paracetamol 1 g every 8 h without the need for opioid administration.

Postoperative pain: NRS 0.

Perioperative complications or adverse events: None.

Patient satisfaction level: Excellent.

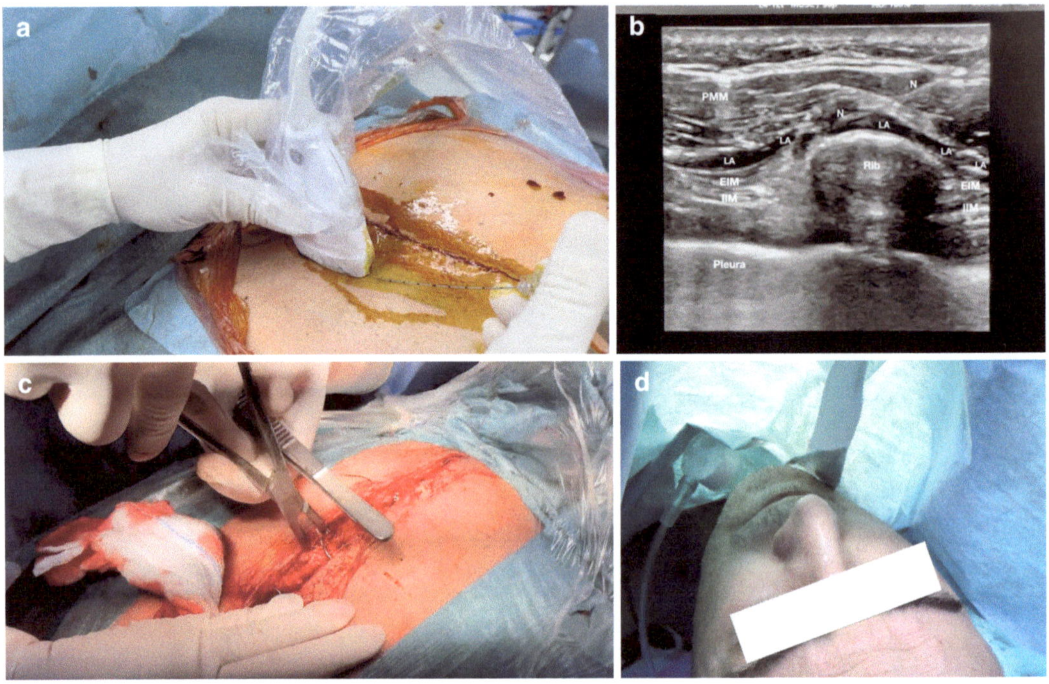

Fig. 25.10 (**a**) Patient and probe position. (**b**) Modified superficial parasternal block. The local anesthetic is injected between the pectoralis major and external intercostal muscles. (**c**) Sternal resynthesis. (**d**) Spontaneous breathing. *PMM* pectoralis major muscle, *EIM* external intercostal muscle, *IIM* internal intercostal muscle, *Rib* rib, *N* needle, *LA* local anesthetic, *Pleura* pleura

25.6 Erector Spinae Plane and Single-Shot Deep Serratus Plane Blocks for Right Minithoracotomy Atrial Septal Defect Closure

The following is the case of a young man affected by several previous transitory ischemic attacks due to the presence of a large atrial septal defect undergoing its closure through right minithoracotomy [11–13] (Fig. 25.11).

Medical history: Man, 38 years old, large atrial septal defect and previous transitory ischemic attacks.

Anesthetic technique:

1. Preoperative continuous erector spinae plane block performed with a high-frequency linear probe and a catheter inserted through a Tuohy needle at the level of T4 transverse process via an in-plane approach and caudal-to-cranial direction (Fig. 25.12).

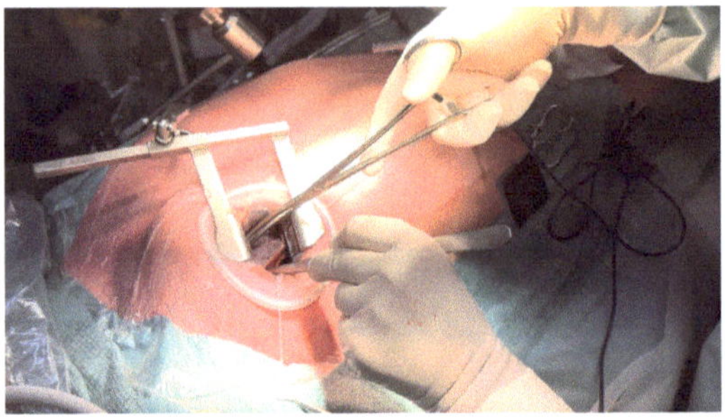

Fig. 25.11 Right minithoracotomy atrial septal defect closure

2. Postoperative single-shot deep serratus plane block performed with a high-frequency linear probe and a 100 mm needle inserted at the level of fourth rib (Fig. 25.13).
3. Interpectoral plane (PECS I) block performed by the injection of local anesthetic between the pectoralis major and minor muscles to manage pain deriving from the chest tube passing through the muscles (Fig. 25.14).

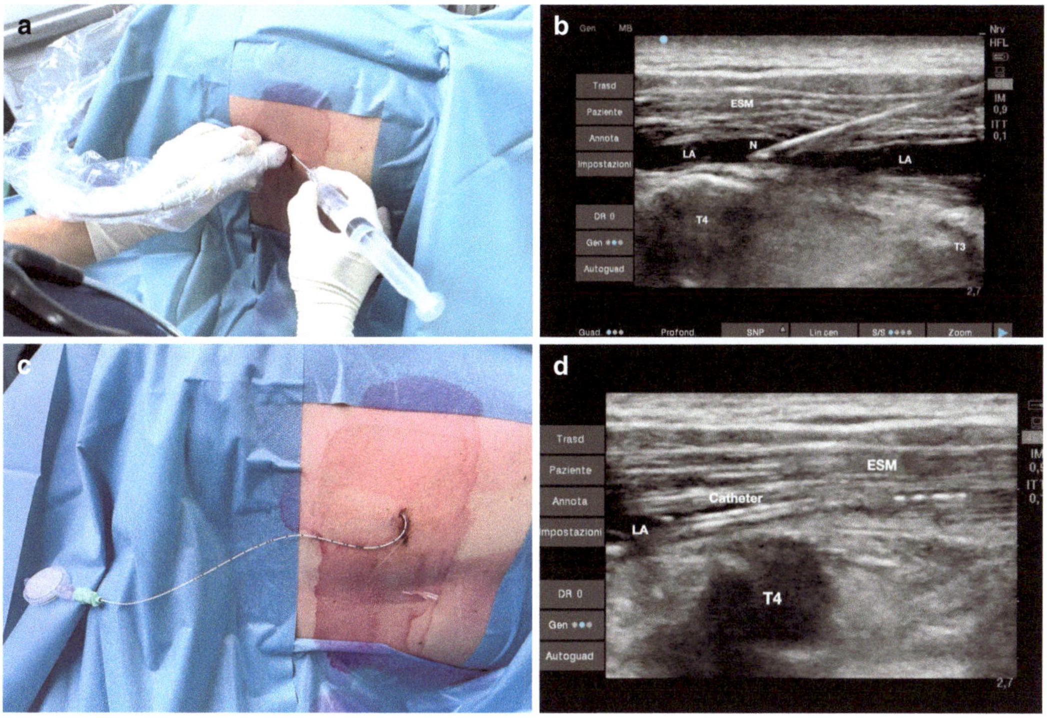

Fig. 25.12 Continuous erector spinae plane block. (**a**) Patient and probe position. (**b**) Local anesthetic is injected between the erector spinae muscle and the T4 transverse process surface. (**c**) Catheter insertion. (**d**) Catheter insertion at the level of T4 transverse process. *ESM* erector spinae muscle, *N* needle, *LA* local anesthetic, *T4* T4 transverse process, *T3* T3 transverse process, *Catheter* catheter

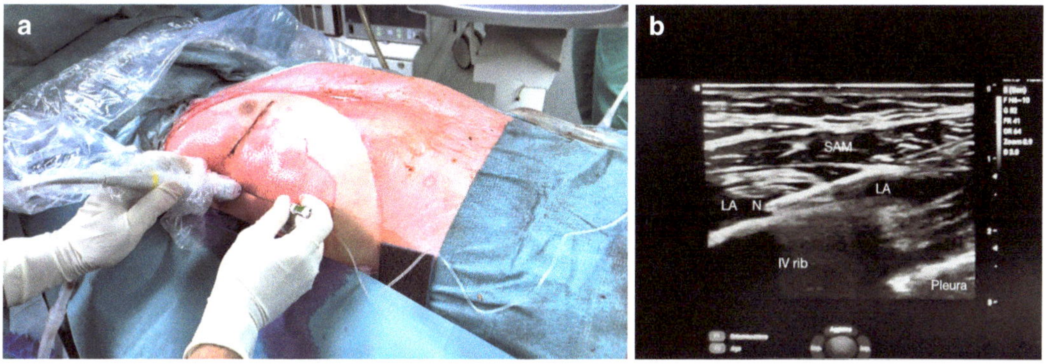

Fig. 25.13 Single-shot deep serratus plane block. (**a**) Patient and probe position. (**b**) Local anesthetic is injected below the serratus anterior muscle at the level of the fourth rib. *SAM* serratus anterior muscle, *LA* local anesthetic, *N* needle, *Rib* rib, *Pleura* pleura

Local anesthetic:

1. ESP block: Preoperative single shot of levobupivacaine 0.25%, 20 mL (50 mg of levobupivacaine 0.25%). Postoperative infusion with levobupivacaine 0.25% (10 mL/h).
2. Postoperative single-shot deep serratus anterior plane block: Levobupivacaine 0.25%, 30 mL (75 mg of levobupivacaine 0.25%).
3. Interpectoral plane (PECS I) block: Levobupivacaine 0.25%, 10 mL (25 mg of levobupivacaine 0.25%).

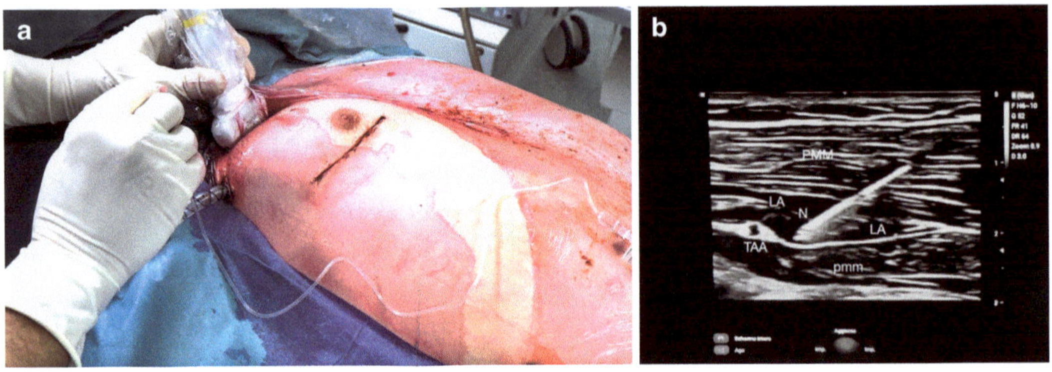

Fig. 25.14 Interpectoral plane (PECS I) block. (**a**) Patient and probe position. (**b**) Local anesthetic is injected between pectoralis major and minor muscles. *PMM* pectoralis major muscle, *pmm* pectoralis minor muscle, *N* needle, *LA* local anesthetic, *TAA* thoracoacromial artery

Adjuvants: Dexmedetomidine 1 mcg/kg (80 mcg) mixed with the whole anesthetic solution.

Intraoperative sedation: General anesthesia.

Postoperative analgesia: Paracetamol 1 g every 8 h without the need for opioid administration.

Postoperative pain: NRS 2.

Perioperative complications or adverse events: None.

Patient satisfaction level: Excellent.

25.7 Superficial Parasternal Block Combined with Deep Serratus Anterior Plane Block for S-ICD Implantation in Spontaneous Breathing Patient

This is a case of a young man affected by Brugada syndrome undergoing a protective S-ICD implantation [14].

Medical history: Man, 45 years old, no pathology referred, no therapy.

Anesthetic technique:

1. Unilateral (left) modified superficial parasternal block performed with a high-frequency linear probe and a 100 mm 21G needle inserted at the level of second and fourth ribs through an in-plane approach and caudal-to-cranial direction. Two injections for the left side (Fig. 25.15a).
2. Deep serratus anterior plane block performed with a high-frequency linear probe and a 100 mm 21G needle inserted at the level of fifth rib through an in-plane approach and caudal-to-cranial direction (Fig. 25.15c).

Local anesthetic:

1. Superficial parasternal block: Levobupivacaine 0.375%, 16 mL (8 mL for each injection for a total of 60 mg of levobupivacaine 0.375%) (Fig. 25.15b).
2. Deep serratus anterior plane block: Levobupivacaine 0.375%, 30 mL (for a total of 112.5 mg of levobupivacaine 0.375%) (Fig. 25.15d).

Adjuvants: Dexmedetomidine 1 mcg/kg (80 mcg) mixed with the anesthetic solution.

Intraoperative sedation: Dexmedetomidine infusion starting at 0.8 mcg/kg in 20 min and then at 0.6 mcg/kg/h.

Airway management: Spontaneous breathing with oxygen 5 L/m (Fig. 25.16).

Intraoperative monitoring: ECG, HR, NIBP, SpO_2.

Postoperative analgesia: Paracetamol 1 g every 8 h without the need for opioid administration.

Postoperative pain: NRS 0.

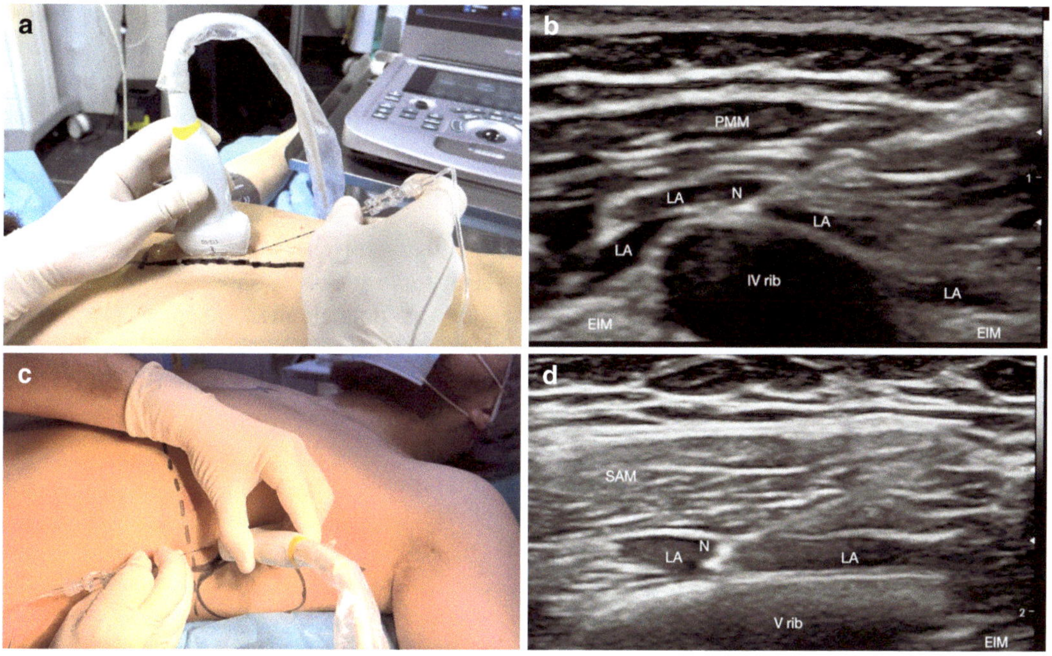

Fig. 25.15 Combined parasternal and deep serratus anterior plane blocks for S-ICD implantation. (**a**) Parasternal block, patient and probe position. (**b**) Modified superficial parasternal block. The local anesthetic is injected between the pectoralis major and external intercostal muscles placing the tip of the needle on the dome of the rib. (**c**) Deep serratus anterior plane block, patient and probe position. (**d**) Deep serratus anterior plane block. The local anesthetic is injected between the serratus anterior muscle and the rib. *PMM* pectoralis major muscle, *SAM* serratus anterior muscle, *EIM* external intercostal muscle, *LA* local anesthetic, *N* needle, *Rib* rib

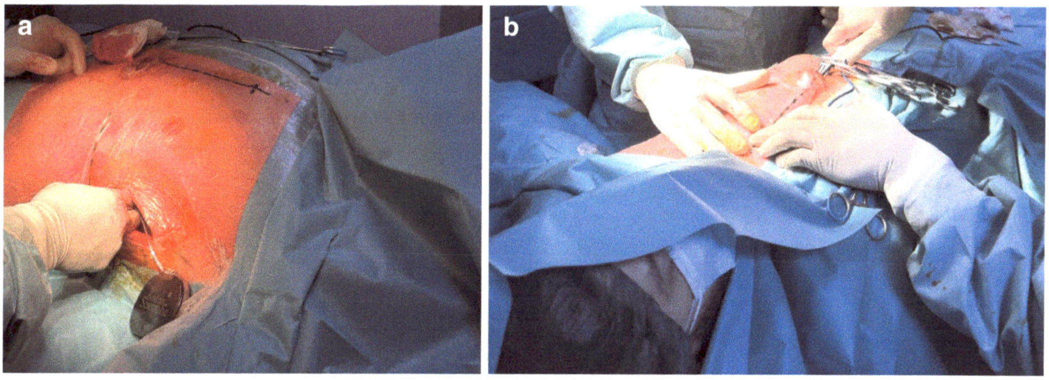

Fig. 25.16 Intraoperative S-ICD procedures. (**a**) Device implantation in the axillary region between the latissimus dorsi and serratus anterior muscles. (**b**) Left parasternal lead insertion and spontaneous breathing

Perioperative complications or adverse events: None.

Patient satisfaction level: Excellent.

25.8 Interpectoral Plane (PECS I) Block for Anterior Chest Tube Insertion After Postoperative Pneumothorax

This is a case of a patient who presented a right pneumothorax 5 days after coronary artery bypass grafting.

Medical history: Man, 78 years old, recent coronary artery bypass grafting, diabetes mellitus type 2, on therapy with insulin and acetylsalicylic acid.

Anesthetic technique: Due to the anterior tube insertion, an interpectoral plane (PECS I) block performed with a high-frequency linear probe and a 100 mm 21G needle inserted between the pectoralis major and minor muscles through an in-plane approach and a lateral-to-medial direction (Fig. 25.17).

Local anesthetic: Levobupivacaine 0.5% 15 mL (75 mg of levobupivacaine 0.5%).

Adjuvants: None.

Intraoperative sedation: Midazolam 5 mg.

Airway management: Spontaneous breathing with oxygen 5 L/m (Fig. 25.18).

Intraoperative monitoring: ECG, HR, NIBP, SpO_2; $ETCO_2$.

Postoperative analgesia: None.

Postoperative pain: NRS 0.

Perioperative complications or adverse events: None.

Patient satisfaction level: Excellent.

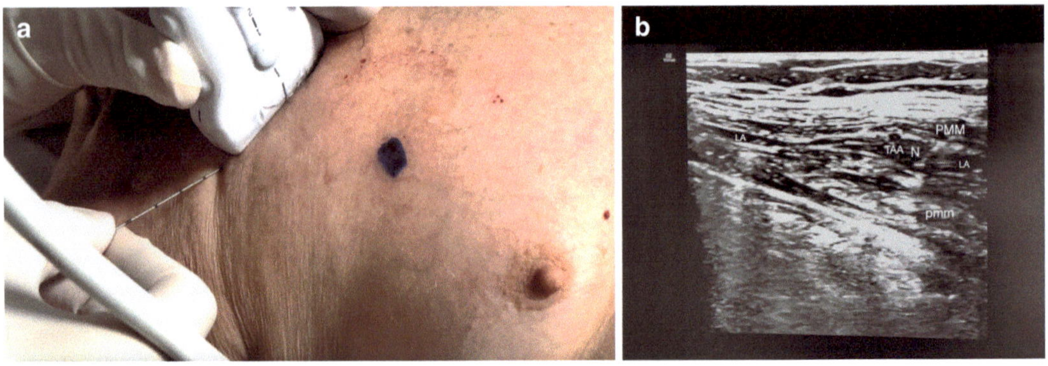

Fig. 25.17 Interpectoral plane (PECS I) block. (**a**) Patient and probe position. The black dot indicates the chest tube insertion site. The needle is inserted in a lateral-to-medial direction. (**b**) The local anesthetic is injected between the pectoralis major and minor muscles. *PMM* pectoralis major muscle, *pmm* pectoralis minor muscle, *TAA* thoracoacromial artery, *LA* local anesthetic, *N* needle

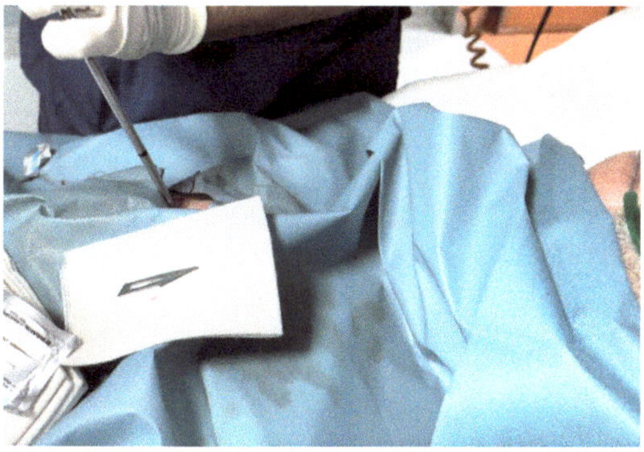

Fig. 25.18 Chest tube insertion and spontaneous breathing

25.9 Single-Shot Serratus Anterior Plane Block for Postoperative Right Minithoracotomy and Rib Fracture Pain Management After Minimally Invasive Mitral Valve Replacement

The following is a case of a patient who underwent minimally invasive mitral valve replacement through right minithoracotomy affected by intraoperative rib fracture due to the dilator. A single-shot serratus anterior plane block was performed to manage the postoperative pain deriving from the minithoracotomy and the rib fracture [15–17] (Fig. 25.19a, b).

Medical history: Man, 67 years old, atrial fibrillation, diabetes mellitus type 2, blood hypertension, chronic kidney disease, on therapy with new oral anticoagulants, metformin and zofenopril.

Anesthetic technique: Single-shot deep serratus anterior plane block performed with a high-frequency linear probe on the midaxillary line at the level of the fourth rib and a 100 mm 21G needle inserted through an in-plane approach and a caudal-to-cranial direction (Fig. 25.19c).

Local anesthetic: Levobupivacaine 0.375%, 30 mL (112.5 mg of levobupivacaine 0.375%) injected between the serratus anterior muscle and the fourth rib (Fig. 25.19d).

Adjuvants: Dexmedetomidine 1 mcg/kg (80 mcg) added to the local anesthetic.

Intraoperative sedation: General anesthesia.

Airway management: Orotracheal intubation.

Intraoperative monitoring: ECG, HR, IBP, SpO_2; $ETCO_2$.

Postoperative analgesia: Paracetamol 1 g every 8 h without the need for opioid administration.

Postoperative pain: NRS 2.

Perioperative complications or adverse events: None.

Patient satisfaction level: Good.

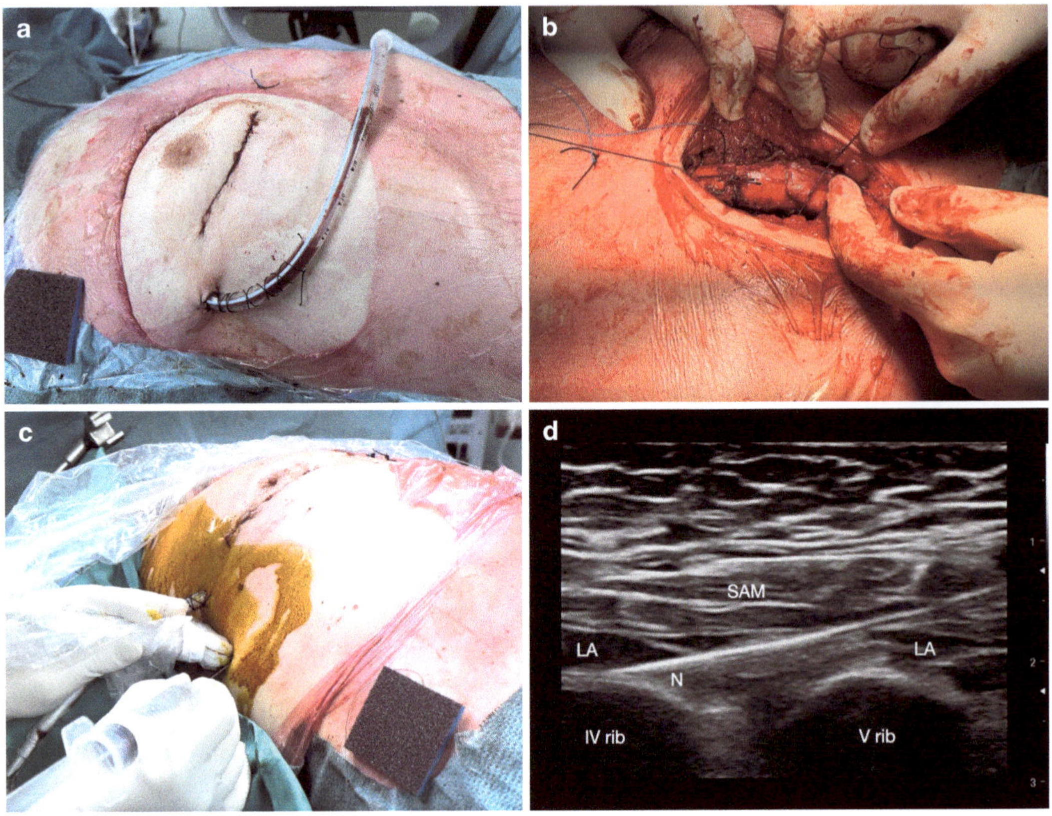

Fig. 25.19 Minimally invasive mitral valve replacement. (**a**) Right minithoracotomy. (**b**) Rib fracture. (**c**) Patient and probe position. (**d**) Single-shot serratus anterior plane block. The local anesthetic is injected between the serratus anterior muscle and the fourth rib. *SAM* serratus anterior muscle, *LA* local anesthetic, *N* needle, *rib* rib

25.10 Ultrafast-Track Extubation in a Patient Undergoing Left Minimally Invasive Thoracotomy Single Coronary Artery Bypass Grafting

The following patient was scheduled for a single coronary artery bypass grafting performed through a left minimally invasive thoracotomy. Given that he presented no further pathologies, he followed the ultrafast-track extubation protocol at the end of the surgery in the operating room [18] (Fig. 25.20a).

Medical history: Man, 75 years old, no noteworthy pathologies, no home therapy.

Anesthetic technique: Left single-shot deep serratus anterior plane block performed with a high-frequency linear probe on the midaxillary line at the level of the fourth rib and a 100 mm 21G needle inserted through an in-plane approach and a caudal-to-cranial direction (Fig. 25.20b).

Local anesthetic: Levobupivacaine 0.5%, 30 mL (150 mg of levobupivacaine 0.5%) injected between the serratus anterior muscle and the fourth rib (Fig. 25.20c).

Adjuvants: Dexmedetomidine 1 mcg/kg (70 mcg) added to the local anesthetic.

Intraoperative sedation: General anesthesia.

Airway management: Intraoperative orotracheal intubation and ultrafast-track extubation at the end of surgery in the operating room (Fig. 25.20d).

Intraoperative monitoring: ECG, HR, IBP, SpO_2; $ETCO_2$.

Postoperative analgesia: Paracetamol 1 g every 8 h without the need for opioid administration.

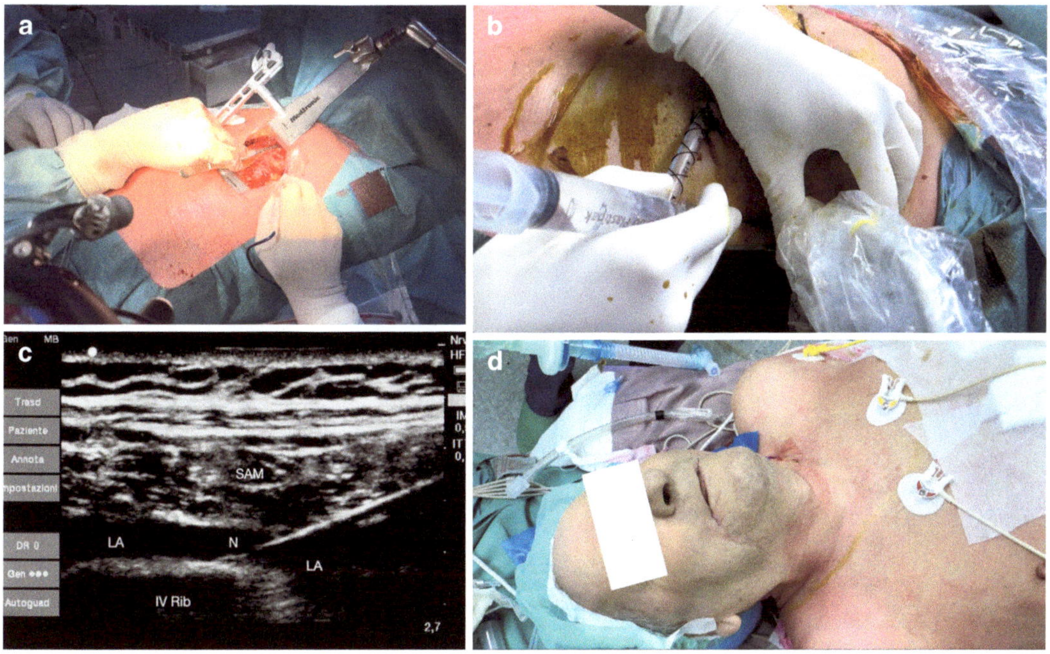

Fig. 25.20 Left minimally invasive thoracotomy single coronary artery bypass grafting. (**a**) Internal mammary artery harvesting. (**b**) Patient and probe position. (**c**) Left single-shot deep serratus anterior plane block. The local anesthetic is injected between the serratus anterior muscle and the fourth rib surface. (**d**) Ultrafast-track extubation at the end of surgery in the operating room. *SAM* serratus anterior muscle, *N* needle, *LA* local anesthetic, *Rib* rib

Postoperative pain: No pain at the end of the surgery. NRS 2 during the 24 postoperative hours.

Perioperative complications or adverse events: None.

Patient satisfaction level: Good.

25.11 Parasternal Block for Sternal Resynthesis in Spontaneous Breathing Patient Affected by Previous Relapsing Postoperative Pneumothoraces

The following is a case of a patient who underwent coronary artery bypass grafting who developed several relapsing postoperative pneumothoraces treated with Heimlich valve for 30 days. When the pneumothorax was solved, he was scheduled for sternal resynthesis. To avoid a risk of a new pneumothorax due to a general anesthesia and orotracheal intubation, a parasternal block was planned to manage the sternal dehiscence [19–23] (Fig. 25.21c).

Medical history: Man, 79 years old, severe chronic obstructive pulmonary disease, blood hypertension, on therapy with albuterol.

Anesthetic technique: Bilateral modified superficial parasternal block performed with a high-frequency linear probe and a 100 mm 21G needle inserted at the level of second and fourth ribs through an in-plane approach and caudal-to-cranial direction. Two injections for each side for a total of four injections (Fig. 25.21a).

Local anesthetic: Ropivacaine 0.5%. 15 mL (75 mg of ropivacaine 0.5%) for each side and a total of 150 mg of ropivacaine 0.5% and a volume of 30 mL (Fig. 25.21b).

Adjuvants: Dexmedetomidine 1 mcg/kg (80 mcg) mixed with the local anesthetic.

Intraoperative sedation: Dexmedetomidine infusion starting at 0.8 mcg/kg in 20 min and then at 0.6 mcg/kg/h.

Airway management: Spontaneous breathing with oxygen 8 L/m (Fig. 25.21d).

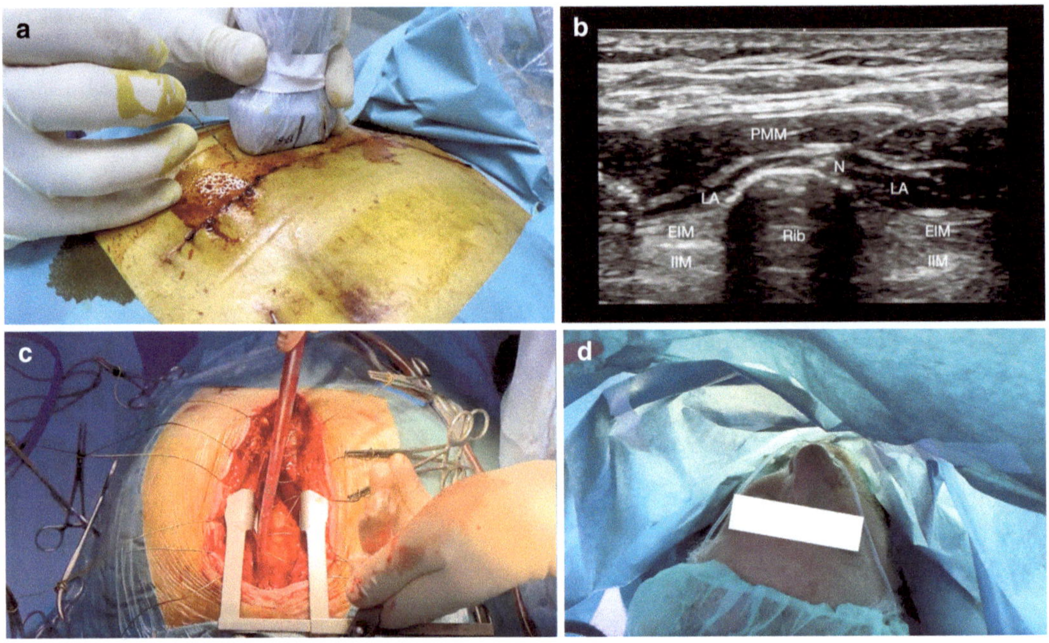

Fig. 25.21 Parasternal block and sternal dehiscence in awake patient. (**a**) Patient and probe position. (**b**) Modified superficial parasternal block. The local anesthetic is injected between the pectoralis major and external intercostal muscles. (**c**) Sternal wire insertion. (**d**) Spontaneous breathing. *PMM* pectoralis major muscle, *EIM*: external intercostal muscle, *IIM*: internal intercostal muscle, *Rib* rib, *N* needle, *LA* local anesthetic

Intraoperative monitoring: ECG, HR, IBP, SpO_2.

Postoperative analgesia: Paracetamol 1 g every 8 h without the need for opioid administration.

Postoperative pain: No pain.

Perioperative complications or adverse events: None.

Patient satisfaction level: Good.

25.12 Serratus Anterior Plane Block for Right Minithoracotomy Revision and Pectoralis Muscle Retraction

Below the case of a patient who previously underwent mitral valve replacement via right minithoracotomy, undergoing wound revision and pectoralis muscles plasty [24] (Fig. 25.22a).

Medical history: Man, 56 years old, blood hypertension, no therapy, mitral valve insufficiency.

Anesthetic technique:

1. Single-shot deep serratus anterior plane block performed with a high-frequency linear probe and a 100 mm 21G needle inserted at the level of fourth rib through an in-plane approach and caudal-to-cranial direction (Fig. 25.22c).
2. Interpectoral plane (PECS I) block performed with a high-frequency linear probe placed at the level of deltoid-pectoral sulcus and a 100 mm 21G needle inserted between the pectoralis major and minor muscles through an in-plane approach and a lateral-to-medial direction (Fig. 25.22e).

Local anesthetic:

1. Serratus anterior plane block: Ropivacaine 0.5%, 20 mL (100 mg of ropivacaine 0.5%) (Fig. 25.22d).
2. Interpectoral plane (PECS I) block: Ropivacaine 0.5%, 15 mL (75 mg of ropivacaine 0.5%) (Fig. 25.22f).

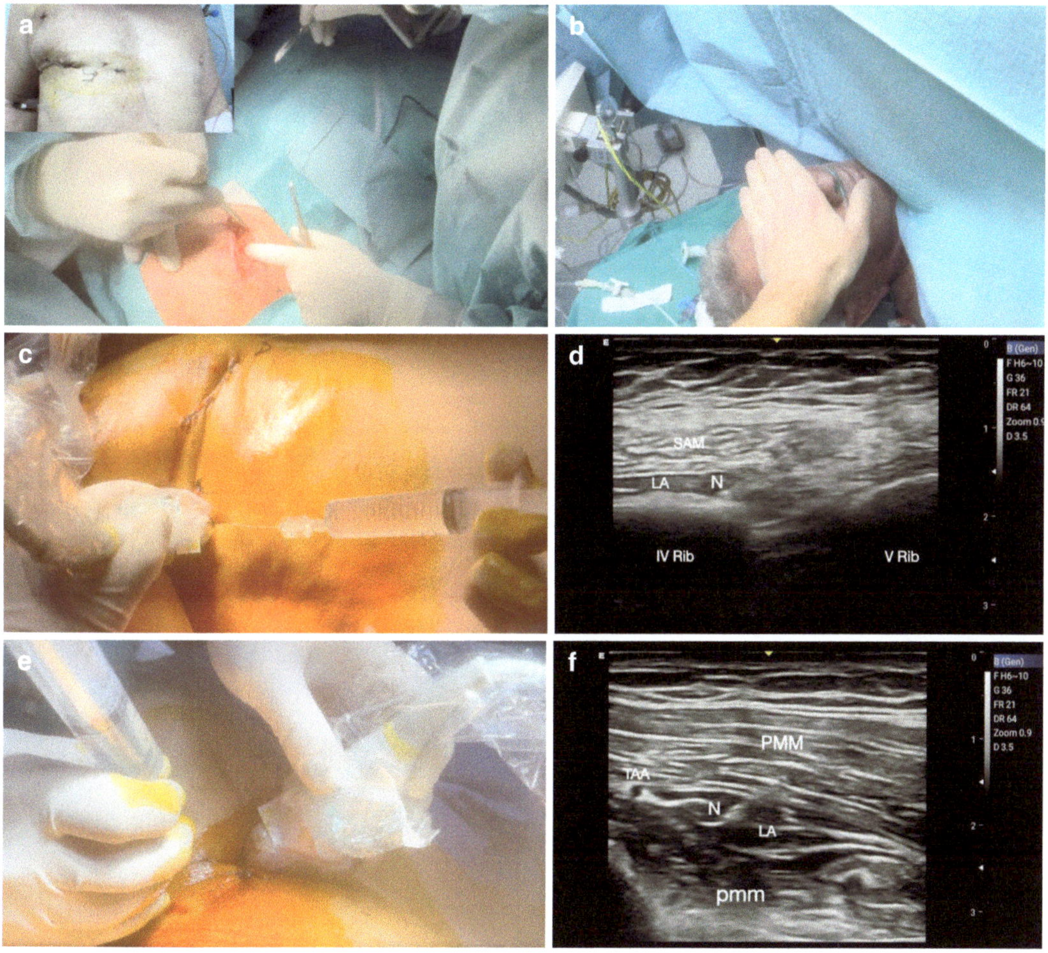

Fig. 25.22 (**a**) Right minithoracotomy wound revision. (**b**) Spontaneous breathing. (**c**) Single-shot serratus anterior plane block. Probe and patient position. (**d**) Local anesthetic is injected between the serratus anterior muscle and fourth rib surface. (**e**) Interpectoral plane (PECS I) block. Probe and patient position. (**f**) Local anesthetic is injected between pectoralis major and minor muscles. *SAM* serratus anterior muscle, *PMM* pectoralis major muscle, *pmm* pectoralis minor muscle, *TAA* thoracoacromial artery, *LA* local anesthetic, *N* needle, *Rib* rib

Adjuvants: Dexamethasone 4 mg mixed with the local anesthetic.

Intraoperative sedation: Midazolam 10 mg.

Airway management: Spontaneous breathing with oxygen 3 L/m (Fig. 25.22b).

Intraoperative monitoring: ECG, HR, NIBP, SpO_2.

Postoperative analgesia: Paracetamol 1 g every 12 h without the need for opioid administration.

Postoperative pain: No pain.

Perioperative complications or adverse events: None.

Patient satisfaction level: Good.

25.13 Continuous Erector Spinae Block for Left Middle Lobe Lung Segmentectomy

The following is the case of a woman affected by lung neoplasia undergoing left middle lobe lung segmentectomy (Fig. 25.23c).

Medical history: Woman, 68 years old, blood hypertension, diabetes mellitus type I, on therapy with metformin and telmisartan.

Anesthetic technique:

1. Preoperative continuous erector spinae plane block performed with a high-frequency linear

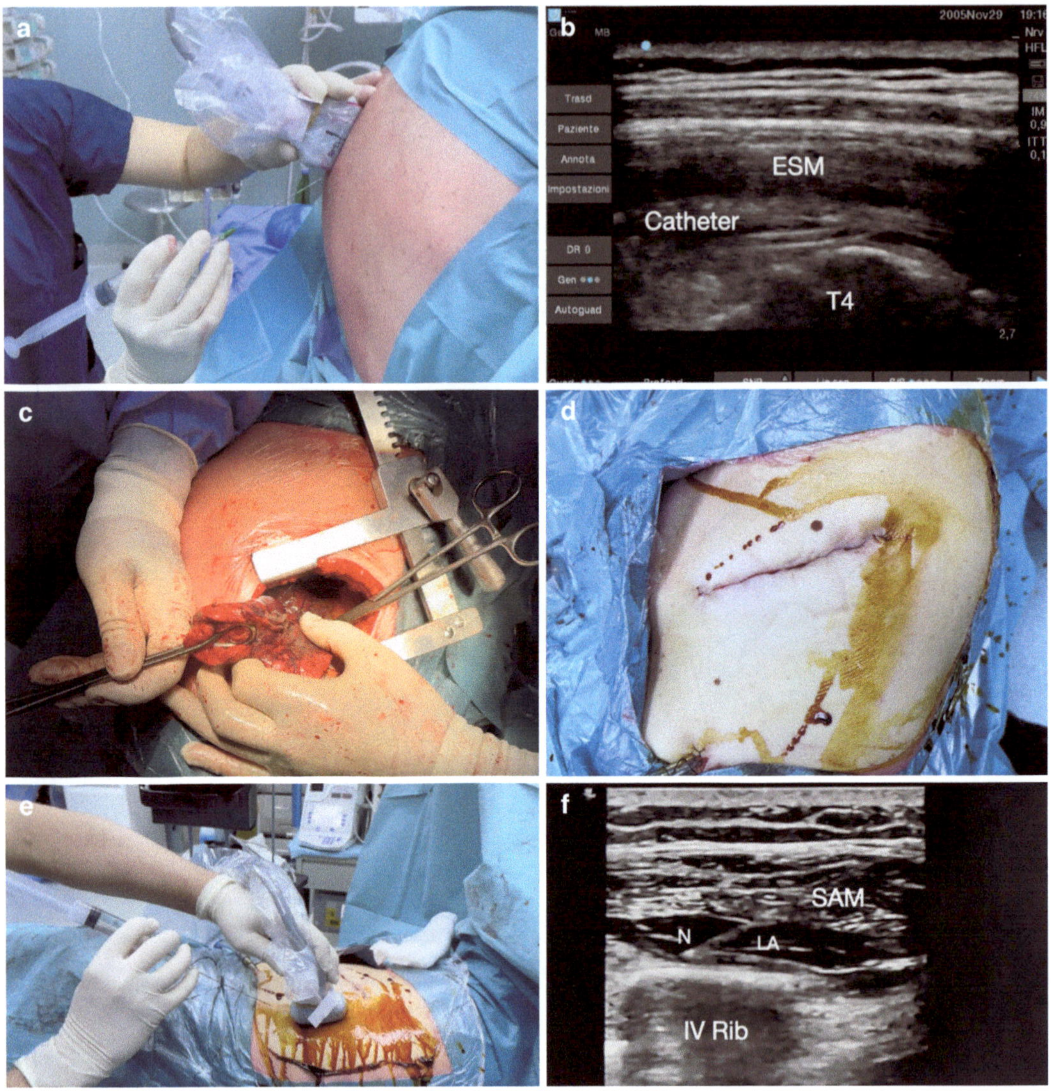

Fig. 25.23 Erector spinae and serratus anterior plane blocks. (**a**) Erector spinae block, patient and probe position. (**b**) Local anesthetic is injected between the erector spinae muscle and T4 transverse process. (**c**) Left middle lobe lung segmentectomy. (**d**) Left minithoracotomy. (**e**) Single-shot serratus anterior plane block, patient and probe position. (**f**) Local anesthetic is injected between serratus anterior muscle and the fourth rib surface. *SAM* serratus anterior muscle, *ESM* erector spinae muscle, *T4* T4 transverse process, *Rib* rib, *LA* local anesthetic, *N* needle, *Catheter* catheter

probe and a catheter inserted through a Tuohy needle at the level of T4 transverse process via an in-plane approach and caudal-to-cranial direction (Fig. 25.23a).

2. Postoperative single-shot deep serratus plane block performed with a high-frequency linear probe and a 100 mm needle inserted at the level of fourth rib in a caudal-to-cranial direction (Fig. 25.23e).

Local anesthetic:

1. ESP block: Preoperative single shot of levobupivacaine 0.25%, 20 mL (50 mg of levobupivacaine 0.25%), followed by catheter placing. Postoperative infusion with levobupivacaine 0.25%, 10 mL/h (Fig. 25.23b).
2. Postoperative single-shot deep serratus anterior plane block: Levobupivacaine 0.25%,

30 mL (75 mg of levobupivacaine 0.25%) (Fig. 25.23f).

Adjuvants: Dexmedetomidine 1 mcg/kg (60 mcg) mixed with the whole anesthetic solution.

Intraoperative sedation: General anesthesia and orotracheal intubation.

Postoperative analgesia: Paracetamol 1 g every 8 h without the need for opioid administration.

Postoperative pain: NRS 2.

Perioperative complications or adverse events: None.

Patient satisfaction level: Good.

25.14 Interpectoral Plane (PECS I) and Superficial Cervical Plexus Blocks for Pacemaker Implantation in Patient with Carotid Stenosis

The following is the case of a man who previously underwent CABG and was affected by third-degree atrioventricular block and scheduled for pacemaker implantation (Fig. 25.24).

Medical history: Man, 79 years old, blood hypertension, smoker, previously underwent coronary artery bypass grafting and left carotid stenting, on therapy with clopidogrel.

Anesthetic technique:

3. Interpectoral plane (PECS I) block performed with a high-frequency linear probe and a 100 mm 21G needle inserted through a lateral-to-medial direction and in-plane approach between pectoralis major and minor muscles (Fig. 25.25a, b).
4. Intermediate cervical plexus block performed with a high-frequency linear probe and a 100 mm 21G needle inserted through a lateral-to-medial direction and in-plane approach between the sternocleidomastoid muscle and C4 transverse process and prevertebral fascia (Fig. 25.25c, d).

Local anesthetic:

3. Interpectoral plane (PECS I) block: Levobupivacaine 0.375%, 15 mL (56.25 mg of levobupivacaine 0.375%).
4. Intermediate cervical plexus block: Levobupivacaine 0.375%, 20 mL (75 mg of levobupivacaine 0.375%).

Adjuvants: Dexmedetomidine 1 mcg/kg (50 mcg) mixed with the whole anesthetic solution.

Intraoperative sedation: Dexmedetomidine infusion at 0.6 mcg/kg/h and spontaneous breathing (Fig. 25.26).

Postoperative analgesia: Paracetamol 1 g every 8 h without the need for opioid administration.

Postoperative pain: NRS 2.

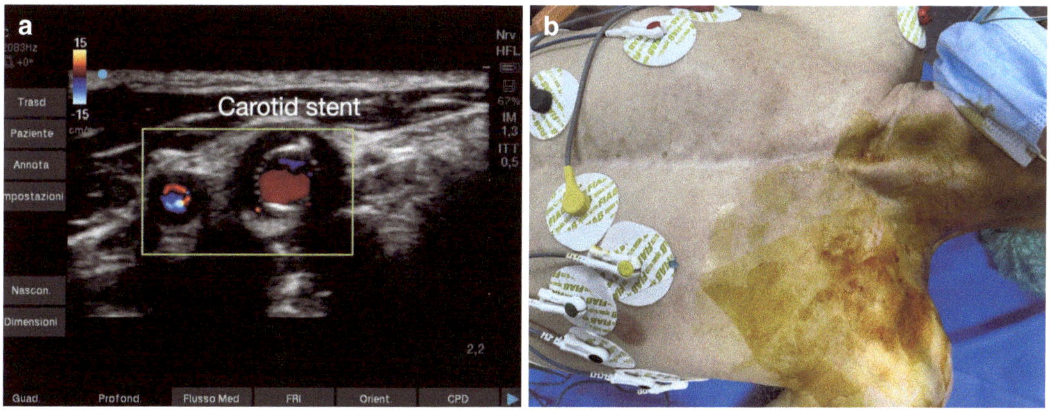

Fig. 25.24 (**a**) Carotid stenting. (**b**) Severe chronic obstructive pulmonary disease, previously underwent coronary artery bypass grafting and left carotid stenting

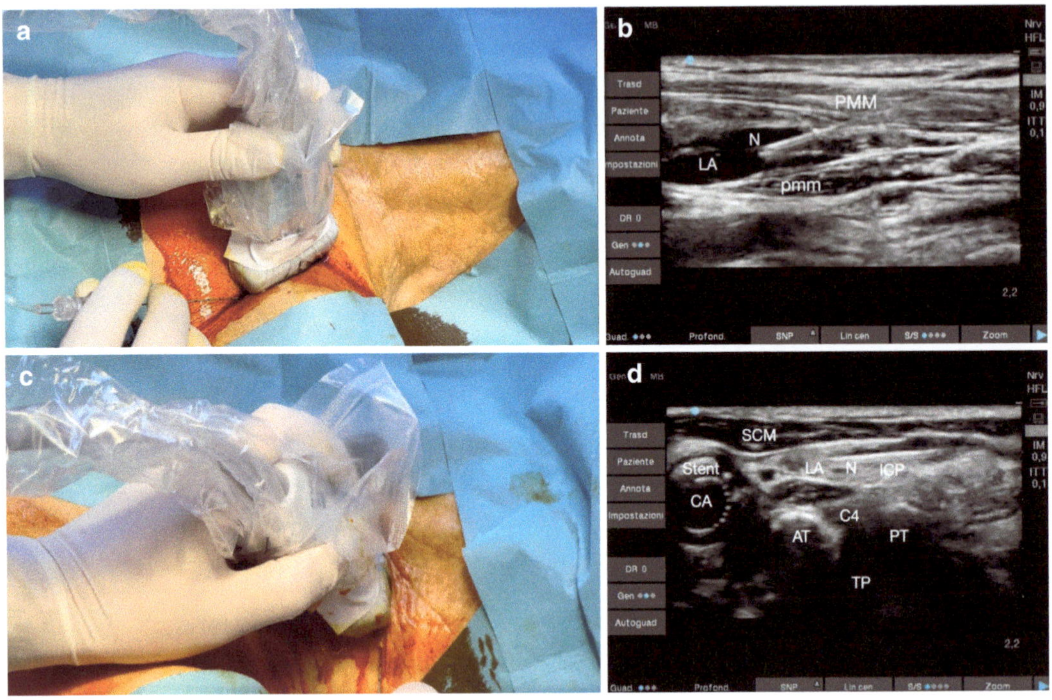

Fig. 25.25 (**a**) Interpectoral plane (PECS I) block: patient and probe position. (**b**) Interpectoral plane (PECS I) block: local anesthetic is injected between pectoralis major and minor muscles. (**c**) Intermediate cervical plexus block: patient and probe position. (**d**) Intermediate cervical plexus block: local anesthetic is injected into the posterior cervical space between the investing layer of the sternocleidomastoid muscle and the prevertebral fascia of C4 transverse process. *SCM* sternocleidomastoid muscle, *CA* carotid artery, *ICP* intermediate cervical plexus, *N* needle, *LA* local anesthetic, *TP* C4 transverse process, *AT* C4 anterior tubercle, *PT* C4 posterior tubercle, *PMM* pectoralis major muscle, *pmm* pectoralis minor muscle

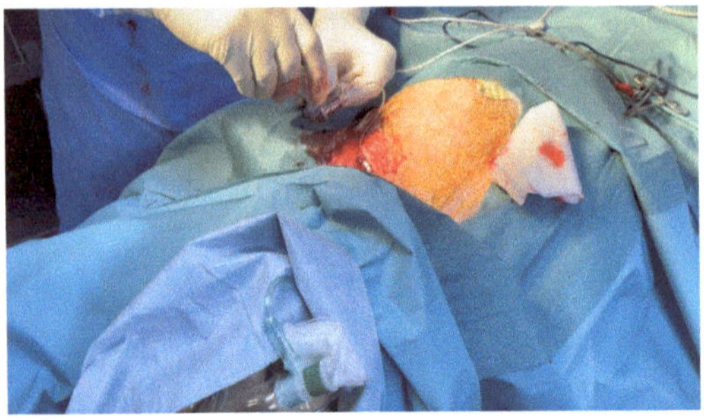

Fig. 25.26 Pacemaker implantation and spontaneous breathing

Perioperative complications or adverse events: None.

Patient satisfaction level: Good.

25.15 Conclusion

Chest wall fascial blocks allow both the management of critically ill patients in awake surgery and the perioperative pain relief aimed at fast-track extubation. The clinical cases previously described aim to broaden the own knowledge and expertise and better focus on the potential of these anesthetic techniques. Sharing daily practice and individual experiences in theatre room is the basis for a personal and team growth.

References

1. Nuove prospettive anestesiologiche ed antalgiche nella moderna chirurgia della mammella. Paolo Scima, Giuseppe Sepolvere. Editore: Explora (30 gennaio 2021).
2. Khalil PA, Becker E. Point-of-care ultrasound-guided serratus anterior plane block for chest tube placement in a spontaneous pneumothorax. Pediatr Emerg Care. 2022;38(8):406–8. https://doi.org/10.1097/PEC.0000000000002663.
3. Toscano A, Capuano P, Costamagna A, Burzio C, Ellena M, Scala V, Pasero D, Rinaldi M, Brazzi L. The Serratus anterior plane study: continuous deep serratus anterior plane block for mitral valve surgery performed in right minithoracotomy. J Cardiothorac Vasc Anesth. 2020;34(11):2975–82. https://doi.org/10.1053/j.jvca.2020.05.021.
4. Mavarez AC, Ripat CI, Suarez MR. Pectoralis plane block for pacemaker insertion: a successful primary. Anesth Front Surg. 2019;6:64. https://doi.org/10.3389/fsurg.2019.00064.
5. Bozyel S, Yalnız A, Aksu T, Guler TE, Genez S. Ultrasound-guided combined pectoral nerve block and axillary venipuncture for the implantation of cardiac implantable electronic devices. Pacing Clin Electrophysiol. 2019;42(7):1026–31. https://doi.org/10.1111/pace.13725.
6. Sepolvere G, Tedesco M, Cristiano L. Ultrasound parasternal block as a novel approach for cardiac sternal surgery: could it be the safest strategy? J Cardiothorac Vasc Anesth. 2020;34(8):2284–6. https://doi.org/10.1053/j.jvca.2020.03.014.
7. Sepolvere G, Fusco P, Tedesco M, Scimia P. Bilateral ultrasound-guided parasternal block for postoperative analgesia in cardiac surgery: could it be the safest strategy? Reg Anesth Pain Med. 2020;45(4):316–7. https://doi.org/10.1136/rapm-2019-100872.
8. Sepolvere G, Tedesco M, Cristiano L. Ultrasound guided parasternal block with dexmedetomidine as effective approach for postoperative analgesia in cardiac surgery. Minerva Anestesiol. 2020;86(7):789–90. https://doi.org/10.23736/S0375-9393.20.14356-6.
9. Costa F, Caruso S, Pascarella G, Nenna A, Grande S, Sarubbi D, Chello M, Agrò FE. Sternotomy debridement in critical patient with difficult predicted airway: can regional anesthesia be the labyrinth exit? Minerva Anestesiol. 2020;86(4):462–3. https://doi.org/10.23736/S0375-9393.19.14133-8.
10. Sepolvere G, Coppolino F, Tedesco M, Cristiano L. Ultrasound-guided parasternal blocks: techniques, clinical indications and future prospects. Minerva Anestesiol. 2021;87(12):1338–46. https://doi.org/10.23736/S0375-9393.21.15599-3.
11. Hoogma DF, Van den Eynde R, Al Tmimi L, Verbrugghe P, Tournoy J, Fieuws S, Coppens S, Rex S. Efficacy of erector spinae plane block for minimally invasive mitral valve surgery: results of a double-blind, prospective randomized placebo-controlled trial. J Clin Anesth. 2023;86:111072. https://doi.org/10.1016/j.jclinane.2023.111072.
12. Borys M, Gawęda B, Horeczy B, Kolowca M, Olszówka P, Czuczwar M, Wołoszczuk-Gębicka B, Widenka K. Erector spinae-plane block as an analgesic alternative in patients undergoing mitral and/or tricuspid valve repair through a right mini-thoracotomy—an observational cohort study. Wideochir Inne Tech Maloinwazyjne. 2020;15(1):208–14. https://doi.org/10.5114/wiitm.2019.85396.
13. Tedesco M, Capuano P, Toscano A, Sepolvere G. Combined erector spinae plane block and serratus anterior plane block for thoracic surgery: is two better than one? Minerva Anestesiol. 2023;89(9):842–4. https://doi.org/10.23736/S0375-9393.23.17348-2.
14. Droghetti A, Fusco P, Marini M, Harizai F, Scimia P. Ultrasound-guided serratus anterior plane block and parasternal block in cooperative sedation for S-ICD implantation. Pacing Clin Electrophysiol. 2019;42(7):1076–8. https://doi.org/10.1111/pace.13727.
15. Sepolvere G, Tognu A, Tedesco M, Scialdone VR, Cristiano L. Successful use of continuous deep serratus plane block for pneumothorax and rib fractures management. Minerva Anestesiol. 2021;87(6):733–4. https://doi.org/10.23736/S0375-9393.20.15309-4.
16. Sepolvere G, Scialdone VR. Single shot serratus anterior plane block for post-thoracotomy pain management in cardiac surgery: could it be enough? Minerva Anestesiol. 2022;88(9):748–9. https://doi.org/10.23736/S0375-9393.22.16467-9.
17. He Y, Li Z, Xu M, Du B, Zuo Y. Single-injection serratus anterior plane block for cardiothoracic surgery via thoracotomy in children: a systematic review and meta-analysis of randomised controlled trials. BMJ Paediatr Open. 2023;7(1):e001912. https://doi.org/10.1136/bmjpo-2023-001912.
18. Parody Cuerda G, Jiménez Del Valle JR, Fernández López AR, Barquero Aroca JM. Ultra-fast track extubation protocol following cardiovascular surgery: Predictors of failure and outcomes. Rev Esp Anestesiol Reanim (Engl Ed). 2023;70(5):259–68. https://doi.org/10.1016/j.redare.2023.05.002.
19. Scimia P, Gentili L, Tedesco M, Fusco P, Sepolvere G. A modified approach to a parasternal block: a case report. A A Pract. 2023;17(1):e01644. https://doi.org/10.1213/XAA.0000000000001644.
20. Sepolvere G, Tognù A, Tedesco M, Coppolino F, Cristiano L. Avoiding the internal mammary artery during parasternal blocks: ultrasound identification and technique considerations. J Cardiothorac Vasc Anesth. 2021;35(6):1594–602. https://doi.org/10.1053/j.jvca.2020.11.007.

21. Sepolvere G, Di Zazzo F, Merola L, Tedesco M, Cristiano L. The correct internal mammary artery anatomy: a topic for ultrasound parasternal block. Saudi J Anaesth. 2021;15(2):233–4. https://doi.org/10.4103/sja.sja_1028_20.
22. Capuano P, Toscano A, Sepolvere G, Tedesco M, Martucci G, Burgio G, Arcadipane A. Parasternal intercostal blocks for cardiac and breast surgery: less is more? J Cardiothorac Vasc Anesth. 2023;37(12):2688–9. https://doi.org/10.1053/j.jvca.2023.09.003.
23. Toscano A, Capuano P, Perrucci C, Giunta M, Orsello A, Pierani T, Costamagna A, Tedesco M, Arcadipane A, Sepolvere G, Buono G, Brazzi L. Which ultrasound-guided parasternal intercostal nerve block for post-sternotomy pain? Results from a prospective observational study. J Anesth Analg Crit Care. 2023;3(1):48. https://doi.org/10.1186/s44158-023-00134-2.
24. Costa F, Nenna A, Barbato R, Benedetto M, Del Buono R, Agrò FE. Serratus anterior plane block for right minithoracotomy revision after mitral valve repair. Minerva Anestesiol. 2017;83(12):1333–4. https://doi.org/10.23736/S0375-9393.17.12186-3.

Correction to: Risks and Benefits

Simona Silvetti, Giuseppe Sepolvere,
Antonio Salsano, and Andrea De Martino

Correction to:
Chapter 18: G. Sepolvere, S. Silvetti (eds.), *Fast-Track in Cardiac Anesthesia*, https://doi.org/10.1007/978-3-031-70899-2_18

This book was inadvertently published missing two contributors in Chap. 18.
The authors Antonio Salsano and Andrea De Martino have been added to Chap. 18.

Antonio Salsano
Cardiac Surgery Division, Ospedale Policlinico San Martino, Genoa, Italy
Disc Department, University of Genoa, Genoa, Italy.

Andrea De Martino
Cardiac Surgery Division, Ospedale Policlinico San Martino, Genoa, Italy

The updated version of this chapter can be found at https://doi.org/10.1007/978-3-031-70899-2_18

G. Sepolvere, S. Silvetti (eds.), *Fast-Track in Cardiac Anesthesia*,
https://doi.org/10.1007/978-3-031-70899-2_26

MIX
Papier aus verantwortungsvollen Quellen
Paper from responsible sources
FSC® C105338

If you have any concerns about our products,
you can contact us on
ProductSafety@springernature.com

In case Publisher is established outside the EU,
the EU authorized representative is:
Springer Nature Customer Service Center GmbH
Europaplatz 3, 69115 Heidelberg, Germany

Printed by Libri Plureos GmbH
in Hamburg, Germany